How and Why People Change

How and Why People Change

Foundations of Psychological Therapy

IAN M. EVANS

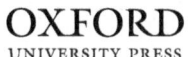

OXFORD
UNIVERSITY PRESS

Oxford University Press is a department of the University of Oxford.
It furthers the University's objective of excellence in research, scholarship,
and education by publishing worldwide.

Oxford   New York
Auckland   Cape Town   Dar es Salaam   Hong Kong   Karachi
Kuala Lumpur   Madrid   Melbourne   Mexico City   Nairobi
New Delhi   Shanghai   Taipei   Toronto

With offices in
Argentina   Austria   Brazil   Chile   Czech Republic   France   Greece
Guatemala   Hungary   Italy   Japan   Poland   Portugal   Singapore
South Korea   Switzerland   Thailand   Turkey   Ukraine   Vietnam

Oxford is a registered trademark of Oxford University Press in
the UK and certain other countries.

Published in the United States of America by
Oxford University Press
198 Madison Avenue, New York, NY 10016

© Oxford University Press 2013

All rights reserved. No part of this publication may be reproduced, stored in a
retrieval system, or transmitted, in any form or by any means, without the prior
permission in writing of Oxford University Press, or as expressly permitted by law,
by license, or under terms agreed with the appropriate reproduction rights organization.
Inquiries concerning reproduction outside the scope of the above should be sent to the Rights
Department, Oxford University Press, at the address above.

You must not circulate this work in any other form
and you must impose this same condition on any acquirer.

Library of Congress Cataloging-in-Publication Data
Evans, Ian M., 1944–
How and why people change : foundations of psychological therapy / Ian M. Evans.
p. cm.
Includes bibliographical references and index.
ISBN 978–0–19–991727–3
1. Behavior therapy.   I. Title.
RC489.B4E96 2013
616.89'142—dc23
2012024756

1 3 5 7 9 8 6 4 2
Printed in the United States of America
on acid-free paper

For
RUBY
Remembering our play dates, treasure seeking in Central Park,
and the Thursday family dinners in Manhattan, 2010

CONTENTS

Preface ix

1. Setting the Scene: Why We Need a Theory for Change 1
2. What Is Therapeutic Change? 25
3. Motivation to Change 53
4. Individual Differences in Ability to Change: Personality and Context 73
5. Conditioning: Changing the Meaning and Value of Events 97
6. Contingencies: Reward and Punishment in Therapeutic Change 115
7. Response Relationships: The Dynamics of Behavioral Regulation 137
8. Cognition: Changing Thoughts and Fantasies 157
9. Self-Influence 179
10. Social Mediators and the Therapeutic Relationship 201
11. Culture as Behavior Change 225
12. Conclusions: How and Why People Can Change and Be Changed 249

References 269
Index 293

PREFACE

This book presents a unified account of behavior change as the result of any purposeful, planful intervention—those typically falling within the aegis of clinical psychology. It is about therapeutic change rather than all of the many possible contexts in which change happens. Human beings change all the time; we are in a constant state of flux as we grow, mature, learn, and adapt to a myriad of physical, environmental, social, educational, and cultural influences. "Nothing is meant to remain the same" is a central tenet of Buddhist philosophy. Dramatic events such as natural disasters, wars, and revolutions cause overwhelming change in the way of life for millions of people. Chance meetings, new employment, and financial loss are among the countless circumstances that cause unpredictable changes in lifestyle. Travel brings a heightened sense of awareness of our world surroundings, and challenges realities we take for granted (Hiss, 2010). Cultural and artistic experiences—literature, movies, theatre, rousing sermons, even dreams—all cause profound inspirational cognitive and emotional change in understanding our society and ourselves. Justice Sonia Sotomayor, the first Hispanic-American to serve on the U.S. Supreme Court, provided a nice example when she described how seeing the movie "12 Angry Men" (Sidney Lumet, 1957) persuaded her to pursue a career in law (Semple, 2010). Of course, in human behavior there is a big difference between a trigger, a catalyst, and a cause.

Many factors motivate and determine psychological development, but only some of them are able to be mobilized within a time-limited therapeutic context. Thus, my focus is on the change that comes about as a result of deliberate intervention, usually initiated by a troubled individual and aided by another person, typically a professional. Furthermore, my focus is on changes that might be thought of as reflecting emotional, or at least interpersonal, needs. It does not attempt to include, for example, how a child acquires reading skills at school, nor the change that comes about because someone decides to learn Italian cooking, nor the effects of an advertising campaign on consumer behavior. The emphasis is on how people's current functioning might change, not how their basic personality dispositions evolved over time. Change can be thought of as planful when it is motivated by the desire to be and feel different; it does not include the rapid change in basic habits required by circumstances, such as moving to a country in which people drive on the other side of the road.

Collectively, whole societies sometimes experience a need to change. In his presidential address to the American Psychological Association, Alan Kazdin (2009a) outlined the many ways in which we should all change our behavior for the sake of planet Earth. Community psychologists have always been interested in big picture social change—how do groups or even whole populations come to make deliberate alterations in their patterns of conduct? In addition to polluting our environment, there are many social phenomena that are psychological or at least public health concerns that we would generally wish to see less of: bullying, teenage binge drinking, school dropout, graffiti, child abuse, and eating junk food. There are others that we would like to be able to encourage: wearing seat belts, inoculating children, using condoms, preparing for natural disasters, saving more, exercising regularly, sleeping under mosquito nets, and putting litter into rubbish bins. Such examples come to mind because there have been at least partially successful attempts to intervene at the community level to effect change in all these sorts of activities. Over longer spans of time social norms can be deliberately changed and patterns of behavior can be significantly altered by community action, legislation, and custom. No one smokes on planes anymore, but before boarding all passengers now have to remove their shoes. Seat belt use in cars is the custom, and today it is far less acceptable for young people to boast about driving while drunk or having unprotected sex than it was just a generation ago.

As these are examples of changes in behavior, and as groups and societies are made up of individuals, ultimately any sound perspective on change will have to be able to accommodate the changes seen in social movements—methodological individualism (Elster, 1989). It is likely that all behavior change, regardless of the circumstances, has features in common, as any change depends on learning and adaptation, motivation and contingencies, and intentions and goals. Improved understanding of the mechanisms of change might reveal the relative futility of some of society's better intentions, such as public good media campaigns designed to encourage people to install smoke detectors, drive sober, tolerate mental illness in others, or go for health check-ups. Altering lifestyles and everyday habits in global society is not in principle different from individual behavior change. Although the analysis of social change is relevant to individual change, limits need to be drawn in order to have some degree of containment. Instead of including all community interventions, the context of my theoretical account of change is essentially that of psychotherapy: there is motivation to be different, the focus is usually on emotion, there are both internal and external contingencies that control actions, and there is a professional agent who is integral to the process of achieving identified goals.

So why did I not just say so from the beginning? The answer is simple. "Psychotherapy" typically suggests a voluntary client with the intention to change entering into a restorative relationship with a therapist. But in mental health services, or wherever clinical, counseling, and health psychology is practiced, those conditions are by no means universal. Clients are often persuaded to seek treatment by some other party, for example, or are subjected to treatments against their will, perhaps by a court order. And although an individual designated as a client might receive a diagnosis of an emotional disorder, and is typically distressed, this is not inevitably so with respect to all the conditions in which processes of change are of interest. Young people considered to be "at risk" for future problems are often exposed to preventive activities. Programs are introduced across entire educational districts that are designed to decrease depression and anxiety in children. Modern society relies heavily on positive individual change being orchestrated by people whom we call mediators: mentors, teachers, parents, peers, ministers of religion, and Supernanny (Frost, 2006). In addition, treatment can be delivered by a computer program rather than a live therapist, or learned from a self-help book (Kazdin & Blase, 2011). Any unified account of change has to accommodate these necessary variants, rather than being a theory only of conventional forms of individual or group psychotherapy. With such a small minority of individuals desirous of change likely to be able to access a psychotherapist or other formal treatment program, a better understanding of how people change is eminently practical.

Because this book is an enquiry into clinical change, my examples will be drawn from the types of issues that engage clinical and counseling psychologists working in the field of mental health and rehabilitation, and, to a lesser extent, related fields such as behavioral medicine and special education. If you wanted to improve your golf swing or learn ballroom dancing such endeavors would clearly involve change. But they are not the domain of mental health treatments. This is despite what are likely to be similarities with training clinically relevant skills, such as teaching a person with an intellectual disability how to prepare a meal or teaching a person with limited social skills to improve his or her interpersonal interactions. The latter two activities are the province of clinical and rehabilitative interventions and are fully relevant to behavior change in the present context. Principles of coaching, instruction, and practice are very germane to planned behavior change in clients showing skill deficits and will be analyzed, whereas golf and ballroom dancing will happily never be mentioned again.

Extracting the most relevant principles of change from the broad field of modern psychology and then lumping them together is more than a bit ambitious. Almost any aspect of psychological research and understanding is potentially germane to the design of a planned program of change. However, there do appear to be certain areas of psychology that are especially relevant as opposed to other areas that are more tangential. Behavioral genetics, for example, is an important area of innovative research and provides new insights into causes of behavior, but for clients the principles come a little too late to bring about change. Other areas of psychology, conversely, have traditionally taken center stage in designing and understanding therapy, such as early development and motivation theory for psychoanalysis, interpersonal processes for humanistic psychotherapy, learning and conditioning for behavior therapy, and information processing for cognitive therapy. My overview of the most relevant concepts will focus on those selective psychological principles that seem to underlie planned change most specifically.

I am certainly not the first person to emphasize change as the essential issue in psychological therapy. Arthur Staats' (1981) work on unifying learning principles and their significance for behavior, development, and clinical treatment is absolutely seminal. Marvin Goldfried (1980) has consistently emphasized that there are commonalities across various orientations that can be identified at the level of clinical strategies or principles of change rather than similarity among specific techniques. The late Fred Kanfer and I used to meet annually at conventions of the Association for Advancement of Behavior Therapy (AABT, now ABCT, the Association for Behavioral and Cognitive Therapies) and stand around and bemoan the rush to empirically validated formulaic treatments. Kanfer's book on behavior change (Kanfer & Schefft, 1988) is still an influential guide, as is his edited text on helping people change (Kanfer & Goldstein, 1991). Goldstein, Heller, and Sechrest (1966) wrote the very first account of psychotherapy as social influence, a brilliant analysis of therapy process, building on the classic *Persuasion and Healing* by Jerome Frank (1961) and later updated by Higginbotham, West, and Forsyth (1988). Tharp's work on self-change, behavior change in the natural environment, and culturally sensitive educational change has been inspirational to many (O'Donnell & Yamauchi, 2005).

More recently there have been well-articulated calls for evaluating principles of change rather than packaged treatments (e.g., Ablon, Levy, & Katzenstein, 2006; Kazdin, 2007, 2009b; Rosen & Davison, 2003). Michie, van Stralen, and West (2011), concerned about population level change (like public health), wrote that "we need to develop the science and technology of behavior change and make this useful to those designing interventions and planning policy" (p. 43). In their important work on change processes in child psychotherapy Shirk and Russell (1996) called for a move away from "name brand" therapies for diagnostic entities to an understanding of treatment processes in the context of case conceptualizations that identify the pathogenic processes that cause or maintain symptoms in children. The latest trend in cognitive–behavioral therapy for emotional disorders is to recognize the commonalities among these phenomena and to distil treatment strategies to a small set of dynamic principles, a synthesis called transdiagnostic treatment (Barlow et al., 2010). And there are serious efforts to unite the empirically supported treatment perspective (Chambless & Hollon, 1998) with the empirically supported therapy relationships movement (Castonguay & Beutler, 2006).

Because so many different "schools" of psychotherapy have flowered since the first seeds of psychologically based treatment were sewn—Freud's "talking cure"—there have been frequent attempts to integrate the various perspectives and to unify the field (e.g., Stricker, 2010). This is often approached through a kind of consensus process—finding common ground, seeing which terms might really carry much the same meaning, or attributing all effects to a shared prerequisite, such as the relationship between client and therapist or changes in the brain. That sort of eclecticism is a worthwhile endeavor, but this book makes no attempt to unify the different schools of psychotherapy. Instead I will try to pare away the superficial and idiosyncratic terminology and see if the underlying principles that are discussed across a wide range of psychological methods can be distilled to their common elements for the benefit of more effective practice. It is about deconstructing the nature of effective therapy by understanding the foundational principles of change—answering the two questions: how and why do people change?

How and Why People Change

1

Setting the Scene
Why We Need a Theory for Change

> But I know a change gonna come, oh yes it will.
> (Sam Cooke, 1964, "A change is gonna come")

The words of Sam Cooke's single "A change is gonna come" provided the opening theme of Barack Obama's victory speech on November 4, 2008. His resonant campaign slogan "Change we can believe in" had been parodied too often to be repeated directly, and yet it provides a meaningful maxim for an exploration of planful personal change. Although this book is about psychological treatments, it is not an attempt to explain how psychotherapies work. Many previous authors have tried to analyze—forgive the pun—the reasons that psychotherapy is effective, to the extent that it is. Most researchers have attempted to examine the mechanisms underlying a specific form of therapy: they are called process studies. There is also a long tradition in psychotherapy research of suggesting that there are emotional influences common to all therapy and that it is these universals that bring about change, not the explicit techniques or methods of the therapy. It has been suggested that the experience itself of being in therapy allows beneficial personal changes to occur—a sort of "nonspecific" expectancy effect. Others have claimed that all the effects of psychotherapy are a direct consequence of the attachment relationship the client forges with the therapist. Thus, some would argue that the treatment strategy has little to do with therapeutic effectiveness, and good outcomes depend on the characteristics of the therapist, not on the validity of the technique used.

Why Change?

I adopt a different perspective by explaining how and why people change. Perhaps people do change simply *because* they have entered into a therapeutic relationship with a caring, well-intentioned, self-confident, charismatic professional, but we still need to understand why. Conversely, if we find that there is more to behavior change than that, we should be able to understand why people change under a host of different conditions and therapies, *including* what it is about entering into an alliance with a therapist that enables change, and what sort of change that is.

This latter point—that there are different types of change resulting from even the most positive of treatment experiences—is central. In the early 1970s, as a rather inexperienced behavior therapist, I was told a valuable story by Jack Annon, who had pioneered behavioral treatments for sexual problems (1977). He described how he had been seeing a young man at the University of Hawaii Counseling and Testing Center who came in complaining of erectile dysfunction. In the course of the assessment it was determined that the man was quite anxious and Jack started selected anxiety management procedures. It was soon recognized that the client's relationship with his wife was stressful, so she was brought in and much time was spent on enhancing communication and problem-solving skills. Their marriage improved greatly and the client's self-esteem increased. He gained considerable insight into how his strict upbringing had made him unassertive and self-critical, which gave him a much healthier awareness of his own strengths as a person, new coping skills, and effective strategies for combating depression. After almost 2 years of therapy, in the last session the client thanked Jack for a truly enlightening, valuable, voyage of self-discovery. But as the couple had decided to leave Hawaii and return to the mainland, he asked Jack if he knew of a good referral in California for someone who could help him overcome his erectile dysfunction.

The more explicit the nature and type of change a person wants to achieve, the more explicit will the method of achieving it have to be. When desired outcomes are very general, perhaps defined by subjective feelings of fulfillment, relief from distress as measured only by a questionnaire, or the achievement of loose, personal goals, it is possible that a variety of general, broadly based treatment approaches will all produce favorable outcomes that are satisfactory from the client's perspective. But psychological therapies targeting explicit, intractable problems must be made of sterner stuff. If psychologists are challenged to improve the social behavior of a child with autism and also alleviate the hallucinations of schizophrenia, in addition to eliminating anxiety in worried people, and reducing criminal activity in offenders, then we will need reasonably deep and certainly consistent explanations of how and why all such change might come about.

The general public's understanding of what is likely to cause beneficial change can be quite unsophisticated. A recent story in my local newspaper caught my eye as an illustration of the psychological naiveté of common sense. The headline was "Drink-driver fails to learn from daughter's accident, say police" (New Zealand Herald, 2010). The story was about a 34-year-old woman arrested for drunk-driving, whose daughter had been seriously injured the previous year in an accident caused by a driver over the alcohol limit. "This woman's family had been directly impacted by a drunk driver, but unbelievably she decided to drink and drive" the police officer was quoted as saying. Although experiences that are very meaningful or traumatic *can* affect your whole subsequent behavior, for them to do so requires that certain processes of change occur. The consequence of a previous tragedy on a "decision" to drink and drive cannot be assumed to be direct. We might even think that previously distressing experiences could *increase* someone's tendency to abuse alcohol: the tendency to act rashly increases when a person is in a very negative mood (Cyders & Smith, 2007). That too is simplistic, but points to the need to understand complex influences on our behavior.

Why a Unified Account of Change?

There are many explanations in clinical psychology as to why a particular treatment is effective. Even with evidence-based cognitive–behavioral therapy (CBT) interventions there are completely different treatment approaches for apparently similar problems. Because we have lived so long with fundamentally different "schools" of psychotherapy we have come to accept these wildly divergent views as inevitable. We fail to see the intellectual limitations of having different groups within the same profession present conflicting views about appropriate treatments and claiming empirical support for each. There are surprising numbers of seemingly different methods that have been shown to work for identical problems (with children's disorders, for example, see Chorpita et al., 2011). This makes psychotherapy less like a science and more like a political campaign among rival contenders for recognition.

At the conceptual level of how and why change occurs, there is a need to try to reduce all these differences to some unifying principles. Having a unified account essentially means that the concepts, explanations, causes, and constructs making up the explanation cannot be inherently contradictory. You do not have a unified theory if you attribute some change to social support and other similar change to restructured cognitive schema, unless you can specify when one source of influence will pertain rather than another. If one model of intervention asserts the relevance of classical conditioning and another relies exclusively on outcome expectancies, we need to have some notion of whether these are different terms for the same thing or whether one is subsumed by the other. This necessitates a basic deconstruction of terms and principles so that the fundamentals are revealed.

Any attempt at deconstruction must be at a deep level if the kind of unitary principles being considered are to relate with equal validity to totally dissimilar types of human psychological complaint. The factors that result in and maintain a person having auditory hallucinations will obviously be quite different from the factors that result in and maintain binge drinking. However, at a certain functional level there may be commonalities; for example, both patterns of behavior may be ways of managing highly distressing thoughts and experiences. Principles of change that could apply equally to both patterns must therefore be rather basic. Because the variety of human disorders amenable to psychotherapy and considered the province of clinical psychology is so varied, it is perhaps understandable why we have varied, unrelated therapies to deal with them, even within the same school of therapy, supposedly working around the same psychological principles. However, it should be possible to find underlying processes able to account for most positive change. This perspective is different from that of Goldfried (1980), or from Kendall's (2009) reexamination of his argument: both envisage change principles specific to defined syndromes, so their focus remains on treatments (the therapist's behavior) rather than change (the client's behavior).

All research in psychopathology accepts the principles of *multifinality* (a given potential causal variable will result in multiple possible outcomes depending on the organizational context within which it operates) and *equifinality* (the same outcome can result from many different causal pathways) (Vasey & Dadds, 2001). Given this reality, many therapists would argue that change plans need to be based on a particularized assessment of an individual's sources of past, current, and future influence, not on standardized treatment protocols for specific diagnostic categories (Eifert, Evans, & McKendrick, 1990; Evans, 1996). Even so, some generalizations open many possibilities; for instance, fear of a negative evaluation might underlie social phobia, test anxiety (actually all forms of performance anxiety), unassertiveness, and loyalty to a criminal gang.

I will offer one more detailed example here of how apparently unconnected topics may share underlying processes. In child psychology there has recently been considerable interest in "emotion talk." This refers to the way adults (usually parents, but also teachers and other meaningful grown-ups in a child's life) engage in conversations with young children so that the child's emotion is identified and labeled. The parent sees a child who is upset as a teachable moment, and may give examples of times she or he also experienced similar feelings and offer suggestions about how such feelings were managed or coped with. We now know that parents who engage frequently in naturally occurring conversations of this kind have children who are particularly competent in managing feelings and demonstrating knowledge of their own feelings and the feelings of others (Van Bergen, Salmon, Dadds, & Allen, 2009). Parents can be encouraged or taught to have these conversations more often, with benefits to their children's emotional competence (Salmon, Dadds, Allen, & Hawes, 2009).

What is conventional verbal psychotherapy if it is not emotion talk? Much of counseling involves the therapist doing precisely what the emotionally skilful parent does—listen to, identify, and validate feelings in an uncritical way, give them labels, suggest causes, provide self-disclosing examples of their own or others' feelings in similar circumstances, and propose possible coping strategies for managing them. Feelings are not just expressed in therapeutic contexts, they are recognized and acknowledged—even more so in group therapy. In other words, much therapy, irrespective of the specific problem, is designed to enhance clients' emotion knowledge and competence. Suggesting a parallel between the interesting child development forays into emotion talk and the events experienced in adult psychotherapy is not exactly an explanation of the latter's effectiveness. But the underlying mechanisms would seem to be so similar that whatever we learn about the processes between parent and child would be directly relevant to the processes between therapist and client.

Shane Harvey and I have also taught teachers to engage in more emotion talk—before, during, and after a possibly emotionally arousing classroom situation—and they do so and like doing so (Evans & Harvey, 2012). We have evidence that teachers who are responsive to children's feelings in this way have classrooms with fewer disciplinary problems, less bullying, and closer student–teacher relationships. Teachers, just like therapists, need to maintain boundaries by limiting self-disclosure, but can still share emotional experiences, thus validating or normalizing those feelings. Better yet, the role of teacher as acknowledged expert encapsulates local cultural norms (standards) for emotional expression and regulation. When we ponder the therapist–client relationship, here is one way in which it is enacted (Strong & Matross, 1973).

Change Does Not Mean Cure

Some of the changes sought during and following treatment are very general, such as the increase in emotional competence just described. Some are very specific, such as being able to sustain an erection sufficient for satisfactory and satisfying sexual intercourse with a partner. For a child client with a significant intellectual disability a very specific outcome might be the elimination of self-injurious head hitting, and a more general transformation might be the ability to interact socially with friends. Unless we are reasonably clear about what positive changes are desired, the debate over which procedures are the best is not very meaningful. Treatment outcome researchers often make claims and counterclaims of effectiveness before first agreeing on the outcomes desired. Maybe the Dodo bird verdict (Luborsky et al., 2002; Rosenzweig, 1936) was wrong and no one should get prizes, yet.

Behavioral psychologists explain that no behavior is intrinsically and unambiguously good or bad, desirable or undesirable, normal or abnormal. But for various reasons this message has not served to radically shape the way we think about clinical change. One explanation for this continued ambiguity is that within the discipline there exists an intellectual continuum from the perspective at one end that all psychological "disorders" are social constructions, having no reality base outside of subjective and cultural judgment, to the perspective at the other end that recognizable and universal forms of psychopathology exist that are genuine entities, with clear-cut physical embodiment and (nowadays) precise neurological representation in brain functioning.

There are numerous apt clinical examples of the confusion caused by this continuum, but let us consider just two of them: adult obesity and attention deficit hyperactivity disorder (ADHD) in children. At one end of the continuum, obesity is described as an "epidemic" similar to an infectious disease that can be precisely defined according to physical measures such as weight or body mass index (BMI). Causes are attributed to genetic variables, brain chemistry, erroneous satiety signals, or hormonal imbalance. Physical treatments are recommended, such as gastric bypass surgery and appetite suppressants. Good critiques of these assumptions can be found in Campos and colleagues (2006) and in Mann and her colleagues (2007). At the other end of the continuum is the perspective that body weight is a socially defined, culturally specific standard that has fluctuated over centuries. Norms and desirable levels are partially created by the media, so we need to be reminded that "real women have curves" (Saguy & Gruys, 2010). The only question of interest is whether a person's weight is directly causing secondary health problems, since it is quite possible to be "fat but fit." Somewhere in the middle of this continuum is the argument that modern industrial societies have, by virtue of prepared convenience foods and minimal calorific energy expenditure required to acquire them, created conditions making it difficult for individuals to regulate the balance between energy in and energy out and to have healthy levels of physical activity. The goal for people in such societies should be "health at every size" (Bacon & Aphramor, 2011). There are tangible implications of these different assumptions for understanding what to change and how to change it. Should we be looking for changes in ventromedial hypothalamic activity, BMI, weight, walking to school instead of being driven, bingeing, physical appearance, approximation to our desired weight, quality of school lunches, increase in general health, less distorted advertising and air-brushing, or more varied fast food menu choices? All of these have been proposed and monitored in one study or another, showing that the question "What should change?" has not yet been agreed upon.

ADHD is considered a real thing by many experts. Children are diagnosed as having the illness, and it is mostly treated with psychotropic medication (methylphenidate) in Western societies. It is deemed a syndrome, with characteristic symptoms of overactivity, inattentiveness, and impulsivity. These can occur in various combinations, thus supposedly producing distinct subtypes, or even two completely different disorders, one of inhibition and one of boredom (e.g., Diamond, 2005). At the other end of the spectrum is an argument that accepts that activity levels and concentration abilities are variable across children and are probably normally distributed traits. The level that can be tolerated or judged to be abnormal depends on the requirements and demands of the setting, related skills such as meta-cognition that children have or have not learned, and the forbearance of the parents and teachers for high activity levels, which if described as "over-" or "hyper-" implies that we know what a proper activity level should be. Teachers tend to judge children as hyperactive when they display characteristics relevant to managing a class full of children, such as interfering with other students' work or rushing through academic tasks (Kenney, Ninness, Rumph, Bradfield, & Cost, 2004). A middling position on the continuum is that although it is true that there is normal variability, there is a tipping point after which the child's behavior causes widespread distress and disruption, interfering with teaching and learning as we usually structure it. It is better for a child to be given the ADHD label than to be judged naughty, disobedient, or a slow learner, as intervention can then be targeted toward the key skill deficits (e.g., self-regulation).

When commenting on psychological models of problematic behavior versus the classic categories of tangible syndromes, Krasner and Ullmann (1969) made the nice distinction between those of us who are credulous (believe that diagnoses from the *Diagnostic and Statistical Manual of Mental Disorders* are real things like pneumonia) and those who are skeptical (think they are socially and culturally defined, like table manners). Except for those few at the extreme end of either continuum, the difficulty is that most psychologists I know are somewhere in the middle, recognizing when pushed that diagnoses are just labels, but at the same time resigned to having to work within a widely accepted classification system for purposes of communication.

It is easy to see that where you sit on the credulous–skeptical continuum will influence how you would go about structuring a therapeutic treatment program. What has not been so obvious is that the continuum also has a fundamental impact on how you make sense of, document, and evaluate change. If obesity and ADHD are specific clinical disorders, then treatment should make them go away, in roughly the same way an antibiotic will cure pneumonia. But if they are not, then what is the expected purpose and outcome of treatment? Should we hope for a degree of change such that a person's weight or activity level moves closer to a socially accepted norm, and if so then whose norm and how close is enough? Stigma (weight discrimination) may be the real public health threat (Puhi & Heuer, 2010), so should social expectations be changed? What changes are needed for a very active child to be judged positively as "spirited," or an impulsive one to be judged as "adventurous," or an inattentive one to be judged as "creative"? Moderate drinking rather than total abstinence is a viable outcome for people who are alcohol dependent, given the demonstrated success of many people who are able to reduce their drinking to low-risk levels (Sobell, Sobell, Leo, Agrawal, Johnson-Young, & Cunningham, 2002). By adopting a "problem-focused paradigm" (Bentall, 2003), clinical psychologists have been able to make considerable headway in reducing distress, improving coping, and humanizing the experiences of people diagnosed with schizophrenia.

Change Is Judged According to the Client's Goals

When people actively seek therapy it is because they want their circumstances to be different (Strong & Matross, 1973). They do not typically express this goal as being free of some syndrome or another. In fact they may not even be aware that they have a syndrome until given a diagnosis by the professional. This means that a client's own personal goals need to be expressed and in turn understood or accepted by the therapist, a process that takes considerable negotiation because many therapists, and certainly behavior therapists, prefer to have explicit treatment goals both agreed upon and also expressed in operational terms. We basically ask clients to state as precisely as possible how they want their lives to change as a result of the therapy—an optimistic request when our assessment is that anxiety, depression, or delusional beliefs expressly distort their ability to make calm, rational, or realistic choices.

There is a further more expansive meaning to client-articulated goals and these are the more personal strivings—the life projects that people seek to accomplish to make existence meaningful (Emmons, 1986). To discover these, we question clients much more broadly about their ultimate goals as they pursue these across the domains of their lives—work, family, health, religion, and so on. Ideally, we would assume, planful change should meet both treatment goals and life goals. The latter contribute to global life-satisfaction; the former are often expressed either as feelings to avoid and be rid of, or positive feelings to acquire (Busseri & Sadava, 2011). In a very interesting analysis comparing avoidance goals with approach goals, Elliot and Church (2002) pointed out that therapy goals can always be expressed one way or the other. Examples they give are "To accept feelings and learn from them" (approach) versus "Not be so moody all the time" (avoidance), or "To have closer relationships with my friends" (approach) versus "Avoid feeling alone and isolated" (avoidance) (Elliot & Church, 2002, p. 244). These authors then showed that clients with more avoidance goals experienced smaller increases in subjective well-being over the course of treatment. Furthermore, when therapy goals were avoidance oriented, the clients reported lowered satisfaction with their therapists, based on questions such as helpfulness of feedback given or degree of insight they thought their therapists demonstrated.

Different Treatments Assume Different Causes of Change

If we consider just one "school" of therapy, the very dominant cognitive–behavioral therapy (CBT), we can see several of the ways in which different methods to tackle different clinical problem areas have evolved. CBT is presented as though it were a single entity or at least a coherent approach. Professionally there appear to be commonalities, with journals, organizations, conferences, and so on, all bearing the same general "CBT" title. This is despite the fact that in terms of their basic epistemological foundations behavior therapy and cognitive therapy are often contradictory. The behavior therapy that was developed, taught, and practiced in the 1970s is very different from the CBT practiced today. Is this because there are new principles replacing the old? Have there been major new discoveries? Is it because the practices of the 1970s have been found to be wrong and new ones have been found to be right? Essentially the answer is "no" to all of these questions. Modern, contemporary CBT is the uncomfortable hybrid it is because of social and intellectual preferences and the persuasiveness of scholarly trend-setters. Within the structure of CBT as an applied discipline there are no prescribed methods for replacing one approach with another, or for deciding whether one set of constructs must be formally modified in the light of new scientific discoveries. The attempt to set a standard by giving the seal of approval to certain treatment protocols (Chambless et al., 1998) was a noble endeavor. But it has backfired by adding newly approved products without taking possibly outdated ones off the shelf.

A striking example of this mushrooming of ideas and knowledge instead of building new concepts on the basis of well-established older ones can be seen in the field of applied behavior analysis (ABA). Historically ABA was part of CBT, but it now sees itself as a quite distinct therapeutic discipline. ABA is the application of Skinnerian principles of a more "radical" behaviorism (devotees call it the "experimental analysis of behavior") to everyday practical problems (Evans, 2005). Although the principles are good and appear to be universal, their translation into practice has not always been sound. For instance, it is clearly effective to teach a simple operant response to an animal through frequent, repeated learning trials. However, this may be neither practical nor humane when teaching a skill to a child with autism (Prizant & Wetherby, 1998). Or it may be that in the laboratory it matters very little whether the operant of interest is a lever press (for rats) or a key peck (for pigeons). But in the classroom, the selection of the most appropriate behavior to reinforce depends on many factors, including the guarantee that the new response will be acceptable in the child's social milieu (Voeltz & Evans, 1983).

In response to these and other criticisms, adaptations of standard ABA programming emerged called positive behavior support (PBS; Carr et al., 2002). PBS interventions strive to be holistic, and socially valued activities are taught in context, without drills. The reinforcers are more natural, often being social or intrinsic rewards rather than primary rewards such as food. In PBS there is a major emphasis on the teaching of alternative behaviors with the same function as the undesirable ones to be reduced. However, and this is the point for the moment, PBS has not *transformed* ABA—it is not the new, modern version of ABA. They just coexist, side by side, advocated by different groups of clinical researchers and practitioners and supported by different training workshops, journals, and conferences. In fact there is even some degree of antagonism, with ABA purists believing that the standards that define PBS are based more on values than on hard data (e.g., Mulick & Butter, 2005). So an opportunity to move ABA forward, based on new scientific insights rather than Skinnerian dogma, has stalled.

It is not an original allegation that in developing psychological treatments we have spread outward rather than built upward. All of psychology is "preparadigmatic," Staats (1990) lamented, by which he meant that our science is similar to pre-Newtonian physics in which a raft of different perspectives, ideas, or analyses could all coexist even though they could not possibly all be correct. We have, he asserted, no agreed upon mechanism in psychology for replacing limited ideas with more correct ones, other than fading professional memories. He also claimed that almost identical bodies of research and conceptual analysis cooccur in our field, sometimes without any of the proponents of one approach recognizing the proponents of another. We have overlapping bodies of work in motivation, personality, social psychology, and child development—spreading but not ascending.

Staats attempted to rectify this disunity by proposing a broad "social behaviorism," with theoretical constructs allowing for hierarchical building of explanations as the topic area demanded different levels of analysis. It was, and to my way of thinking still is, a desirable effort (Evans, Eifert, & Corrigan, 1990). But it has not caught on. Many readers, even those well versed in CBT, may barely recognize his name or be able explain his philosophy of science. Perhaps he was before his time, perhaps he is not the Newton of psychology, perhaps his ideas were insufficient, or perhaps psychology is not really a natural science at all. Hans Eysenck (1967) also realized that although different phenomena required explanation at different levels of abstraction, each level had to be logically linked to the others. Thus, different brain processes could be linked to different learning and conditioning mechanisms, yielding different traits resulting in different personality dimensions and from thence to different attitudes, social behavior, and even political beliefs. Today, however, we have rampant reductionism. For example, complex and subtle features of adolescents' social behavior are "explained" by reference to the construct *the adolescent brain* having heightened responsiveness to incentives and socioemotional situations (Casey, Jones, & Hare, 2008). Such perspectives offer no apology for ignoring any of the intermediate explanatory requirements when accounting for wide individual differences in adolescent behavior across families, communities, and cultures.

To permit a simpler, more prosaic influence on the way clinical psychologists think about change, the present attempt at a unifying perspective is going to be much humbler and more limited in scope than the grand theories of Staats or Eysenck. The advantages of this attempt are purely practical. Practitioners do struggle nobly to make sense of new methods of psychotherapy, despite the opprobrium heaped on them by critics such as Dawes (1994) and Baker, McFall, and Shoham (2009). They conscientiously attend workshops, they learn innovative techniques, and they acquire new words to use with clients. Some may also become ardent believers and advocate their ideas in journal articles, popular media, web sites, academic conferences, and through their teaching, training, and supervision. Perhaps they are a little too ardent at times; regrettably there are rather too many gurus in psychotherapy (Rosen, Barrera, & Glasgow, 2008). Given our constant desire to present clinical psychology's interventions (especially in the CBT tradition) as "rigorous," "evidence-based," or "scientific," it must surely be recognized by anyone who has watched these methods fade away as fast as they emerged that clinical psychology's techniques are largely taught and promulgated through social influence processes, not scientific discovery. This can be seen at conventions of any professional group—one year a topic is hot and the next year it is history. These are more like new fashions in clothing than paradigm shifts.

Searching for Basic Principles

In this complex intellectual environment a relatively simple and coherent set of principles of how and why people change could provide practicing clinicians with a steady, empirically based foundation from which fancier and more complex therapeutic strategies can be built. A review of the principles could be even more valuable for students and novice therapists. A reason for this can be seen by looking back at the history of behavior therapy or of CBT. When behavior therapy began it drew almost entirely on basic principles of conditioning and learning. This meant anyone familiar with learning theory could deduce, for any given client or type of problem, a possible treatment strategy that maximized the client's prospect of change, either through learning something new and adaptive or unlearning something old and maladaptive.

But as different protocols emerged, it became possible for trainees to use the protocols without fully appreciating the principles underlying them. At about the same time these protocols materialized, the emphasis on formal empirical validation of specific treatment packages became ever stronger. The upshot of this was that the protocols themselves were manualized. And because the outcome data supporting a given package were based on its delivery only in that explicit form, there was less room for novices to be able to modify the manual on any grounds other than a few trivial details about client preferences. Different problems demanded different packages, so the packages were customized for specific syndromes, those characteristic of the clients who had been in the original validation trial. It is now clear from the writings of many distinguished clinicians that experienced practitioners do modify these protocols with impunity. But for students this is not so easily done, especially if they are unsure of the underlying principles.

Valuable as treatment manuals might be for consistency, they are rarely able to accommodate individual and cultural differences in clients. This is because similar sets of symptoms can have completely different causes (functional relationships). Furthermore, people with different developmental levels, education, life experience, and culture do not share the basic skills and values that are assumed when treatments are developed. Many contemporary treatment protocols, for example, require reflective thinking—mindfully introspecting on our own cognitions and emotional sensations. Obviously we would be cautious about assuming that a young child can do this (Alfano, Beidel, & Turner, 2002). But this is also a skill that adults with difficulties such as Asperger's Disorder or early signs of dementia are unlikely to come into therapy possessing. Certain limitations in meta-cognitive and meta-emotion skill are to be expected in many other people. Every practicing clinician knows that you cannot assume all clients will be able to engage equally successfully in therapy techniques that require mindful self-awareness, whether the technique has been empirically validated or not. An elderly participant in a Massey University study of anxious veterans of the atom bomb trials in the South Pacific described mindfulness training as "airy fairy nonsense" (Jourdain, 2010).

A further complication is the way in which therapeutic procedures are commonly described in the professional literature. Therapy techniques are not usually presented as principles of change (Doss, 2004). Weersing, Weisz, and Donenberg (2002) made a list of techniques used in child and adolescent treatments. Many of them describe things a therapist might claim to be doing, such as "Trying to understand the original circumstances that led to the current problems," or "Identifying and challenging irrational beliefs, attributions, and schemas." Spirito and colleagues (2011) used this checklist to find out what a group of therapists in America most commonly offer adolescent outpatients after discharge from a hospital for suicide attempts. Methods rated as "frequently" used identified the professionals' goals, not mechanisms of change: "Trying to enhance the adolescent's cognitive or affective perspective-taking skills." Of those few items in the checklist that seem to be clearly about change, the one most frequently used by the therapists in the sample was "Training in problem-solving skills," but only by 58% of them. Of these varied professionals 28% reported that they "never" used rewards or praise in adolescent outpatient therapy.

There are other reasons why treatment protocols will inevitably come and go. The most realistic is that the social and philosophical contexts within which clinical psychology designs services are also in a state of constant flux and change. Trends in service philosophies might be mildly influenced by psychological insights, but generally they happen quite independently. Deinstitutionalization of psychiatric patients occurred as a result of complex economic and political forces, including civil rights and greatly improved medications. It had little to do with the wonderfully clear demonstration that social learning principles generated programs significantly benefiting the lives of hospitalized patients (Paul & Menditto, 1992). Because traditional contingency management programs were based on the organizational structure of the hospital ward, they became largely irrelevant as interventions once the patients were integrated into community care (Wakefield, 2006). This occurred despite solid evidence that the underlying principles themselves were sound. The task for psychologists interested in treatments for people with persistent psychiatric disorders is to devise ways in which positive social learning, reinforcement and cognitive principles, and social support can be used constructively in natural community environments in which access to rewards is not restricted. That requirement essentially eliminates the formal protocol once called "the token economy" (Kazdin, 1977). It is now largely an historical curiosity.

Unfortunately there are an awful lot of potentially relevant principles to address and the challenge is to isolate the most central ones. Because my topic is actually how and why people change their *behavior* (actions, feelings, thoughts), the answers have to be consistent with known behavioral principles. I use the term behavioral quite loosely and it is not an attempt to privilege any special theory of learning such as neobehaviorism, social learning theory, or cognitive theory. In fact, all of these approaches will be drawn upon if they seem to help us understand processes of change in practice. Some principles, such as reinforcement and association, are so fundamental they will crop up without further justification. Others, such as whether changing cognitive content directly alters feelings, are in need of more careful scrutiny. However, I will start the analysis at the level of measurable outputs (things people do or say or emote) and measurable inputs (contexts, settings, stimuli, consequences, and, of course, other behaviors), and in this sense the meta-theory is essentially small "b" behaviorism.

Finding unifying explanatory principles is not the same as judging all therapies to be basically the same. It has become a popular idea in psychotherapy research that seemingly any and all therapies bring about some degree of change in clients (Wampold, 2001). It is also claimed that the self-reported benefits expressed by clients in verbal psychotherapy are experienced quite early in the therapeutic process (Hansen & Lambert, 2003). Early rapid improvement (Ilardi & Craighead, 1999) could be due to "nonspecific" positive expectations (placebo effects) and what Carl Rogers (1958) described as "loosening of feelings." If many different approaches and forms of therapy all result in early benefit, it is understandably tempting to conclude that the specific forms of treatment are unimportant compared with entering into an alliance with a therapist (Strupp, 1986). From there it is a small step to the argument that what makes therapy work must, therefore, be some underlying mechanism common to all. The common element of most "talking therapies" is the engaged positive relationship between client and therapist, so this might be considered the source of all change. On the other hand, careful studies of the sequences of change that occur during therapy strongly suggest that early alterations in key maintaining patterns of behavior are more predictive of good outcome than the therapeutic relationship. For example, behavior theory proposes that constantly trying to restrict our dietary intake is what sustains the binge–purge pattern of bulimia nervosa, and it is early change in dietary restriction that proves to best predict overall clinical improvement in such clients (Wilson, Fairburn, Agras, Walsh, & Kraemer, 2002).

I hope to show, therefore, what therapists have to arrange in order to induce change. A useful metaphor is that of "kernels" (Embry, 2004; Embry &

Biglan, 2008), the ideas at the heart of any intervention plan. One reason the search for such kernels or elemental principles is so appealing is that when we look closely at treatment manuals they are invariably multifaceted. That is to say, the better-established, validated protocols have a whole series of different components or strategies—they are ears of corn, not simply a collection of kernels (Weisz, Ugueto, Herren, Afienko, & Rutt, 2011). Psychological syndromes are complex, and complex strategies targeted at different elements of a syndrome may be essential. But what is unusual is that treatment protocols designed for completely different types of problems and syndromes share many strategies in common. There might be, for instance, a stress management kernel in the treatment of posttraumatic stress disorder (PTSD), chronic pain, binge eating, generalized anxiety disorder, hypertension, autism, and irritable bowel syndrome.

Psychotherapy as a Framework

It is an inconvenient truth that therapists are not essential for therapeutic change. Most people change of their own accord, with no therapist involved. Even quite significant and distressing personal problems can be altered by people's own efforts. This is fortunate, as there would never be enough psychotherapists to deal with the range of all possible human psychological needs (Kazdin & Blase, 2011). In the 1960s, when behavior therapy as a field first emerged, if people made significant improvements on their own it was still being labeled "spontaneous recovery." Today we tend not to think this kind of change is truly spontaneous at all. We now accept that people find strategies that work for them from many different sources—family, friends, rabbis, general practitioners, books, television dramas, and so on. So pervasive are such social, cultural, and media forces that it behooves professional therapists to pay close attention to these powerful influences.

Where does that leave the very popular domain of formal self-help and professional advice delivered through books and videos? Undoubtedly this is a relevant topic since the reputable guidebooks are planful, they are deliberately embraced by the "client," and generally they are based on sound psychological principles. If learning deep muscle relaxation is a useful strategy for managing stress and anxiety, it matters little whether the client is taught the technique in person by a therapist, or reads about it in a self-help book, or models it from an informative video. The only true difference is that the author of the self-help manual has to anticipate the range of possible needs of almost any random person who picks up the book and tries to follow it. A self-help book has to present the guiding material in a way so generic that the essential principle is clearly spelled out. Good self-help books do exactly this (Watkins & Clum, 2008).

We know why people want to change. People seek or enter therapy because they are unhappy with their lives and their experiences as they are and because they have a social-cultural understanding that psychological therapy ("counseling," "analysis"—clients are not always clear on what it is called) represents a possible solution to their troubles. A whole host of people are referred for therapy because someone else of importance or in control thinks the individual's behavior is harmful, annoying, or distressing to others in the immediate social milieu. People rarely enter therapy because they have a distinct and recognizable condition for which some form of psychotherapy is the correct treatment needed to restore them to health. Syndromes may be a convenient way of categorizing many of the types of distress or annoyingness that we in Western society have decided are amenable to psychological intervention. But people do not come to therapy because they have the syndrome—they have the syndrome because they have come to therapy—or at least to professional attention.

Don Baer (1997), the most articulate pioneer in applied behavior analysis, famously argued that people enter psychological treatment because someone is complaining about them; that someone could be themselves. Only when the person is no longer complaining or being complained about, Baer concluded, have they been successfully treated. The goal of psychotherapy is to change clients' behavior so that no one of social relevance complains about them anymore. What makes this proposition interesting is that it suggests that we could get equally good outcomes by changing the people doing the complaining. The individual may not be doing things very differently, but the *acceptance* of the identified problem behavior, or the person's own tolerance for it, has been altered.

When first assessing a client's motivation for therapy, most psychologists will ask the individual why he or she has come to see them. This is not exactly the same query as "what is troubling you?" The real questions are, what do you expect therapy can do for you, what alternatives do you know about or have tried, and what triggered the referral? These are contextual issues surrounding all planful change, and, as we will see when examining motivation to change, they can be highly influential. Clients, by definition, are seeking help; we need to know what that means for them before negotiating goals.

There is one very major difference between carefully designed and controlled treatment outcome studies and the use of the same treatment strategy to provide help in routine clinical practice. In the former, the clinical researcher has a treatment and needs to recruit people on whom it might be tried out; in the latter, the practitioner has a person, a client, and needs to find a treatment that might help him or her. Often individuals in research trials are volunteers or people not yet seeking treatment, since they cannot already be in any form of clinical treatment or that would be a major confound for the trial. Practitioners have no such luxury. Their clients usually have a host of relevant and related problems, will inevitably have tried different treatment approaches already, or may even be undertaking other treatments at the same time.

When someone finally presents to a clinical service with a request for treatment, the referral route might have been quite elaborate. It starts with some alteration, whether biochemical, social, societal, or natural disaster, which has destabilized their usual adaptive functioning or exceeded their ability to cope. In all likelihood there will have been a subjective moment of urgency, of desperation, or of extreme need that has triggered the process of professional or formal help seeking. This is because consulting a professional for therapy is not, even in our modern society, the very first thing people think of when they are distressed. A combination of a perceived urgent need along with recognition that psychological intervention is plausible and the psychologist is an expert will result in a service contract. Thus, the process of psychotherapy often has to begin with crisis management before a complete formulation of the client's requirements can occur and treatment targeted to the individual's more fundamental and recurrent needs can begin. Inevitably, therefore, change theory, like treatment, must address short-term change as well as long-term, more permanent changes.

Therapeutic Treatment of Syndromes

Within apparently similar diagnostic categories (American Psychiatric Association, 2000), good description can reveal major differences suggesting different change needs. For example, within the pattern of obsessive–compulsive disorder (OCD), some people's obsessions are aversive, unrealistic thoughts that are themselves threatening (sexual, aggressive, scatological, and blasphemous). Others' obsessions are potentially realistic concerns about accidents, contamination, mistakes, creating order, and so on—not intrinsically threatening but triggered by threat cues (Lee & Kwon, 2003). Clients with the same OCD diagnosis can thus require very different interventions to reduce distress. If someone has repetitive thoughts about spreading feces over a church altar, you cannot expose them to (confront them with) the situation the way you might if they feared catching germs from the communion chalice.

Psychological research on the identified forms of psychopathology has provided many insights into what maintains these abnormal patterns. It might be expected that if a pattern can be explained, then it would be only a short step to finding an effective treatment. That has been the main story in the history of medicine. It has only partially worked for psychiatric disorders, where many biological treatments, from brain surgery to lithium, have been discovered by accident. Psychologically, however, if it is recognized, say, that one reason for the restricted eating of a client with anorexia is because of a distorted perception of her own body, then a rational therapy to change anorexia might involve correcting that erroneous image. Similarly, if anorexia is seen as an unconscious strategy for exercising control over parental and family dynamics, then a rational treatment would include family therapy designed to reduce family conflict and improve relationships. For individual clients a very clear formulation or conceptual model of interacting variables leads logically to individually tailored designs for change (Persons, 2008). Potentially there should be a close relationship between understanding the dynamics of psychopathology and the design of specific therapeutic treatments.

Syndromes also reveal all-important patterns of change as they themselves were acquired or evolved into a serious problem. Even if an emaciated adolescent client were judged by her family as having always been a "fussy" eater, she must have at some stage changed from being an essentially typical eater to one who we describe as anorexic. Other clients had at one time typical abilities to venture out into the environment or mix in society and then something occurred, either gradually or suddenly, to change them, so now they fear such experiences and have what we describe as agoraphobia or panic disorder. People who were generally happy and contented began to change at some point to being disconsolate, melancholic, generally sad, and participating in fewer and fewer of life's pleasures to emerge with what we describe as depression. Words such as "cure" imply reversion back to the preclinical stage; how far back we must go is unchartered territory.

When discovered, the origins of many well-known syndromes do, therefore, provide us with insights into the principles and processes of individual change. It may be necessary to take some liberties with these insights and to simplify them somewhat, but the hypothesized mechanisms causing clinical distress provides one of the best tests of any unified theory of underlying change. Thinking of the client with anorexia we might be able to see that family influences are important, but so too are erroneous beliefs, and so too are peer pressures. Are all these principles going to be necessary for understanding how to bring about change, and if so, how, if at all, do these mechanisms relate to each other? Or we could ignore causes entirely and argue that the key change required for anorexic clients is simply that they eat more and restore their weight—however that can be achieved (see Chapter 10 for a discussion).

Must We Always Know Causes in Order to Produce Change?

This book is not about psychological difficulties per se. Even when we know precisely what has caused a problem, these may be historical realities that cannot be reversed, such as early trauma. And because many clients have "comorbid" disorders (more than one form of psychopathology present at a given point in time), it suggests that there may be causes that relate to distinctive features of the client's basic temperament or personality. Despite these challenges, is it really possible to discuss how people can change without probing how they got to where they are now? If we want to understand how people can quit smoking, do we need to know all the factors that caused them to smoke in the first place? Teenage smoking, drinking, and hard drug use have been linked to exposure to community violence (Vermeiren, Schwab-Stone, Deboutte, Leckman, & Ruchkin, 2005). But is that how it starts or how it is maintained? Do substance abuse treatments need to consider the role of trauma following witnessing of and victimization by violence in inner-city youth?

A simple answer is yes, of course, it would be easier to change someone's behavior if we knew exactly how the behavior developed. However, the reality is that even though we do not have that knowledge, we can bring about change. Consider autism. Despite a few promising leads, we do not have the slightest idea about what causes it. Yet there is very strong evidence, based on systematic literature reviews, that an early and fairly intensive regimen of structured learning opportunities can impart skills that improve outcomes for young children with autism (Makrygianni & Reed, 2010). There are many causes for behavior patterns and they all vary in the level of directness of their influence.

Let us stay with smoking to illustrate this. Nicotine has addictive properties, generating strong urges. Also smoking cigarettes, for whatever reason, helps people emotionally—the habit makes them feel good or at least less bad, so we need to see it as a coping strategy. Ah, but surely young people started smoking because it was perceived to be a grown-up thing to do, so maybe we need to consider media influences? But probably their parents smoked, so modeling is relevant, or their friends encouraged it, so we have to analyze peer group influence. Then again, stores that sell cigarettes to minors and the low cost of cigarettes both relate to ease of access. In Indonesia where there is no minimum age for the sale of cigarettes, the average starting age for boys is 7 (Hodal, 2012). I could go on, but the point is hopefully clear: behaviors that are of interest because we hope to change them are caused and controlled by many factors. Anyone involved in planning their change needs to recognize the varied causes from the most distal to the most immediate. We also need to differentiate initial causes, such as wanting to appear cool to friends, from maintaining factors, such as the calming effects of cigarettes. As a 14-year-old boy in Jakarta stated when interviewed: "When I have a problem to solve—and I have so many problems at school—I have a smoke. It relaxes me and makes me forget" (Hodal, 2012, p. 21).

If we were now to plan an intervention for current smokers, most of the distal causes cannot be changed and most of the maintaining variables are the inevitable consequences of the behavior. So the solutions for the problem are simply going to have to be very different from the causes. Understanding the causes could help to plan a preventive intervention, as happened in California and Florida when public health campaigners suggested *not* smoking was the cooler lifestyle choice, with smokers portrayed as the puppets of the tobacco industry (Rosenberg, 2011). A possible solution for stopping smoking might be to foster the behavior of *desistance*, but lack of will-power is not one of the original causes of the smoking habit. When contemplating the dynamic factors that maintain particular behavior patterns, knowing about response interrelationships and the effect of one response pattern on another offers a conceptual framework for thinking about planful change (Chapter 7). Ideally the plan would incorporate elements from all the different levels (distal versus immediate; initiating versus maintaining), but could not address all of them directly.

An additional example might help cement this argument. Think about youth crime, a major social problem. Even the most cursory analysis of factors increasing a young person's probability of committing a crime immediately reveals multiple causes within five broad domains. (1) *Individual factors* include cognitive deficits, hostility, impulsiveness, and antisocial attitudes. (2) *Family factors* include harsh and inconsistent parental discipline, domestic violence, parental criminality, and sexual abuse. (3) *Peer-related factors* include antisocial associates, gang membership, and lack of positive leisure activities. (4) *School factors* include failure to develop meaningful relationships with teachers, being bullied, disengagement from learning, and early suspensions and expulsions. (5) *Community and neighborhood variables* include overcrowded, underresourced neighborhoods with high crime rates, economic deprivation and unemployment, poor housing, and easy access to drugs and weapons.

No intervention could modify all of those influences. But if we understood what promotes *change*, perhaps interventions can be devised that would be able to significantly alter the life trajectory of a young person currently engaged in criminal behaviors, *despite* those influences. The source of this optimism comes from a second fundamental truth about causes of problems. Although problem behaviors are multiply determined, those same underlying risk factors do not inevitably lead to the same undesirable outcomes. Many young people are exposed to the same causal personal, family, and school variables as described above, but do not become criminals. There are preventive influences as well as causal ones: inspirational teachers, strong mothers, celebrity role models, and positive peer friendships. Factors that put a young person at risk are not the mirror opposite of the influences that combine to determine a positive outcome.

Change Not Treatment

Other scholars examining psychotherapy have also come to the realization that change is the central issue (e.g., Strong & Claiborn, 1982). Miller and Hubble (2004), in their tongue-in-cheek envisioning of the future for psychotherapy, wrote, more seriously:

> the decades-long debate between this or that model, specific versus common factors, technical versus theoretical integration, and so on misses the point because it focuses almost exclusively on the means of production (e.g., theories and methods) rather than the product of therapy—that is, the creation of meaningful and lasting personal change. Simply put, it has proceeded as if the field were in the therapy business rather than in the business of change. (p. 62)

This book is not a guide for how to do psychotherapeutic treatments—the "means of production." But if the basic mechanisms of change are outlined as clearly as possible, coming to appreciate them should allow the deduction of many strategies for producing meaningful outcomes (Evans & Meyer, 1990) for individuals, groups, and communities. Some of these arrangements might be entirely novel and never previously attempted in those particular forms. What the psychological literature has to say about conditions and variables that make change more likely is not the same as a how-to-do-therapy manual, since therapies almost inevitably confound the principles of change with the manner in which these principles are delivered or communicated. And, as already said, that difference in translation (the difference between ABA and PBS, for instance) masks the common underlying principles. Two therapies that appear to have similar goals may rely on very different rationales; yet these may be differences in their proponents' talk rather than representing fundamental differences in achieving change.

Happily there are several helpful generic accounts of how to be a good therapist. The best ones drill down to the essential features common to many therapies based on interpersonal interaction: (1) That the relationship between client and therapist is an affirming, positive one. (2) That both client and therapist expect a beneficial outcome. (3) That there is a therapeutic "story," such that the problem is recast and understood in a new conceptual framework. (4) That some aspects of the problem and the negative emotions are confronted directly, often through instruction, modeling, and actively testing reality. (5) That mastery is encouraged by the acquisition of new skills. (6) That the focus tends to be on the present and the future rather than dwelling exclusively on the past. (7) That there is an emphasis on ensuring, maintaining, or increasing the client's autonomy (Argyris, 1970). Each of these, however, requires clients to change, which is not restricted to therapist influence.

Not all psychotherapy has to be about change. It can be about receiving permission to stay the same, as in the early days of sexual therapy when much of the focus had to be on normalizing practices that elements of society had declared to be taboo (Annon, 1977). Psychotherapy may involve gaining acceptance of yourself as you are. I once had a client in my private practice in Hawaii, Gloria, who burst into tears when I asked her what her goals for treatment were. "Can't you just let me be myself? I don't want direction. I just want to think and reflect and feel supported." As a teenager, a brilliant student and a talented pianist, Gloria had felt dominated by her overprotective parents. She had deliberately gone away to California for college to escape, but in her second semester she experienced a severe viral encephalitis that resulted in her being hospitalized in a coma for 6 months. During that time her parents came to help take care of her, asked her new boyfriend to cease all connection, and destroyed all personal items such as love letters that were in her student apartment. When she recovered enough to return to Hawaii she had memory difficulties and other cognitive limitations and was now even more controlled by her parents than ever before. Frustrated, moody, lonely, and having academic difficulties at the University of Hawaii where she was now enrolled, Gloria persuaded her parents to let her see a psychologist and I blundered unwittingly into the very conflict she was fighting against. Naturally, some change did happen, eventually. I was her ally negotiating with her parents, advocating for her to be able to live on her own, make friends, and establish her independence. But I constantly had to be wary of any hint that she should be indebted to me for gains achieved.

Nardone (2004), in analyzing clients' requests for therapeutic help, came to realize that there is often an unspoken demand: "change me without changing me." Marsha Linehan (1994) has superbly described the fundamental dialectic of acceptance and change and of working with people to help them change when what they crave most is acceptance. How can a therapist communicate to clients that he or she accepts them unconditionally, and in the same breath recommend strategies designed to alter them? If you have to change you cannot be acceptable as you are. Luckily, only a minority of clients demand unconditional acceptance. These tend to be people whose personal sense of themselves as acceptable is compromised, or people who believe that they cannot be both loved and criticized at the same time. Such dynamics are particularly characteristic of individuals who attract the diagnosis of Borderline Personality Disorder. But many people have difficulty feeling secure as a person, or in their relationships with romantic partners, or with others who they feel should be unequivocally on their side, such as a parent or a therapist. When this type of insecurity is severe, it creates demands on their relationships and emotional expectations that cannot easily be fulfilled—especially by those therapists who try to maintain some degree of detachment in their relationships with clients.

It has been noted frequently that psychotherapy is not about personal discovery so much as persuasion to a new perspective. Wittgenstein (1980), for example, argued for a version of acceptance rather than resolution—namely that it is necessary to live within life's constraints. He saw the problems of life as unhappiness, feelings of sorrow, and fears. To remove these feelings and replace them with positive alternatives requires changes in a person's life and, in particular, requires establishing an agreement with the forms (mould) of living; as a result it becomes possible to experience life as a joy. "The fact that life is problematic shows that the shape of your life does not fit into life's mould. So you must change the way you live and, once your life does fit into the mould, what is problematic will disappear" (p. 27). Two meanings of acceptance have crept into this discussion: self-acceptance of oneself as one is (roughly the meaning used in Acceptance and Commitment Therapy, to be explained later) and acceptance of differences, lifestyle choices, and eccentricity by one's immediate society.

Neither of these meanings precludes taking action. I experienced a resonance of both when as an academic professor of clinical psychology in rural upstate New York I was very cautiously approached by a number of people who met together as a support and self-advocacy group. Calling themselves "The Butterfly Club," they were transgender and transsexual individuals who essentially interviewed me rather than the other way around. Their request was for someone professional who might be able to assist them in a variety of emotional areas as the need arose—like anyone else they could experience anxiety, depression, relationship difficulties, and marital tensions—but who would not attempt to change their sexuality or their cross-dressing, trample on their identities, or attribute their emotional concerns to their transgender status. There are various groups of people whose experience of conventional psychiatric and mental health services has been extremely negative and destructive (Corrigan & Penn, 1999). For me at the time, 30 years ago, it was an eye-opening request, but one to which I could easily acquiesce. Today there are Butterfly Clubs of transgendered and transsexual people all across the world, providing information and awareness, combating discrimination, and supporting change—but not change grounded in conventional, statistically normal behavior.

Implications

In the area of public policy and evaluation, problems of the kind I have been using as examples—smoking and youth crime, and complex relationship dynamics—have become known as wicked problems (Rittel & Webber, 1973). Wicked is not used in the moral sense, but in the mathematical sense of being convoluted and highly resistant to resolution. Wicked problems are interdependent and always multicausal, as I have been illustrating. We are all familiar with the fact that attempts through social policy to solve such problems often have limited benefits and unintended consequences. We might try to reduce dependence on carbon fuels, but by promoting biofuels we see destruction of native forests and loss of farmland that was previously used to produce staple food crops in third-world countries.

From a public policy perspective there are clear criteria for problems being designated as wicked. For instance, the problems are unstable, they often do not really have a clear solution, there are disagreements among stakeholders as to their basic nature, they are socially complex, and at the institutional level often have different agencies and organizations responsible for attempting to manage them. When change is achieved it is often not sustained. Because of this, researchers and evaluators have come to recognize that conventional linear attempts at solutions are unlikely to work. In fact, most of the wicked problems we would all like to address—such as climate change, crime, unemployment, disaster preparedness, and chronic illnesses—have been marked by rather spectacular policy failures.

If we think for a moment about the characteristics of wicked problems we will see that they are not terribly different from many problems that come to the attention of clinical psychologists, counselors, and therapists. Marital difficulties, for example, are likely to be multiply caused, their definition depends on who is describing the problem, their successful resolution is not likely to involve complete elimination of all further difficulties, and they are influenced by ecological, social, and physical factors over which the protagonists may have little control—family pressures, job insecurity, children with disabilities, household accommodation, and health. And so it seems likely that the sorts of nonlinear methodological approaches that have been required of policy makers may need to be considered in psychotherapy research as well.

There is a final irony to this analogy between individual treatments and public policy interventions. In the public policy arena it is now clearly recognized that the solution to all wicked problems requires changes in *individual* behavior. The intervention tactics available to governments and social agencies are quite limited—increasing taxes (on cigarettes and alcohol), legislation (raising the drinking age), and public service announcements (information and advertising campaigns). Institutional and governmental change efforts usually focus on attempts at punishment—penalties, fines, and loss of privileges. We do not reward drivers for obeying the speed limit; we punish them if they exceed it. We all know how useless that has proved to be as a strategy. All these methods are designed to change behavior, but it is increasingly realized that they rarely do so without the commitment and acceptance of individuals.

Change can be immensely difficult, but sometimes can be very easy. It has been reported in a number of psychotherapy studies that about 25% of clients improve significantly after just one session (Barkham, 1989; Howard, Kopte, Krause, & Orlinsky, 1986). If we accept that finding at face value it is perhaps a testimony to the power of psychotherapy. But if we think about it from the perspective of measured change, questions immediately arise. What changed after one session? What was the original targeted concern? Was it a wicked problem? What degree of change constitutes improvement? Defining what we are interested in according to change concepts lays bare many of the concepts in outcome evaluation that have a great deal of surplus meaning: cure, recovery, improvement, treatment, and therapy.

When our focus is limited to psychotherapeutic outcomes, it is natural to think of symptoms disappearing and syndromes ameliorated. But psychologists recognize that changes of this kind occur against a finite pattern of daily activities—how people are spending their time and their lifestyle (Walsh, 2011). Change should convey that the full complement of those typical daily patterns of life quality is improved. To judge a clinical outcome as positive requires that the new pattern is better than the old, by many possible criteria. Recognizing that clinical change takes place against the backdrop of everyday variation and growth, Karoly (1999) proposed that it be construed as pattern interruption or destabilization, with effortful attention to the establishment of alternative patterns, followed by the restabilization of these alternative patterns. To understand this shift in perspective, we now need to examine in much greater detail what psychologists conducting treatments mean by change.

2

What Is Therapeutic Change?

A cartoon in *The New Yorker* (August 2, 2010, p. 27) shows a patient on the couch turning to his therapist and saying "As far as your bill is concerned, I've finally learned to say no." The joke works because most people recognize that teaching people to be more assertive is a common focus of psychotherapy. In clinical work with clients, however, it is rather easy to take for granted that we all understand the target of change and even what we mean by change. This chapter could as easily be called "what changes?"

In psychotherapy we talk about clients "working through" their problem, moving further down the path, overcoming the past, gaining insight, achieving personal fulfillment, or becoming self-actualized. Stiles and his colleagues (1990) theorized that in successful psychotherapy clients' painful thoughts, memories, and feelings are *assimilated* into schema, a familiar pattern of ideas and constructive ways of thinking. Engaging in psychotherapy is sometimes compared to embarking on a journey, perhaps one of exploration and self-discovery. Karoly (1999), knowing that life is already a journey, characterized psychotherapy as correcting "ineffective life-course management (ineffective self-regulation or psychological wayfaring)" for those of us "travelers" who are "moving falteringly toward vaguely understood destinations" (p. 284). All of these images have the value of creating an expectation that in treatment something new or the restoration of something old is to be experienced. Psychologists typically do not talk about curing psychological disorders, but growth is still a commonly used metaphor, particularly in humanistic contexts. Achieving or maintaining "wellness" is regularly used in mental health nursing and psychiatric settings. Even though psychologists repudiate the idea that clients literally have an illness, the fact that psychiatrically defined syndromes are widely accepted as the target for treatment means there is an unrecognized bias in the way we think about the change that will result from treatment. There is a rarely challenged assumption in outcome evaluations that clients have "got" something bad (just like a virus or a growth) and when treatment is over that something should be gone and will not come back. An even stronger assumption is that in the process the client should not have picked up some other bad thing. In medical treatments it is not uncommon to have to worry about patients having surgery to remove something and coming away with a new infection, or getting a treatment to combat an illness in one organ resulting in harm to another. These are commonly referred to as the iatrogenic effects of treatment and surgeons and psychotherapists try to avoid them.

One of the visions of what psychotherapy, counseling, or any other formal psychological intervention does to you is that of tension release, often called catharsis. This was originally a central feature of Freudian psychoanalysis. In the very first case Freud was involved with—treatment actually carried out by his colleague Josef Breuer—the striking discovery was that when the client, Anna O., talked openly about recent upsetting events and experiences, she enjoyed some immediate symptomatic relief. Many religious experiences and rituals similarly purport to drive out the inner demons. Persistence of the concept may be related to the everyday experience that venting about a problem, having a good cry, or releasing pent-up emotion in some other way seems to leave you feeling better afterward. Guerin (2001), challenging the concept of catharsis as the release of tension (grief, anger), has argued that it is "how one talks about the events with other people and the social consequences of this approach that are important" (p. 49). This "interbehavioral" (Kantor, 1969) analysis of change mechanisms helps us think about the terminology of change as socially constructed metaphors rather than factual accounts of a known behavioral phenomenon.

A troubling metaphor, very common in the area of sexual abuse and trauma generally, is the image of clients being damaged, mentally wounded, or emotionally scarred, so the purpose of psychotherapy or counseling is to heal, rather than bring about behavior change. The trouble with words is they begin to create their own reality. It is very common among my local media or TV news anchors or print journalists, when discussing some horrendous accident or assault, to say that the physical scars will eventually heal, but "the emotional ones will stay with the victim forever." Clients and counselors often share this kind of dramatic language, thus lowering expectations that positive change is possible. Although not wishing to minimize the sequela of traumatic experiences, reversing these effects has been shown to be possible, using a variety of different techniques (Taylor & Harvey, 2009). Are there emotional scars following trauma? Is there some sort of shadow left by past experience, and if so how do we ensure that it remains as inert as internal physical scars?

Harm Reduction or Recovery?

"Recovery" as an outcome falls uncomfortably close to the cure idea. Much beloved by the mental health community—the recovery model is a philosophy as much as a measurable goal—recovery implies freedom from the disorder or remission of the illness. The connotation of the term is positive and encouraging, and thus helps to promote a valuable sense of optimism. Hope is a major theme. But in reality two-thirds of the people with psychoses do not become completely free of all features of their disorder, although obviously they can and do change and go on to lead happy, productive, and fulfilling lives in their own sometimes benignly eccentric ways (Turkington et al., 2009). People's feelings of well-being are subjective, made up of cognitive elements such as personal fulfillment and perceived quality of life, and emotional elements, such as happiness and satisfaction with life (Diener, Oishi, & Lucas, 2003).

Psychiatrists propose that there is actually a continuum of recovery styles (McGlashan, 1987). At one end is the "integrated" recovery style, in which individuals come to recognize that psychotic experiences originate within the self. Integrated clients are curious regarding their experiences, aware that there is continuity between psychotic experiences and nonpsychotic experiences, and tend to further their understanding by eliciting help and support from others. At the other end of the continuum is the "sealing over" style in which the psychotic experience is perceived as alien, disconnected from the usual experiences of the individual, who is less likely to engage with mental health services. These styles can be measured by a self-report questionnaire, agreeing or disagreeing with statements such as "I liked some of the unusual ideas I had when I was ill" (Drayton, Birchwood, & Trower, 1998). Both styles can lead to positive social and emotional outcomes, but neither guarantees absolute client satisfaction. McCleery and Evans (2001), for example, found that clients showing favorable reduction in symptoms after cognitive–behavioral therapy (CBT) still reported feeling lonely and isolated. One of Hagan and Turkington's (2011, p. 9) clients, diagnosed with a psychotic disorder, poignantly expressed his treatment goals as "having a place to live, someone to live with, and something to live for."

Knowing that some persistent and harmful patterns of behavior may not show major change but can still be modified so as to be somewhat less harmful to the individual or society has led many intervention studies to conceptualize positive change as harm reduction. Reducing the likelihood of harm is especially useful as an outcome goal when dealing with really intractable behaviors such as drug addiction, alcohol abuse, or gambling. In such patterns it is the secondary consequences of the problem that need to be minimized (see the advocacy work of the Canadian Harm Reduction Network, http://canadianharmreduction.com/). Clean needles reduce the risk of HIV infection; receiving methadone at a clinic reduces the risk of crime committed in order to purchase illegal drugs. Teaching clients to inhibit domestic violence when drunk, or limit family financial losses when gambling, might not improve the actual problem but will decrease its negative secondary consequences. Reducing the risk that something harmful might happen to the individual or the risk that others might come to harm is a pragmatic outcome designed more to benefit society than the client, but that is valuable for everyone concerned and should always be considered when designing and evaluating interventions.

Forms of Change

Howard and his associates introduced a useful three-phase sequential notion of the recovery process, based on the metaphor that clients feel ill, show symptoms, and experience a disability in functioning. The outcomes of treatment would thus involve (1) remoralization, which is rapid improvements in well-being; (2) remediation, which is gradual symptom relief; and (3) rehabilitation, which is the eventual "unlearning of troublesome, maladaptive, long-standing behaviors and the establishing of new ways of dealing with...life" (Lutz, Martinovich, & Howard, 1999, p. 572). Measures of each process should provide three different trajectories of client benefit from treatment. However, this notion has to be qualified by the inevitable interactions among these three broad trajectories, as will be further explained in Chapter 7.

Additionally, it must be recognized that the change we are interested in clinically may take a variety of different forms. Rutter and Rutter (1993) proposed five possible types of change according to the core mechanisms: there is (1) an alteration in the biological substrate, (2) establishment of an underlying psychological structure (e.g., acquisition of communicative language or the emergence of attachment), (3) the learning of a specific behavior or skill, (4) the development of new values or expectations that serve broadly to regulate behavior (e.g., the internalizing of parental rules), and (5) change in social interaction patterns that influence later behavior (e.g., being accepted by a particular peer group influences many later social activities from criminal behavior to academic interests). In applied behavior analysis this latter form is referred to as "habilitation," or the degree to which our behavioral repertoire maximizes short-term and long-term reinforcers in the individual's natural environment.

We will encounter additional forms as well as elaborations of these five types. But for now it should be clear that thinking of change just as the difference between two scores on a measure of an attribute is not likely to be sufficient to understand underlying mechanisms and processes. As Serin and Lloyd (2009) expressed it so well: we know the beginning and end points for the caterpillar turning into a butterfly, but the details of the transformation remain obscure.

Research Definitions Versus Clinical Expectations

Measures of Outcome

From this introduction it can be seen that therapeutic change has at least four distinct features. One is that there must be something identified as change worthy for both the individual and society; another is that the person moves discernibly from one state of being to another (literal change); the third is that the final state, the end-point of therapy, meets some social criterion of success or personal satisfaction with the outcome; and the fourth is the pattern (sequence) of alteration over time. All four of these features are acknowledged in the research literature, but not at the same time. With respect to the fourth, clinical psychology research focused on outcomes has been less interested in the nature of change itself. The tradition in most treatment studies is the two-wave measurement at the beginning of the treatment of some dimension thought to be relevant, and then to measure it again at the end of treatment and possibly some period of time after treatment has ended, the so-called follow-up assessment. The difference between the beginning and the ending score represents the degree of change the treatment has achieved, but forms of the alterations underlying this change of status are less often examined.

Target behavior selection. Different terms and concepts have been used to describe these four features. The first is usually subsumed under questions of target behavior selection, or in the compelling question posed by Robert Hawkins (1974): "who decided *that* was the problem?" Just as psychiatric diagnoses can be unreliable (the given labels vary according to who is making the diagnosis), so the selection of the behaviors to be targeted for treatment is a complex professional judgment task producing very varied decisions across experienced professionals (Wilson & Evans, 1983).

Statistical significance. The second feature is analyzed according to many measurement algorithms for representing the magnitude of change, such as the statistical significance of the mean pretest/posttest differences or, more usefully, calculations of effect size. Effect size is an estimate of the degree of change in light of the variability of scores before and after treatment. The metric was an important step forward in research design and publication standards—most journals now do require that effect size be reported, not simply probability values of the significance of the difference between means.

Because the size of anything is always relative, the effect size metric is based on the difference between preintervention and postintervention scores (or the difference between two groups at postintervention) expressed as a ratio of the variability within these scores. This means that if everyone's score is pretty much the same to begin with, very small ending differences between groups or conditions will be judged as representing a large effect (Chambless & Hollon, 2012). Large effect sizes might still mean many clients showed no change, whereas small effect sizes could indicate modest but meaningful gains for almost everyone. So effect size is still a statistical concept and not a measure of the absolute size or importance of an observed difference. In everyday life we are beset with this same ambiguity. Recently a company promoting a fuel additive as increasing gas mileage was charged by the New Zealand Commerce Commission with false advertising. The company's response was that in objective tests, cars fuelled with the additive did travel further on the same amount of gas than those with regular fuel, which was precisely what they advertised. However, for a full tank of gas, the increased distance traveled was only a couple of yards—not exactly what the motoring public was expecting.

Clinical significance. For these reasons the third feature has received a great deal of attention, being represented by terms such as "social validity" (is the change valued by others; can others really notice the difference?), the "clinical significance" of change (is the change large enough to be clinically important, or is it just "a few yards"?), and "meaningfulness" (will the change be sufficient to make a difference in the individual's overall quality of life?). A client's new test score may be statistically different from the original one but still not be very important in terms of practical benefits. A depressed person's Beck Depression Inventory (BDI)-II score might drop by 50%, from 40 to 20. That is a large change, but although it indicates symptomatic improvement, it certainly does not mean that the client is back at work free of depressive moods and melancholy thoughts. If a teenager with anorexia has gained weight, but now feels unattractive and is consciously monitoring everything she eats, is that meaningful therapeutic change? A distressed couple might have half as many arguments after marital therapy, but does their general profile now resemble that of nondistressed couples (Jacobson & Truax, 1991)?

What changes? A fourth consideration, then, is really *what* has changed? The answer is not always obvious. After treating a child with a phobia, let us say a fear of dogs, the successful outcome observed or reported is that the child does not cry when seeing a dog, no longer clings to a parent in the presence of a dog, and may even approach a friendly dog and be willing to pet one. But could this mean that the child has become more courageous—engaging in approach behaviors despite fear—or is managing to control anxious expression despite still feeling some degree of apprehension or threat from dogs? Bravery is a good outcome, but it is not the same as having zero level of fear; in fact, clinically it might be much better and more adaptive than being totally fearless.

Alternative Concepts in Communicating Change

A completely different sort of measurement model is to first define precisely what a desired and desirable outcome would look like for the client—a criterion reference—and then see what sort of treatment is necessary to get the client to this point. Meeting the minimal criterion, regardless of by how much, is the treatment objective. Thus, for example, an investigator might aim to reduce all depressed clients' BDI-II score to 13 or below, which evidence suggests can be considered a valid cut-off score between clinical depression and everyday gloom. Typical body weight for height in a group of clients with anorexia seems like a worthy, if limited, criterion, compared with simply reporting number of pounds gained. When researchers have faith in the validity of the scores on their measure, they will refer to this standard of clinical outcome as remission. The criterion-referenced approach to treatment evaluation has the added advantage that we can specify the outcome for a group of clients in terms of how many of them actually reached the standard after treatment—a useful result that is masked by group averages (Evans, 2007).

Because all criteria have to be defined somehow, clients—as opposed to research participants—often have a chance to specify more exactly what their own desired outcome might be. They set their own benchmarks. The practical reason this is important is that once clients reach their desired outcome they should want to stop treatment. In everyday clinical practice criterion referencing is what is typically in place, if only implicitly. But the model is not used in most research studies. Research studies generally end when the preselected number of treatment sessions required for the experimental protocol has been reached. Progress—desirable change—of some kind will have been reached and that is what gets reported, but how closely this progress matches the actual needs and desires of these participants often remains unknown. Also ambiguous is whether the treatment for those showing the least progress might not have been fully successful had the intervention simply continued for a longer period of time. Thus, declaring one treatment superior to another disguises the possibility that the less successful treatment might have fared better had it been continued over more sessions. In routine practice, in contrast, the client and the therapist together set goals, ideally in definable recognizable terms. When these targets have been achieved, therapy is judged to be successful and is ended, no matter how long that takes (within certain practical limits set by third party insurers or public agency guidelines).

In clinical practice it is the client who tells the therapist that he or she is now feeling less depressed, or is really sleeping better, or that his or her child's teacher is reporting much less disruption in the classroom. We want clients to be able to say "thank you doctor, but I no longer need your help" (Castelnuovo, Faccio, Molinari, Nardone, & Salvini, 2005, p. 242). Outcomes in the clinic are more closely tied to the broader therapeutic goals (consumer satisfaction; subjective well-being), whereas in the empirical literature they are most often reported as changes in scores on a preselected test instrument whose value and importance we are still left to judge.

Real clients always use an unspoken effect size model. They are well aware that their complaint, whatever it was, fluctuated to some extent before treatment, or, like problems such as tension headaches, were getting steadily worse and more frequent. They are also likely to experience variability in their feelings of improvement during and after treatment. Thus, the client has to judge that he or she, although not perfectly improved all the time, now has more "good days" than before. If pretreatment experiences were consistently bad (little variability), small, low-variability gains posttreatment will be more obvious by contrast. Clinicians might remember that when they ask clients at the start of the next session "How was your week?" (or words to that effect), they are requiring clients to make a highly complex judgment. It will be influenced, up or down, by many extraneous factors such as contrast effects, their pessimistic cognitive style, their desire to please the therapist, or their desire to solicit sympathy.

Because treatment research relies on formal measurement to determine change, it raises the immediate problem of how faithfully the instrument is measuring the phenomenon of interest. As these instruments are so crucial for communicating research findings, a huge amount of professional energy is spent on developing, refining, and validating them. But in the end the score on the instrument is a *measure of* a something, not the something itself. A BDI score is not depression. A mother's rating of her own child on the Child Behavior Checklist is not a measure of the child's behavior but her perception of that behavior (Evans & Nelson, 1977). Even direct behavioral measurement may not precisely represent the clinical concern. The number of times in a 50-minute class period that an active child is off task (a nice, easily recorded, precise measure) is not the same as that child's engagement with the learning process, which is presumably what everyone is after. This point was originally made forcefully by Winett and Winkler (1972) when they subtitled their article "be still, be quiet, be docile" to emphasize that classroom interventions were implicitly about academic achievement, but the reported outcomes were only about sitting quietly in class.

The prechange–postchange model is the one most widely used in group research because the goodness of the outcome is conveniently expressed in terms of the mean improvement for the group as a whole. Thus, one criticism of any study purporting to show effective treatment could be that although 50% the clients did show considerable gains in scores, 25% of the clients did not change at all, and another 25% of the clients actually got slightly worse—their scores deteriorated. The overall gains could be quite large, but practicing clinicians deciding to introduce this supposedly well-validated treatment might be very disappointed if their clients performed like the two unsuccessful subgroups in the original study. Long ago, when it was claimed by Eysenck (1952) that psychoanalytic therapy did not really do much for anyone, its proponents suggested that this apparent ineffectiveness was an artifact of many people getting better and a few getting worse. Bergin (1967) coined the term "deterioration effect." Psychotherapy was so powerful, the argument went, that clients could be harmed as well as helped. It is certainly regrettable that various popular treatments such as boot camps for youth are not just inert but can cause further harm (Lilienfeld, 2007). If we start from a change perspective, however, the argument takes on a different hue. Change is change. *How* we judge it—up or down, good or bad, short-term or long-term—is a different issue.

Evaluating Change

Many excellent scholars have recognized that thinking about change requires a value judgment. Thus, descriptive terms such as "clinically significant change," "social validity," and "meaningful change" (Evans & Meyer, 1990) have been introduced and defined. However, from what has just been argued, these kinds of value judgments will be seen to cut across a series of different measurement issues. Because the issues are quite complex, the discussion thus far has been a ramble through many important nuances. It would be helpful here to quickly summarize the basic argument regarding client change. This has nothing to do with the reliability and validity of a measure. It is a given that psychometric criteria have to be met—if we are measuring something it has to be a reasonable estimate of the construct being measured. Essentially there are five completely different aspects of evaluating change we need to consider. Here are the questions:

Have we identified the appropriate thing to measure? This could be about target behavior selection (Evans, 1985), it could be about whether the client's goals were correctly recognized to begin with, or it could be about selecting the defining feature of a complex phenomenon (or response class) as an indicator. One of the great controversies in the treatment of alcohol problems, for example, is whether the appropriate outcome should be total abstinence or controlled drinking. In an entirely different sphere, I am professionally interested in changing (increasing) children's enjoyment of school in order to prevent dropping out. So should I be measuring it by asking students if school feels accepting and they belong, if learning is fun, or if they like their teacher? Or should I assess it behaviorally by giving them a choice between going to school or going camping?

Has the phenomenon we decided to measure actually changed? This is basically a technical measurement issue, and no matter how good your research design it is not easily answered if the pretreatment levels fluctuated or were going steadily up or down. Sidman (1960) had it dead right when he argued that unless a person reveals a "steady state" it is difficult to measure a true change in anything. When trying to interrupt a time series, random variations across different time frames bedevil interpretation as researchers in climate change and traffic accidents know only too well. Note that this question is not at all the usual researcher's question about internal validity: did the treatment *cause* the change? If there is genuine change and that is what was wanted, I am not at this point worried about whether it was the treatment as specified or something else entirely that brought it about.

Is the degree of actual change sufficient to meet treatment objectives? This question is about whether change is sufficient for the client or those around him or her to "stop complaining." Is the change recognizable to the client and is it what the client wanted or expected? This issue is about meeting criteria of worthwhileness.

Is the worthwhile level of change going to last for a reasonable period of time? This is a fairly obvious question about the permanence of change—which cannot always be guaranteed or may not even be a reasonable outcome expectation. Researchers in eating disorders can help clients reduce their frequency of bingeing to zero posttreatment (judged as recovery) and some of them even lose some weight (Grilo, Masheb, & Wilson, 2006), but for how long is this pattern maintained? A young child treated successfully for trauma following sexual abuse might yet experience stress when encountering sexual situations as an adolescent. If children's engagement with schooling is targeted, for example, they cannot really be expected to enjoy school for the rest of their student days. On the other hand, if I am claiming successful treatment of a convicted rapist, society would surely expect the client not to ever offend again. There is also the hope that desirable change will continue to increase still further, long after the treatment has ended. An even better outcome would be if the observed change led to other improvements (positive side effects): the abused child is more resilient, the engaged student plans to go to college, and the rapist is more empathic.

Has the observed degree of change been obtained at a behavioral cost? If I were interested in evaluating a psychotherapeutic treatment I might want to pose this question as one of cost-effectiveness—was the outcome worth the resources used to achieve it? That is a legitimate question, but it is not relevant to the clinical judgment of change. The cost I am referring to here is the possible negative impact the change in the targeted behavior might have on other valued behaviors or on the client's situation. For instance, the increased assertiveness mentioned at the beginning of the chapter might have a deleterious effect on a marital relationship. Could increased enjoyment of school have a negative effect on a child's industriousness (study habits)? This question is about negative side-effects, but that is not quite the same as treatment being harmful—treatment can be harmful because the change was for the worse, whereas this issue is about positive change that comes at a behavioral cost.

Maintaining and Extending Positive Change

Having mentioned the long-term duration or permanence of change, it is now an opportune time to address this issue in detail. Returning to formal clinical treatment studies, in good research design follow-up means the participants are reassessed some time after the therapy has formally ended. Commonly used time intervals are 3 months and 6 months after treatment. What we are interested in is whether the positive changes made by the end of therapy have been sustained—or, even better, that further progress has been made (that is the hoped-for exponential effect). In the most regrettable case the client's functioning may have slipped back to levels seen only early in the treatment process.

In one study of 196 adolescents treated for major depressive disorder, 96% showed an absence of symptoms on the Schedule of Affective Disorders and Schizophrenia for School-Age Children (SADS), regardless of the type of treatment received (medication, CBT, a combination, or a placebo). Five years later, however, 47% had had a recurrence (Curry et al., 2010). Such reversions are called relapses—medical analogies being so very pervasive. The more we know about certain behavioral phenomena, the more we know whether relapses are likely (if there are two steps forward, is one step back to be expected?) or whether with appropriate supports and new coping skills the client's trajectory is likely to be one of steady further improvement. Does the first occurrence of one serious mental health episode, such as major depression, make a subsequent one more likely, and what might be the reasons for such a "kindling" effect?

There are many clinical phenomena in which you might strongly expect a sort of waxing and waning effect rather than an on/off, present/absent kind of distinction. Mood disorders provide a vivid example, for good reason. We know that for anyone, ordinary negative moods come and go with some regularity. People who do not have a disorder can recognize their moods and will have an inkling as to their cause, mange them so they are not too intense, and have strategies for getting themselves out of a funk. Thus for clients with a mood disorder repeated negative moods can be expected, but without those effective self-management skills they will be harder to deal with. Clients worry about reoccurrence. This is a kind of "scarring" effect, as some have called it; a negative mood state reminds the person of past negative mood states, so that future negative moods are dreaded (Alloy, Abramson, Walshaw, & Neeren, 2006). The same downward spiral occurs with anxiety sensitivity or fear of fear, to be discussed later. When trying to understand change, the nature and causes of these variations in trajectory need to be unpacked.

Follow-up measurements, then, assess the continuation of therapeutic benefits. One of the most valuable features of treatments based on cognitive-behavioral models is that since the expected outcome is rarely that of a cure (full remission of all symptoms), the conditions that would allow for behavioral changes to be maintained or generalized have been carefully analyzed and can be built into the design of treatment. In the applied behavior analysis tradition, maintenance and generalization have been given formal definition and status as well-established phenomena, defined behaviorally. *Maintenance* refers to the continuation of a behavioral pattern either in the absence of the therapeutically engineered controlling conditions that caused it or in the transfer of control from therapeutic conditions to comparable conditions in the natural environment. *Generalization* refers to the continuation of the behavior pattern in settings and contexts other than those that were present during the therapeutic phase. There is a degree of overlap between the two ideas, in that maintenance involves behavioral permanence in conditions other than active therapy, but in practice the methods for supporting both continuation of behavior and its occurrence in relevant new contexts are slightly different and merit separate consideration.

Maintenance

What things does a therapist need to do during treatment to promote maintenance? First, we know that behavior that has been reinforced on a partial schedule is more resistant to extinction (more persistent) once reinforcers no longer occur—the partial reinforcement effect (PRE). The partial reinforcement principle would suggest gradually withdrawing any artificial reinforcing consequences, placing the person on a lean, intermittent schedule of, ideally, unpredictable reward. A plausible explanation for the PRE is that the frustration arising from nonreward is extinguished; a nonreward experience does not signal no further reward ever.

If rewards in life are intermittent and unpredictable, learning to perform despite occasional disappointment could be a very useful attribute. But it would be far more obvious and sensible to try to design treatment such that once the therapist was no longer reinforcing the behavior directly there would be some other more natural contingency of encouragement operating, such as from a teacher or parent (a mediator). Compliant behavior might now be rewarded by the gratification of pleasing the teacher, and diligent study might be rewarded by pride in better grades or satisfying feelings of competence. Many effective treatments, in other words, do not really have to end at all. If something is working to maintain positive behavior, maybe it should just be continued. This shifts the emphasis from a unique, bounded therapeutic program conducted by a professional to the idea that therapy consists of arranging natural contingencies and contexts that result in desirable outcomes and that these can be continued without direct professional involvement. This is exactly what Tharp and Wetzel (1969) explained and described: to bring about long-term change, reconstitute the natural sources of reward, usually social, in the child's environment and try to ensure that they continue, which they will if the child's behavior change is equally reinforcing to these "change agents." However, when we learn that contingency management interventions with substance abuse are the most effective of the psychosocial approaches (Dutra, Stathopoulou, Basden, Leyro, Powers, & Otto, 2008), arranging social rather than material rewards for drug-free days is difficult in a natural environment that is hard to access.

On the other side of the coin, if the desired change is reduction of emotional arousal, the process is analogous to the conditioning phenomenon called extinction. We want the response to be eliminated and to stay that way. Sadly, however, a firmly established phenomenon in classical conditioning is that a response that has been extinguished is prone to return—"spontaneous recovery"—after a period of time or if several new learning experiences are introduced. To promote maintenance of a reduced emotional response, therefore, a therapist might be able to arrange the same conditions in the clinic as would produce greater permanence of the extinction effect. These conditions include overlearning, which means continuing the extinction procedure long after the unwanted emotional response seems to have disappeared, and trying to eliminate new reconditioning trials, such as further stressful experiences. In real life things are not as easy. Imagine someone being treated for public speaking anxiety. Assume that this client does have to give a certain number of public speeches. If the client gets through one speech reasonably successfully his or her confidence for the next occasion will be enhanced. If the client performs poorly his or her anxiety regarding the next performance will increase, regardless of within-session gains.

Generalization and Transfer of Training

More often than not, psychological treatment involves shaping new social and emotional skills in the clinic, with the expectation that they will be used by the client in the real world. That is not so much a treatment goal of maintenance but of generalization. Because so much of what is taught in the office is expected to generalize to the outside world, it is not surprising that therapists have given the topic careful consideration.

In applied behavior analysis generalization has come to mean that a response will occur, appropriately, in a context different from that in which it was acquired (Stokes & Baer, 1977). If the stimulus configuration changes, will the behavior continue to occur? Thinking practically, this might indicate that if you have successfully taught greater compliance to directives from a parent at home, for example, then the same willingness to follow directions will occur for a teacher in a classroom. Or if a client has successfully learned to tolerate a feared object such as a spider or a mouse in the therapy room, then the client will be able to go into his or her attic or basement—the decrease in fear has generalized.

One of the fascinating realizations in clinical work is just how specifically certain stimuli can control behavior, especially emotional reactions. The person whose fear of insects—spiders and cockroaches are common phobic objects—has been significantly reduced in the office will often report total panic when encountering the same insect in the natural environment. Why? Because on that occasion the insect was not confined to a glass container, or the insect suddenly moved, or it looked like it was going to run toward the client, or it was just a little bigger than the one used during treatment, or the therapist was no longer present as reassurance. In the days when treating specific phobias was still a common thing to do, clients often gave these altered stimulus configurations as the reason for the failure of the treatment procedure to generalize to all insects or small animals in all environments.

There are various things a therapist can do to increase the likelihood of generalization. They follow logically from what has just been said. In the therapy stage when new skills are being taught or emotional responses to external stimuli are being reduced, it is helpful to vary the stimulus context during the therapeutic procedures. Extinction, if that is the mechanism, must be to all relevant and likely insect stimuli, not just to one. Technically speaking, exposure to many different versions of the feared stimulus in the extinction procedure (nonreinforced presentations of the conditioned stimulus) broadens the *inhibitory* stimulus generalization gradient, which is what we want to ensure. It should be noted that according to experimental studies (Dunsmoor, Mitroff, & LaBar, 2009), fear is very likely to generalize to a wide range of potentially threatening stimuli, as can be seen in clients with posttraumatic stress disorder (PTSD) who become very fearful of events and conditions that only slightly resemble those present at the time of the trauma.

There is an additional meaning of generalization in the behavioral literature and that is not the production of the same behavior in different contexts (stimulus generalization), but the production of different behaviors in roughly the same context (response generalization). We know a great deal about response generalization from a long history of success in teaching people with severe developmental disabilities and acquired brain injuries to perform everyday tasks such as simple self-help tasks or work-related skills. We could, for example, teach a youngster with severe handicaps to wash his or her hands and dry them on a towel after using the toilet. Now the youngster goes to a restaurant, or to school, or to work, and each place is a little different: the soap dispenser requires pulling or pressing, the towels are continuous rolls of cloth that have to be pulled, or paper towels that have to be tugged out of a dispenser, or blow dryers under which hands have to be placed. To combat the possible failure of response generalization, the appropriate learning program for such a client is to train him or her in a variety of settings with all the behavioral variants required by different faucets, soap dispensers, and drying procedures. This type of training in multiple exemplars is called general case instruction, and it is hugely useful when teaching the common elements of slightly different functional skills. Lest you are tempted to dismiss these issues as being of little interest in your own world, think back to a time when you were visiting a foreign country: you might have skills in catching the Hop or the Skip bus in Boulder, Colorado, but still not be fully competent to use the Snapper Card on the Go bus in Wellington, New Zealand, although the general principles of catching a bus are pretty much the same across both cities.

It is from work environments that a broader concept of generalization—known as transfer of learning (or training)—has special application to clinical practice. Just think how often we clinicians or educators try to generate behavior in another environment by means of skill development programs, taught in lectures, seminars, manuals, workshops, and group therapy. Hundreds of hours are devoted to in-service "professional development" by corporations, schools, and government organizations. Most trainers, be they teachers or professors or therapists, are hoping for "far transfer" to dissimilar contexts, but that is harder to achieve than "near transfer" in which the new context is quite similar to the training context. When the novel task is analogous to the training task, transfer is enhanced if the individual is given a cue to use a relevant principle. Transfer is further enhanced when the training is voluntary and the trainee has certain prior characteristics: cognitive ability, conscientiousness, or motivation to learn. It is also helpful for trainees to have some prior knowledge of the domain to which transfer is intended (Barnett & Ceci, 2002; Blume, Ford, Baldwin, & Huang, 2010). A number of very general skills, such as reasoning or research skills taught in formal education, do transfer, but probably far less than many academics would hope for. However, critical thinking skills, higher-order reasoning, hypothesis testing, or simply schooling for children are examples of ways of interconnecting deeper knowledge structures that facilitate transfer. In work settings effective transfer is most likely to be found when the culture supports and rewards the new learning and innovation that might arise from the training, which is precisely what we have already concluded to be true in therapy settings as well.

Preventing or Avoiding Loss of Treatment Gains

Although we often think of change as the acquisition of new, appropriate, functional skills, it is equally important (when concern is with negative behaviors) to understand ceasing a behavior, or desisting from a previous undesirable pattern such as criminal activities. Later I will touch on the role of punishment as a socially sanctioned method to encourage the cessation of antisocial and illegal behavior. It is a topic of considerable complexity because some of the people we hope to change do not fear punishment. For another thing, individuals who have frequently been punished for offences predict the risk of further future punishments to be lower than those who have been punished less or not punished at all. They seem to adopt the "lightning never strikes the same place twice" fallacy and "reset" their estimates of the certainty of punishment (Pogarsky & Piquero, 2003). Just to take one further example, punishment's effectiveness depends on who delivers it: sanctions imposed by people who matter to an individual, such as family or friends, are more effective than those imposed by some remote judicial authority (Braithwaite, 1989). In an oft-cited survey of British youth, teenagers were asked what they perceived as the most serious consequences of being arrested. Only 10% of the respondents said "the punishment I might get," whereas 55% said "what my family or my girlfriend would think about it," and 12% identified "the publicity or shame of having to appear in court" (Zimring & Hawkins, 1973).

So we need to think more logically about conditions supporting the cessation of undesirable behavior. Echoes of Zimring and Hawkins' work were reported by one of my doctoral students, Nick Wilson. His dissertation revealed an interesting finding regarding long-term outcomes, postrelease, for a group of high-risk violent prisoners. These men had spent long periods in prison for repeated violent offences. Their risk to society (likelihood of reoffending) could be assessed to a degree by static predictors, such as the number of previous offences, age when offending started, gender, and even ethnic group. To these predictors, correctional psychologists often try to add more dynamic predictors based on personality characteristics, cognitive style, and criminogenic needs (the degree to which violence satisfies needs for power or domination, for example). Of these various predictors an especially useful one is revealing a psychopathic personality profile—in other words having a callous disregard for the feelings of others, having limited ability to show remorse or express guilt, and having grandiose ideas of your own importance.

Combining static and dynamic predictors allows the psychologist to make better than chance predictions regarding the repeat offender's risk of further violent crime. Wilson was interested in the false positives: men who by every known indicator were likely to commit further serious offences on release from prison, but who in fact had no subsequent periods of reimprisonment. Wilson found a small group of men who had very high indicators of risk, but who had not apparently reoffended seriously for a follow-up period of 5 to 10 years postrelease. He tracked these men down to see what was keeping them on the straight and narrow and thus "beating the odds."

One of the first important findings, as you might well have expected, is that the men were far from being on the straight and narrow. They were not living the lives of model upright citizens and the pillars of their communities, nor had they become particularly likable. Many of them were still abusing drugs or growing marijuana for supply, and committing a range of minor criminal and driving offences. One man described how every time he passed a convenience store he thought about how easy it would be to break in or viciously rob the elderly store owner. His primary cognitions—often the target of CBT-oriented rehabilitative programs in prison—had not really changed, but he was no longer acting on the basis of these thoughts. This is the critical issue. Despite very minor changes in the broader pattern of criminal conduct, these men were successful in not committing any more of the major physical assaults that had landed them in prison.

When probing for the likely cause of this successful maintenance of treatment outcome, Wilson was able to identify a number of factors. Note that these are the conditions to which the men themselves attributed their lack of violent offending; they were coconstructed by Wilson's observations of their social circumstances, lifestyle, and environmental conditions. When I have asked graduate clinical psychology students to deduce what the preventive circumstances might be, they often correctly guess that the men had new, strong women partners who were a positive force in their lives. There exists a great deal of data confirming that marriage, or its equivalent, sustains positive behavior (Waldron, Hughes, & Brooks, 1996). Students sometimes recognize that having a second family of young children in these new domestic arrangements provided the men with an incentive to be a better role model and parent than they had ever been in the past. My students are less likely to come up with any of the real physical causes of change: these men were older, prison conditions had left them infirm and in poor health, and they simply did not have the athletic prowess that had made them so dangerous in earlier years. And finally, few students fully recognize the importance of context, and thus most failed to guess that these men had made a conscious choice to now live in more remote rural communities with many fewer temptations than in the past—fewer bars and brothels, other gang members, or expensive stores and banks (see Chapter 4).

Desistance

The men in Wilson's follow-up had not really changed that much in terms of their basic personality patterns. But their opportunities were reduced and there were certain personal social constraints that were serving to inhibit their old deeds. So to understand change we need to understand why people *stop* doing things they are tempted to do. In the criminal justice literature the mechanism related to the cessation of criminal activity is called *desistance*. A rapidly growing body of research and theory has begun to identify factors that correlate with desistance, the major ones being good marriages, stable work, transformation of identity, and aging.

What is so fascinating about our new understanding of men who have changed from being active offenders to desisted offenders is what it tells us about the outcomes we should be looking for in all clients of mental health and psychological services. Maruna (2001) has described changes in lifestyle from impulsive responding for extrinsic rewards to more thoughtful consideration of the rights of others. Serin and Lloyd (2009) emphasize that change to desistance is not quite the same as removal of the risk factors that originally led to criminal careers. Firm intentions to remain crime free do not lead to change very often either. The motivational influence of anticipating the possibility of a crime-free future is important, as are changes in identity and cognitive factors such as hopefulness, altered beliefs, and recognizing the need to change past associates and habits. Yet these intrapersonal moderators are insufficient to effect change unless supported by new opportunities such as employment, overcoming substance abuse, and stable marital relationships. These variables interact—along with the well-known influence of time alone—in different ways and at different developmental intervals. An attitude shift to stay crime-free may need to precede but then be maintained by acquiring employment, which in turn might satisfy the "criminogenic" need for material reward, but only as long as a cognitive shift toward the value of long-term outcomes has taken place, which will be followed by newly valued social recognition and the intrinsic satisfaction of thinking of the needs of others.

Behaviors that are controlled by impulses necessitate different cessation strategies from behaviors that are controlled by the outcomes they achieve (their function). Behavioral change that requires constant inhibition of action tendencies (urges, impulses) is much harder to maintain than changes in which the dynamic influences have been unequivocally altered. This is why relapse prevention as a purposeful strategy was developed in the context of treating impulse problems such as alcohol addiction or child sexual abuse (pedophilia).

Lapses, Relapses, and Their Prevention

Lapses—failing to implement an acquired skill—occur in all areas of behavior change. A particularly apt example can be seen in parent training. After a teaching intervention, parents will be much better equipped with simple, basic child discipline strategies. Sometimes, however, these take time or need to be practiced in a reflective manner. There will be many occasions in normal family life in which there is little time (sending children off the school, grocery shopping) and parents are pressured (have brought work home) and distracted (on the phone, bathing the new baby). Sanders (1982) defined these as hectic times in which proper program implementation was at risk, so that parents needed to be alerted to these critical periods and to have deliberate strategies for dealing with them.

Many of the changes people hope to accomplish involve stopping current activities that are inappropriate, harmful, illegal, or all three. These are behaviors that are strongly habitual, that are driven by powerful urges, and that have to be actively inhibited. Common clinical examples are consuming alcohol, binge eating, smoking cigarettes, and sexual paraphilias such as exhibitionism or watching child pornography. Given that many treatments teach clients to control these undesirable behaviors but may not eliminate the urge to perform them, it should not be surprising that "relapse" is quite likely. Slipping back into an old pattern of behavior—having a cigarette after quitting smoking, or finishing off a box of chocolates when trying to consume fewer carbohydrates—is a common enough experience for most of us to realize that it presents a challenge to permanent change.

There are two fundamental principles in the many strategies known collectively as relapse prevention (Marlatt & Gordon, 1985). The first is the "what the heck" principle: we need to ensure that one slip-up or violation of a rule for abstaining from a behavior does not indicate to the individual that control is impossible. We know most about this effect from the studies of treating alcoholism. Within the culture of many alcoholism treatment services is a belief that if someone were to violate an abstinence rule, they would then, because of their "illness," be prone, driven in some internal way, to drink more. This is the "one drink then drunk" myth that becomes for vulnerable people a self-fulfilling prophecy.

The second principle is that habits, with their associated urges when prevented, are highly controlled by eliciting stimuli that trigger the undesired response the client is attempting to inhibit. It is harder to control sexual behavior when in the presence of highly arousing erotic cues; the sight and smell of alcoholic beverages trigger the urge to have a drink. One solution, therefore, is to avoid being exposed to these stimuli, as they make desistance so much harder. To this we can add another fundamental principle, confirmed in hundreds of experimental studies: stimuli tend to control behaviors in the contexts in which those behaviors were learned (see Chapter 5). If learning new habits, unlearning old ones, or learning to resist temptations occurs in only one context or setting, a change in that context will result in the person reverting to former ways of behaving (Laborda, McConnell, & Miller, 2011).

Relapse prevention strategies, which were developed around drinking behavior and rapidly adopted by clinicians treating all the urge-based habits, make good use of these two principles. The Alcoholics Anonymous depiction of there being no half way behavior between total abstinence and inebriation is challenged, partly by education and persuasive communication, but even more so by normalizing the idea of relapse so that clients are led to expect that relapse is the norm and if they do break down and engage in the prohibited behavior it is not a disaster but an opportunity to learn where their vulnerabilities lie and to be better able to prepare in the future.

The other principle involves variations of the theme of not being exposed to triggers, which can include rules such as not living next to an elementary school if the client is a child sex offender being released from prison. It also includes more formal efforts to decrease the triggering properties of certain cues. Here the strategy is exposing the client to typical eliciting stimuli in a controlled setting, such as the sight, smell, and taste of alcoholic drinks in the clinic or laboratory where actually drinking them is not possible. The conditioning rationale for this is essentially that of extinction or habituation—the urge should decrease with unreinforced exposure to the stimuli. A third variant is to erode the power of these cues by altering their valence so that they no longer have positive affective value for the individual—we might try to make the sight of someone smoking nearby evoke disgust (yellow teeth and bad breath) and fear (of lung cancer) rather than the urge to light up a cigarette. When this is done verbally it seems like verbal conditioning, if it is done using imagined scenes to create an aversive association it is called covert sensitization, if negative consequences are imagined it is called covert punishment, and if the client is encouraged to think of these negative images when in the actual situation and feeling an urge it is called a self-control strategy (all of which are mentioned again in Chapter 9). A fourth idea is to uncouple the automatic connection between a trigger and an impulsive act (the sequence being experience distress, feel the urge to drink, see a bar, order a drink). It has been proposed that this can be accomplished by intensely shifting attention from that sequence to distracting internal and external cues (Hsu, Grow, & Marlatt, 2008).

Although these are clinically all very useful strategies for ensuring longer term maintenance of change, they do not illuminate the underlying processes of change. Instead they tell us something important about the way change can be sustained. Given that all change is by degrees over some span of time, it might be that so-called relapse prevention strategies are simply a special case of a more general process in which any temporary or transitional change becomes more permanent. This is a very subtle distinction, so it can be made a little more concrete by considering a clinical phenomenon. Let us use bedwetting. Children with a diagnosis of enuresis wet the bed at night outside expected patterns of normative development. Volume of urine is not an important dimension in this phenomenon—we do not look for change being smaller and smaller amounts of wetting each night. We just have a clear goal: dry nights. So as the treatment begins to show an effect, what is the change actually seen? It is more and more regular dry nights. The child does not show slight improvements each night. After X number of dry nights in a row, the child, the parents, and the clinician will start to feel change has been achieved. But lapses are common and after a few dry nights the child might have an accident and wet the bed; then there will be a few more dry nights, then maybe another lapse, and then a long period of dry nights, and so on, until eventually 99% dry nights can be expected. What has changed here is the pattern of dry nights or the ratio of wet to dry nights, and that ratio can be plotted as a cumulative moving average, showing steady change. But what has actually changed is only the probability that any given night will be dry—this should go from zero before treatment to 100% posttreatment. Relapses are not always a failure of change but are integral to the change process. In other words, whether a lapse is judged to be a new state of affairs (a reversal) or simply a further step in the variable change sequence depends entirely on the time frame selected. If you have a 4-month frame for treatment and its follow-up, a reversal (an accident) after 6 months is a relapse; if you have a 24-month time frame for treatment and follow-up, a reversal after 6 months is merely noise in the change cycle.

Measuring Progress, Measuring Change

When someone does change, assuming for now that we know what we want to change, how much of it is meaningful, and across what time frames and contexts we expect to achieve it, we are still left with the rather neglected topic of what the change looks like, over the course of time. Think of the patient in the cartoon described at the beginning of this chapter. He has finally learned to say no. What would have transpired? Was he never able to say no and then one day, after a therapy session, he was always able to say it? Or could he previously say no but only reluctantly and in safe situations, and now he can say it in somewhat more threatening or conflictual situations? Or could he always really say no but when he did so it made him horribly nervous and uncomfortable and now he can say no without those feelings?

The reader may think this is ridiculous hair-splitting. However, for a therapist or any other change agent, including the clients themselves, it is of critical importance to know what change will look like in order to monitor whether it is happening. Even in the case in which there were previously no examples of the behavior that are now there one hundred percent, unseen alterations may have been occurring. Insight is often conceptualized in this nothing or all state. A client can seem to suddenly realize something that was not recognized before—the "eureka" moment in our clients that as therapists we live for. But that is a rarity, and even when it does occur there is a sneaking suspicion that little changes were taking place, little chippings away at the defense mechanisms or growing doubts beginning to form about unsupportable attitudes, cherished beliefs, or the truth of a delusional thought. Almost everything we are interested in changing changes slowly in some measurable amount, and monitoring those values should be tracked for any planned change. Remember too that setbacks are inevitable. Clients often have to do worse before they do better; in developmental psychology we talk about U-shaped development in which a new competence interferes with an old one (Gershkoff-Stowe & Thelen, 2004).

Being able to define change properly is essential for understanding it. Bed-wetting, the messy example I have landed us with, is not actually an all or nothing phenomenon any more than insight. The change taking place is actually the steady change in latency from going to bed until next urination. That time interval gets longer and longer until eventually it is longer than the duration between time to go to bed and time to wake up in the morning. After waking up at the appointed hour, the child can go to the toilet and urinate there—that is a dry night. If the parent wakes the child at 3-hourly intervals and gets him or her to the toilet three times a night, then the child will also have a dry night, but the sleep-to-bed-wetting latency is shorter than the natural duration of a night's sleep.

Will a person being treated for a sleeping disorder gradually be able to spend more and more hours asleep, fall asleep more rapidly, and wake up in the night less and less often? Not really. In fact, if clients are following the stimulus control suggestions of the procedure validated by Richard Bootzin, they will spend less time asleep at night at first. Only until the bed and bedroom become strong cues for natural patterns of sleep will number of hours asleep increase. Eventually the person changes from a disrupted sleep pattern to a natural one (Bootzin, Epstein, & Wood, 1991).

Shaping and Chaining

Some desired behaviors are genuinely novel, particularly sporting skills. Before being trained in an oceanarium, no young dolphin has ever jumped through a hoop before or balanced a ball on its nose. Skinner (1958) was responsible for introducing the concept of shaping new behavior by rewarding successive approximations to the desired performance. Now imagine that the therapist's goal is to teach a young person with a significant intellectual disability to make a sandwich. Right now, the client, Joshua, does not have that skilled behavior in his repertoire—if you ask him to make a sandwich he cannot do so. That is State A. (A very different problem arises if he *can* make a sandwich and you tell him to and he doesn't. Then the behavior to be taught is compliance, the ability to follow instructions, not *how* to make a sandwich.) After a number of teaching sessions, when you ask Joshua to make a sandwich, he washes his hands, goes to the fridge, gets the lettuce, the mayonnaise, the pastrami, and the bread, finds a knife, spreads some butter, puts it all together with bread on the outside and the other stuff on the inside, puts it in a Ziploc bag, and hands it to you. That is State B. How did Joshua get from A to B?

Before answering that let us address the matter of competence. If it takes Joshua 63 minutes to get from A to B, he is not a competent sandwich maker. If he needs to wait to be told instead of initiating the skill when he is hungry or it is lunch time (unless his job is to make sandwiches for someone else), he is not a competent sandwich maker. If he is making the sandwich for someone else who likes mustard rather than mayonnaise, he is not a competent sandwich maker. If he runs out of mayonnaise or the bread is frozen and he does not know what to do about that, he is not a competent sandwich maker. So the mere fact that he has reached State B may have little to do with his true competence in practical, qualitative terms.

Leaving that aside for the moment, we are still asking what changed between A and B. The problem is nothing like an increase in salivary flow when a previously neutral bell rings (Pavlov's measure). It is somewhat like continuing to add correct nonsense syllables to the list you can verbally recall (Ebbinghaus's measure). The reason is that behaviorists, following Skinner's lead, have correctly recognized that routines such as making a sandwich are made up of a series of subskills or coordinated responses, each of which is probably already in Joshua's repertoire. He does not need to be taught how to unscrew the mayonnaise jar or how to slip an object into a plastic bag. He might not know how to spread mayonnaise thinly with a knife or how much to use, so that subskill needs to be broken down into yet more basic movements as well and shaped by steadily raising the requirement for positive feedback. But Joshua, unless he has cerebral palsy, can make all of these movements just as one of Skinner's pigeons was already able to peck at a disc covering a microswitch. Skinner inferred correctly that the way to teach a new complex skill was to chain together a series of less complex skills—to analyze the desired task and identify its component parts, then teach each of these parts one at a time, preferably in backward order. To encourage each component to occur we might have to model it for Joshua (show him) and we might need to provide physical assistance (guide his hand) and gradually fade out that assistance. There are literally thousands of published studies confirming that this is a successful way to teach everyday functional skills, as well as many other routines.

Because that is exactly what we would do to teach Joshua to make a sandwich (no one has ever come up with a better way), the measure of progress is the number of steps in the sequence that he can perform correctly on his own (without being prompted or given some sort of physical assistance). The steps have to be in the right order—you cannot put the slices of bread in the plastic bag until you have put all the ingredients in between them. Clients such as Joshua with developmental disabilities or traumatic brain injuries will steadily acquire more and more components, more or less following a conventional learning curve (little progress at first followed by increasingly rapid progress after a few instructional trials). Now, incidentally, we can return to competence measures that are over and above the basic skill sequences: Joshua needs to be able to do the task at the appropriate time (when it is lunchtime or when he is hungry), and he must do it fairly quickly, reasonable fluently (without making a huge mess), and safely (without cutting himself); in addition, he must be able to select his ingredients (his favorite bread), be healthy (picking healthy lettuce and tomato rather than liverwurst), be socially responsible (not use the last of the bread without going to get more), and be able to solve a problem if the mayonnaise jar cannot be opened or there are no more Baggies to put the sandwich in (Weld & Evans, 1990). All of these other features are important qualities of the routine, the basic sequence of which he has acquired. And this example serves as a perfect model for almost all meaningful change in which the basics that are acquired need to meet societal expectations of quality of performance, or competence (Brown, Evans, Weed, & Owen, 1987).

What Else Changes?

Getting away from mastering sandwich making—although it provides a convenient practical illustration of many issues—and thinking of all the other sorts of things we try to change clinically in ourselves and our clients, we are still not really close to knowing what changes with change. In the physical world most things change in a sort of steady fashion, except for when there is little noticeable change followed by a sudden big change—when a tipping point is reached. Yes, water turns to steam at a precise moment, but until then the water has become steadily hotter, one degree at a time. A tectonic plate may suddenly move, causing an earthquake, but the pressure on the plate has been rising steadily. Human change can be somewhat like this. An early developmental psychologist, Myrtle McGraw (1935), gave one, not the other, of her twin children a great deal of practice in climbing stairs, but when they reached a certain age, both of them went up and down stairs equally skillfully. Supporting components had to mature, after which change was rapid. Practice may make perfect, but not in a linear fashion. So when we say anxiety has decreased, depression has diminished, and assertiveness has been achieved, what has actually changed over time?

For a lot of the things we are interested in we do not really know. If your measure of anxiety is a 20-item questionnaire (which basically asks the client "how anxious are you?" in 20 different ways), we infer change from a decrease in the total score. But each time you administer the scale you do not really expect that fewer and fewer anxiety *items* will be endorsed and that this reflects less anxiety. At the very best, the 20-item scale is a sort of personal barometer, answering the question "How do I feel today? A bit less anxious?" Making that inference might reflect fewer physiological symptoms, the ability to do tasks previously avoided, feeling braver, or sometimes feeling just as nervous but ignoring it. The complication is that all four, and maybe others, of those elements of anxiety (see Chapter 7) might be relevant and accurately reflect the changes desired by the client. If the client does not like the feeling of being anxious, feeling nervous and behaving anyway is not as good an outcome as just not caring about it.

The better the trajectory of a phenomenon is understood, the better its change can be assessed. Ever since Fenz and Epstein (1967) ingeniously measured the heart rate and skin conductance of novice and experienced skydivers we have known that the fear occurs rather differently during anticipation of an event, at the moment of confrontation, and while performing the perilous action. (Novices get more and more fearful until they actually have to jump out of the plane.) Social fears, such as performance anxiety when giving a speech, reveal similar phases: anticipation, confrontation (the moment the speech starts), and performance (giving the speech). In a sophisticated analysis of change, Price and Anderson (2011) showed that after successful therapy for speech phobia, anticipatory anxiety is still present, though lessened, still peaks at confrontation, but, crucially, declines during performance.

Any feature of human performance can be measured, but usually we do not bother to do so. Skinner, for example, was especially fascinated by the rate of the operant response as a measure of its "strength" and started to measure that almost exclusively. That works fine for pigeons, because they peck away in a pretty repetitive fashion, but it does not work so well for dolphins because they like to play around between learning trials, not keep doing the same thing over and over again. Other behavior analysts have measured other features of the operant, for example, the force with which the lever is pressed. If you are interested in infant motor development, for example reaching, you will see that the coordinated coactivation of muscles follows an erratic pattern of slow improvement before fluid, accurate reaching is achieved—shaped by physics, not society (Clearfield, Feng, & Thelen, 2007). If you are interested in ballet dancing, similar fluid grace of the movement is important; if you are operating a crane, number of logs moved per hour is important, which might not require much grace but fewer, less jerky mistakes and dropped loads. I once measured male sexual arousal by increases in the circumference of the penis, the standard metric at the time, only to discover that maximum circumference was reached well before the penis became stiff and erect enough to allow conventional intercourse, which is what clients were really interested in (Farkas et al., 1979).

Subjective Impressions of Change

It is often proclaimed that in order to promote the most beneficial client change therapists need to take the pulse of client satisfaction often and early (Miller, Duncan, Brown, Sorrell, & Chalk, 2006). However, one of the most challenging methodological issues in measuring change is that in so many practical therapeutic contexts the therapist is very dependent on the client's self-report, whether it be his or her responding to a questionnaire, reporting changes seen in everyday life, or keeping formal counts and self-observations. Because such self-reporting and self-rating is so notoriously unreliable, a new discipline developed in the 1970s called behavioral assessment, which was devoted to obtaining a much better understanding of how to develop practical, veridical (true, accurate) measures of the clinical phenomena targeted for change in treatment. At one level it might be argued that who better than the client can tell you whether progress has been made? So self-reported satisfaction should perhaps be the only outcome of interest. Unfortunately there are systematic sources of error in self-ratings and other similar measures. It is revealing that when Tang and DeRubeis (1999) reported sudden gains in clients early in therapy, the measure was their self-reported strength of symptoms on the Beck Depression Inventory (BDI).

Subjective reports of change and self-report measures are not the same thing. By "subjective" we mean reports of feelings, moods, and inner satisfaction, states of being that can be known only to the individual and can ever be known only to the individual. These are experiences that cannot be corroborated or validated by any other source. Concurrent overt manifestations such as facial expressions of emotion can be completely false and easily misjudged: there are tears of joy as well as sadness. However, if you ask the person what they had for breakfast, and they reply "sausage and eggs," that is a self-report of an event that can be verified, at least in principle, even if they ate alone, were not secretly observed or videoed, washed their dishes after they were finished, and had no missing eggs in their fridge—although if all of those conditions pertained absolute verification might require a stomach pump.

In other words, self-report is supposedly of a something that is real but usually private, and subjective report is the report of a feeling or experience that is its own reality. Self-report is frighteningly inaccurate (Smith, Jobe, & Mingay, 1991) and subjective report of client improvement is distorted by numerous interesting and quite well understood factors. I was once very pleased to see the progress being made by an adolescent client having major conflict with his parents. I was encouraged when he told me all about his new part-time job at a fast food restaurant and the special hat he wore and the net to keep his hair out of the food. But when he stole his mother's check book and absconded with $5000 embezzled from her bank account, I found out from the fast food outlet they had never heard of him. People have a desire to please and belong (conformity), they want to appear normal (social desirability), they have a need to justify their actions if they have spent money and resources on treatment programs (cognitive dissonance), and sometimes they see and feel what they think they should see and feel (expectancy effects).

Trajectories and Dynamics

It is now clear that meaningful change does not occur in a simple linear or even a smooth curvilinear fashion, nor should we expect it to. As will be explained later, response interrelationships characterize individuals' repertoires. Clients with an anxiety disorder probably have to feel a little less fearful before initiating changes in difficult approach behavior behaviors. If these are successful their confidence will increase and their appraisal of their own efficacy will be affected, resulting in less anxiety but greater risk for an aversive experience. In terms of measured symptoms they might experience sudden gains (Hofmann, Schulz, Meuret, Moscovitch, & Suvak, 2006). In psychotherapy, a client's subjective sense of well-being usually occurs very early in treatment—within the first few sessions (Hansen & Lambert, 2003). In fact, if that early effect is not experienced the likelihood of a successful overall outcome is greatly diminished: rapid (within the first four sessions) reduction in binge eating strongly predicts feelings of self-control, eventual "remission" (not binge eating at all), and greater weight loss (Grilo, Masheb, & Wilson, 2006).

A seemingly opposite type of effect has also been reported as a "depression spike": after a short period of rapid progress depressive symptoms suddenly increase, although eventually followed by a decrease (Hayes, Feldman, Beevers, Laurenceau, Cardaciotto, & Lewis-Smith, 2007). In writing narratives of their therapy experience, rapid responders expressed more hopefulness that the other clients. For those clients revealing a spike in depression symptoms, if these symptoms reflect mood, it is not hard to imagine that as a client engages in deeper cognitive self-analysis it will exacerbate negative moods although ultimately it will facilitate change in a more positive directions.

Implications

In clinical work, change is usually not what you think it is—if you have thought about it at all. We have been somewhat misled by the confines of the experimental research literature into thinking of change as an alteration in a parameter or the score on some measure. Clinically meaningful change requires that an individual, as a result of treatment, be different, and that that difference is noticeable, desirable, and enduring. We have also been led to think that change means no longer showing symptoms—recovery. But that is not correct either.

Therapy does not result in cures, although if someone has had an experience or a condition that has been disabling in some way, the impact of this disability can be dramatically reduced.

Psychometric measures, relying so heavily on ratings, self-report, and subjective judgment, are much easier and more convenient to use in both practice and research than more veridical measures of actual change. Contemporary treatment research literature is overly dependent on the perception of others with a vested interest in the outcome, such as parents, teachers, or referring clinicians. Being able to gauge accurately how much something has changed remains very elusive. Ironically, in a few contexts subjective impression is the reality. If a client who was previously unhappy now says that he or she is much happier, what other index of change do we need to care about? If an angry teacher or a parent is confident that a child's conduct has improved, there may be no real need for a more objective outcome. However, when these subjective judgments are overly influenced by factors such as wanting to please the therapist, or cognitive dissonance arising from the cost of treatment, or being too self-satisfied with unchanged behavioral patterns that may not be so readily tolerated by others (peers, partners, managers, friends), then subjective estimates of change have severe limitations.

When the target of treatment is the reduction of undesirable behaviors, clearly identified as harmful to all concerned, such as criminal conduct, the importance of desisting is great, even though the individual's overall change may be less than hoped for. When the negative behavior is more ambiguous, such as possibly serving a function for a person with very few or limited skills, ceasing the behavior entirely is not such a clear marker of desirable change. In such instances the acquisition of alternative, more appropriate life skills is the outcome that should be emphasized. If the focus is on individual behavior change, the resultant improvement in quality of life is an important outcome to document.

Change is not a simple linear process. Change can be spontaneous, dramatic, or minimal like an advancing glacier. With many behaviors, change in the consequences of the behavior for the person's social context may be more important than radically altering the course of the behavior. Social criteria determine the level at which most behaviors will be considered acceptable and tolerated. Our exploration of how and why people change requires recognition that we need to be as clear and consistent as possible in defining what change is and the psychological processes whereby a person's life trajectory becomes meaningfully different. It is complex because behavior is complex, interrelated, and intertwined with changing environmental systems. This will become more obvious when we examine motivation to change.

3

Motivation to Change

Everyone has heard the old joke about how many psychotherapists does it take to change a light bulb? Answer: Only one, but the light bulb must want to change. The idea that clients of psychotherapy have to want to change before therapy has a chance of being successful is an old one. But it is erroneous. In cognitive–behavioral psychotherapy there are endless examples of clients who have no particular interest in changing or a desire to act differently. Children with autism, toddlers with compliance and conduct problems, school children with challenging behaviors, teenagers generally, but those with anorexia in particular, sex offenders, and people with early-onset psychosis, who may be in distress but are unaware that changing something about their cognitive and emotional actions is what is needed, are all obvious examples of clients who are not explicitly motivated to change or be changed.

On the other hand, of course, when individuals are motivated to change, therapy is both easier to implement and more likely to be successful. In this chapter I will examine what is meant by motivation to change, how the practitioner can raise that motivation in clients, and how therapists can mobilize clients' motivation in order to increase the likelihood of their achieving successful outcomes. Remember that the research and evaluation literature often concentrates on the idea that therapies must be successful, whereas in fact the important result of therapy should be that clients are successful. Hopefully all therapists will have an understanding of their client's true goals and motivation to change, but may not be implementing strategies to enhance motivation in a strategic and planful way. This chapter will explain why that is so important and will suggest how it can be done. I will also explain the value and importance of establishing an awareness of change in the sorts of people already mentioned who may have no apparent motivation to perform differently. Such clients are merely at the end of a continuum of motivation to change, not a completely different species.

It is important to recognize the distinction between motivation to *change* and the motivation that sustains either the old behavior or the motivation that may be needed to sustain the new behavior. There are subtle differences. To clarify them, consider a former client of mine, Carla, a financially well-off graduate student in a professional doctoral program, who shoplifted expensive items from stores once or twice a week. She had been caught and confronted a couple of times, but until this point had never been charged. She was adamant that she wanted to change this behavior, mostly on the basis of her fear of being arrested and having to go to court and the humiliation she would feel. Interestingly she was less motivated to change by the fact that she was defrauding the owners of the stores.

Carla's motivation for stealing seemed to derive from two sources of reward. One was that although she insisted the items she stole were of little value, they were in fact very costly and were sustaining a quality of material lifestyle she would not otherwise have been able to afford. The second was more intrinsic. Prior to a shoplifting episode she felt a great deal of tension, but after successfully getting out of the store without being apprehended, she experienced an enormous sense of relief. (We will encounter this phenomenon later when considering two-factor theory of avoidance of punishment.) The motivation for engaging in the more socially correct behavior—walking into a store and paying for a purchase—was weak. Most of us do not feel a great sense of pride in the fact that we paid for the items we have taken out of a store, but we might enjoy shopping.

Affective and motivational processes operate in parallel so that individuals can have strongly conflicting feelings toward the same person or situation. These processes then motivate them in opposing ways, which in turn leads to solutions that are compromises between opposing forces. In Carla's case there were three sources of motivation relevant to her treatment. Her motivation to steal was strong, the motivation not to steal was minimal (requiring something like taking a new-found pleasure in normal shopping), and the motivation to *change* was moderately strong, but based on fear of public embarrassment and potentially serious legal consequences (avoidance), rather than a desire to do the right thing (approach). In the office, telling me about what she called her "kleptomania," Carla would sob and talk about how she had to overcome it. When walking into a store, highly tense and thinking of something she wanted but could not afford, her determination to change was completely overridden. This is one of the fundamental dilemmas of real life clinical change that will be explored in this chapter.

Enhancing Motivation in the Context of Treatment

Motivation theories tend to be divided into two frameworks in psychology. One is drive theory in which a person's actions are pushed forward by internal forces and needs—Michael Jordan, the great basketball player, wrote a book about himself entitled "Driven from within" (Vancil, 2005). The other frame encompasses goal theories, in which a person's actions are seen as pulled forward by desired outcomes—with insight and honesty Michael Jordan actually wrote:

> It was so easy for me to find ways to motivate myself. It didn't matter whether it was the seventh game of a playoff series or the 60th game

of another season... my driving force, my passion, was to impress people with what I could do. (Vancil, 2005, p. 181).

It is self-evident that when clients deliberately seek therapy they are both driven from within by the desire to be different and are propelled forward by desired outcomes. However, every therapist has encountered clients who appear reluctant to follow therapeutic advice and suggestions, seem resistant to implementing previously agreed upon strategies, and prevaricate in pursuing a new direction. This should come as no real surprise. Everything we do as human beings, even the things we do not like about ourselves, we do for a reason. To change that pattern and do something else is fundamentally difficult, especially if that something else is completely new and different and thus daunting.

This is true whether others, such as parents, have to make the changes for the sake of a child client, or whether whole societies have been encouraged to change. In the United States, despite intensive public health efforts, people are still more likely to eat French fries than fruit and vegetables (Centers for Disease Control and Prevention, 2010). The reasons for this represent a textbook case of the issues concerning individual motivation to change: fries taste better, vegetables are more expensive and take time to prepare, and neither the immediate nor longer-term health benefits of vegetables make themselves obvious. Now add to everyday obstacles to change a likely assumption: most clients come to therapy expecting to be helped, to be cured, and to have their problems solved for them. They do not necessarily see therapy as a requirement that they change, any more than change has been the explicit focus of treatment by professional psychotherapists in the past.

Clients' difficulties with therapeutic change have given rise to many theoretical concepts and explanations, all of them underestimating that not changing really is the default option and it is why anybody ever changes that needs to be explained, not why they do not. Despite this, there are four major and comprehensive ideas that have become prominent in the clinical treatment literature. These are (1) the stages of change model, originally developed in public health contexts related to smoking, diet, and exercise; (2) the closely related concept of motivational interviewing, originally developed in the context of alcohol and drug counseling; (3) the theory of reasoned action and its morphed version, the theory of planned behavior, originating from health psychology; and (4) the function of behavior, originally developed in the context of changing challenging behavior in people with severe disabilities. These different origins have shaped the kinds of ideas developed. But so dominant are these models that it is now necessary to describe them and to examine the extent to which their basic principles overlap or the extent to which they are all equally relevant to any change endeavor.

Stages of Change

The stages-of-change theory acknowledges the position concluded in the previous chapter—clients trying to change their lives do not follow a linear path. It proposes that people go through a series of stages in which they first are barely focused on the need to change, then they think about it (contemplation), then they undertake some planning and preparation indicating a greater level of commitment, and finally they embrace change, take action, and perform the necessary behaviors that will bring change about. If they are successful a fifth and final stage involves actions that are designed to sustain long-term change. Since first articulated with reference to smoking cessation by Prochaska and DiClemente (1982, 1983), their Transtheoretical Model has achieved widespread acceptance and their early paper in the *Journal of Consulting and Clinical Psychology* is among the most frequently cited articles in the history of clinical psychology. The model has been taught to physicians to assist them in encouraging their patients to alter health-related behaviors, and appears on countless blogs and self-help web sites to help people keep their New Year's resolutions. It has generated commercial products to encourage change (e.g., Pro-change Behavior Systems, Inc.) and is used in marketing, the travel industry, sport and exercise programs, nutrition, and many others. Clearly Prochaska and DiClemente have struck a responsive chord for researchers and practitioners dealing with the fact that in any group of clients there always appear to be some for whom change is very difficult.

The Transtheoretical Model is considered here as a motivational paradigm because the precontemplative and contemplative stages involve a shift toward greater commitment and determination to change. The essence of the idea is that clients go through various stages before reaching a level of motivation representing willingness to implement specific strategies for change. For example, clients may come to therapy—for whatever reason—and talk about how they want to be different, but are in fact only contemplating being different. They say the right things but seem unable or unwilling to take the necessary hard steps to bring about change. Only later is there a serious commitment to change. An important implication is that therapeutic planning needs to be matched to the client's stage of change.

Not surprisingly, Prochaska and DiClemente developed this model in the context of people with habit problems—unhealthy eating habits, overeating, being too sedentary, engaging in inappropriate sexual behaviors, smoking, or other more serious addictions such as alcoholism and abuse of illegal drugs. The common element in these problems is the person engaging in a repetitive action that although harmful to self or others is nevertheless reinforced by some mechanism and so the behavior is hard to inhibit or to desist from doing. The client has the desire to stop these behaviors, but finds it difficult to do so. To change will require effort, practice of alternatives, management of contexts to reduce temptations, and a host of difficult maneuvers we will be exploring soon. Prochaska and DiClemente argued that it is possible to judge clients' motivation to change from their engagement in these alternative behaviors.

Because the model is not really about stages of change, but is about stages in the processes that lead to change, it seems to me that the model would be better described as a stages-of-commitment model. What the stages-of-change model identifies so well is the fact that because some behavioral phenomena have such potent intrinsic rewards attached to them they are difficult to cease at will. The model has its most promising support when applied to addictions: psychological patterns marked by short-term gain at the expense of longer-term costs. Because many of us know the feelings of compulsion that drive behaviors such as drinking alcohol to excess, smoking, and abusing prescription or illegal drugs, it is common for society to dub intrinsically rewarded behaviors as addictions. This conveys a sense of biological control that we are unable to regulate by willpower and connotes decreased responsibility for our continued engagement in the behavior despite serious consequences. The congressman who sends sexually explicit Tweets, the governor who visits brothels, and the president who has oral sex with an intern seem so bizarrely self-destructive that the explanation can only be that they must be "addicted" to these forms of behavior.

In the next chapter I consider a wide range of internal (personality) and external (environmental) variables that make change difficult. I do not find it entirely convincing that people inevitably go through a predetermined sequence, and agree with Bandura (1997) that dividing complex interactional sequences into stages is arbitrary. There are also a number of significant critiques of the strength of the evidence; Whitelaw, Baldwin, Bunton, and Flynn (2000) is one of the best examples, focused on lack of complexity, and there are other criticisms of the available empirical evidence as well as difficulties in measuring any of the stages, or separating them from general beliefs about someone's ability to change. But as a metaphor it is clearly useful: do not contemplate change, contemplate the results; taking some action, however small, is better than not.

Motivational Interviewing

Throughout this book we will encounter three particularly important ideas: that change is often difficult; that clients can be reluctant or unable to even recognize that the solution to their distress *is* to change; and that as a rule, clients do not like to be told by someone else that they need to change. These three ideas are closely linked, especially during the first interview in which the therapist tries to establish the nature of the problem, what the client hopes to achieve, and some sort of expectation as to what therapy is all about (Walitzer, Dermen, & Connors, 1999). The way the therapist asks the questions to obtain this information is thought to impact the degree to which the client becomes a collaborator in the process of change. Referred to in a number of schools of psychotherapy as the "strategic dialogue" (Nardone & Salvini, 2007), the ideal style of questioning clients is one in which the clients themselves begin to reach certain conclusions regarding the importance of change. As the Spanish philosopher Solomon Ibn Gabirol said: "a wise man's question contains half the answer" (Pessin, 2010).

In contemporary cognitive–behavioral therapy, this type of strategic questioning is known as motivational interviewing. Despite the word "interviewing," it is considered treatment, or part of treatment, designed to change clients, in this case facilitating their change. Developed by Miller (1983) in the context of working with clients with alcoholism, motivational interviewing has been interwoven with the stages of change model, but focuses specifically on the early stages of interviewing clients who either might have been referred by someone else—someone complaining—or have not yet fully accepted that they have a problem requiring change. The basic interviewing techniques have become widely adopted and entire books have been devoted to the methods (e.g., Miller & Rollnick, 2002). The objective is for the client to come to recognize and voice, without being told or confronted, that he or she has a problem (countering any denial or minimization) and needs to change (countering resistance, or making excuses, or delaying action). The originators are modest in their claims and recognize that client ambivalence does not simply disappear.

Motivational interviewing is a component of the broader topic of the therapeutic alliance and the relationship between therapist and client (Chapter 10). It specifies a number of very useful tactics for creating expectancies regarding change and placing the responsibility for change on the client. Having the client list the costs and benefits of continuing current behavioral practices is a useful way of differentiating short-term pleasures from longer-term harm. It is educative rather than coercive. It encourages the client to present the case for change, sometimes through role-playing or paradoxical argument. It promotes good interview techniques such as asking open-ended questions and affirming the client, especially when they engage in "change talk."

It can be somewhat disconcerting to realize that within different schools of psychotherapy and descriptions of different psychotherapy techniques very similar strategies to increase motivation to change have been introduced with different names. In Solution-Focused Brief Therapy (De Jong & Berg, 2008), for example, clients are asked the "miracle question." What would life be like if you woke up the next morning and while you were sleeping a miracle occurred and the problems you have been discussing have been solved? What changes, large or small, would you notice? The therapist and client than use this interview technique to coconstruct the goals for therapy in a positive, context-relevant, solution-focused way, using as a guide examples of past successes in coping or dealing with problems. Israel Goldiamond (1974), one of the innovators in behavior analysis, always began by asking clients what life would be like for them 6 months after "L Day"—that being the day they felt liberated from their problems.

Theory of Planned Behavior

The theory of planned behavior is another model that has received a considerable degree of recognition in behavioral and cognitive–behavioral circles. One reason for this was the long-standing realization that people's attitudes are very poor predictors of their actual behavior. Saying and doing are not the same things. Ajzen and Fishbein (1973) formulated their theory of reasoned action in an attempt to explain this discrepancy. A better predictor of someone's behavior is their intention to perform it, but the road to hell is still paved with good intentions. Intention in their model is a cognitive representation of the action preceding the actual behavior. Intention is a function of attitude toward the behavior and subjective norms. Ajzen (1991) later added the construct of perceived behavioral control and the expanded model was called the theory of planned behavior.

Attitudes about a behavior are the person's positive or negative feelings about performing it. These are influenced by behavioral beliefs concerning the desirability of the perceived consequences of performing the behavior. Subjective norms are the person's judgment regarding how the behavior will be perceived by people important to that individual. Behind this judgment are normative beliefs. Because attitudes and perceived norms can be easily confounded, there are ambiguities in the model. But of greater concern is that the model assumes individuals have the freedom to act once the intention is formed. By adding perception of the ease with which the behavior can be performed (beliefs about behavioral control), however, the theory of planned behavior does accommodate constraints on action, such as limited time, resources, ability, and environmental barriers. If perceived control is accurate then that variable has a direct effect on behavior rather than going through the mediating variable of intention.

The implication of the theory for therapeutic change is that the individual's underlying beliefs (attitudes, subjective norms, and control beliefs) all need to be changed. When proposing a strategy or other action for a client to engage in, you could estimate the behavioral beliefs by asking the person to suggest the benefits or value of the behavior—and you would be excused for thinking this sounds a lot like parts of motivational interviewing. Similar questioning (which can be accomplished by the use of various questionnaires) should reveal the client's normative beliefs ("I couldn't go to the gym five times a week because my friends would think it rather odd") and control beliefs ("I can't afford gym membership, and I don't have time to go during the day"). If the control beliefs are more around personal ability ("I'm not really good at lifting weights") they are essentially the same as those that Bandura called "self-efficacy beliefs," to be discussed again later.

Quite apart from other insights provided by the model, it does explain why to some extent simply providing information to clients can effectively change their behavior for their benefit, especially toward a healthier lifestyle (Hardeman et al., 2002). The beliefs that individuals express are not judged to be dysfunctional core beliefs, as in cognitive theory (Chapter 8); they may be perfectly rational (the client cannot actually afford the gym membership), and they may be unique to the person ("my wife would be really pleased if I started going to the gym"). So to get from beliefs to intentions, and from intentions to performing new actions, the therapist's task is to provide new and alternative information, or encourage the client to seek it, which will allow beliefs to be tested, challenged, or experientially disconfirmed (this being a bit like the behavioral experiment we will encounter in cognitive therapy).

A widely accepted model in health psychology that is basically quite similar proposes that whether an individual adopts a health-related behavior depends on perceived threat, perceived barriers (to change), and specific triggers that cue a new behavior. This Health Belief Model (see Conner & Norman, 1995), as it is called, suggests that perceived threat is a function of someone's sense of susceptibility to, and someone's understanding the consequences of, a particular disease. Perception of barriers is based on a balance of the costs and benefits of the behavior change. As defined by Glasgow (e.g., Glasgow, Toobert, & Gillette, 2001), a perceived barrier is a client's estimate of the challenge provided by social, personal, environmental, and economic obstacles to a behavior at the desired level of achievement. In their example, applying the model to self-management in diabetes, both the required behavior (correctly administering insulin) and a typical barrier (fear of hypoglycemia) are syndrome specific. Change principles are universal, but their translation into many domains of practice often requires specialized, problem-specific knowledge.

In the health belief model appraisals of potential risks and gains precede the determination to change unhealthy lifestyles. In the theory of planned behavior motivating change requires targeting three types of belief. Neither has much to say about how appraisals and beliefs are to be changed, except that the beliefs of interest are not seen as deep-seated, largely unconscious, or irrational. Thus, it is assumed, such beliefs are fairly easily altered by rational discourse, new information, and alternative perspectives on the client's situation. If it were that simple, however, why don't people just routinely take action and do more of the things they know are good for them: eat healthier food, exercise more, recycle, put up the storm windows before the winter snow, study hard to get good grades that will facilitate college entrance, or send that check to the Salvation Army's earthquake appeal? Behavior theory has a simpler answer: the less desirable but more convenient alternatives are often powerfully reinforced.

Function of Behavior

The idea that all behaviors have a function is widespread across a variety of apparently totally different areas of psychology. Thus, functionality might be quite a useful unifying concept for thinking about motivation to change. In trying to understand the emotional development of children, particularly how emotion regulation develops adaptively for most children, child psychologists have argued that emotion itself is functional (Thompson, 2001). By this is meant that emotion serves a purpose. Emotion is therefore good, or adaptive, or desirable, according to how well it does so.

Young children might be playing an imaginary game in which they are pretending to be dangerous creatures and they are running around roaring and shrieking and chasing each other all in good fun. To stay part of the game with all the other children it is necessary to get excited, to be aroused, and to show general pleasure. The function of this emotional arousal is that it maintains the game. A child who gets overexcited (cannot modulate his or her arousal) might get aggressive or belligerent or dominate the play. This is considered "over"emotional because it interferes with continuing the fun game. Other children are no longer having fun and the game ends. The overreactive, underregulated child's emotional expression was dysfunctional for that context. Another child who finds the game intimidating and is not having fun might show distress, switching from being excited to being fearful and perhaps crying or withdrawing. Although that stops that child's participation in the game, the anxiety does serve the function of allowing the child to withdraw from an activity that is no longer pleasurable. The best regulated children eventually tire of the game and find something else to do: by managing their emotional arousal they are able to sustain a broader function, which is continuing to be friends with each other and preserve the positive social relationships. Children who get overexcited and become aggressive or children who become overly anxious and withdraw are not considered socially skilled by teachers, parents, or peers because their emotional reactions are not functional for the longer-term goal, which is maintaining positive, fun, friendly relationships with other children.

In one of my own research projects we saw very good illustrations of exactly this kind of process (Galyer & Evans, 2001). We played an imaginary game with an empty box, in which we as the grown-ups pretended that there was something inside the box (either a growling monster or a purring kitten). A few children became so overexcited by this game that they could not contain their curiosity and they grabbed the box out of our hands and ripped open the lid, only to confirm petulantly that there was nothing inside. That pretty much ended the fun game; not much more could be done with an empty box. Other children became so fearful that there might be something in the box that they withdrew and refused to continue the game. Many children, however, were able to manage their emotions so that the interaction could continue. Some changed the valence of the monster in the box, telling us that it was actually a friendly monster, or just a baby monster with no teeth. Others said the kitten was sleeping, they could hear it purring, and that we should keep very quiet so as not to wake it. So the imaginary game continued and the enjoyable interaction with the adult was maintained.

In a totally different context and a very different literature, applied behavior analysts have explained how what appears to be purely negative, socially inappropriate behavior on the part of children with significant disabilities actually serves a function for these children. What teachers and parents and therapists consider to be "challenging" behavior, such as self-injurious head banging, is functional, because it often allows the child to escape a negative situation, perhaps being told to do something he or she does not want to do. Aggressive behaviors such as pulling another child's hair or grabbing their toy away from them has the function of obtaining something desired: being left alone or getting the toy that they want to play with. Behaviors such as this might seem hard to explain, until we realize that what characterizes children with autism or other developmental disabilities is that they lack other, more common or acceptable forms of communicating their wants and needs.

Mark Durand (1990) made an important contribution to understanding such challenging behavior by arguing that very often these negative behaviors had communicative intent. They were designed to achieve some outcome, such as gaining a material object, getting social attention, avoiding a task demand, or escaping from an aversive situation. It is not necessary to confirm that the behaviors are deliberately planned to obtain these outcomes. It is simpler, and makes fewer assumptions, just to recognize that as these behaviors do serve those functions, they will occur in situations in which the outcomes are desired. If children with autism can escape from unwanted interactions with peers by exhibiting a self-injurious behavior, then that behavior will be reinforced by the consequence of being removed from the situation.

From that example it can be seen that a "treatment" procedure such as time-out would not be an effective deterrent to self-injury, since the time-out achieves precisely the goal of the challenging behavior—escaping social demands. Behavior analysts are therefore totally correct in insisting that it is not possible to change inappropriate behavior unless its function is understood. Thinking even more deeply about this it is possible to argue that instead of trying to understand the "cause" of a behavior we should try to understand of which variable or influences the behavior is a function. Functional analysis is thus a better way of thinking about causes. This is precisely the argument that Skinner (1953) made years ago. He did not like thinking about the causes of a behavior at all. He argued that the proper task of a science of behavior was to specify the antecedent and consequent events, which are generally environmental, of which the behavior of interest was a function. When that is known, it would become possible possible to manipulate these variables and change the behavior: predict and control.

Changeworthy Behaviors Fulfill Needs

There is an important practical implication of recognizing that all behavior serves some kind of function. If the function is meeting important psychological needs (self-esteem, social attention, sexual satisfaction, and so on), then it will be hard to change the behavior that serves that function unless we can find an alternative, more socially acceptable behavior having the identical function. If a child with autism is banging his head in order to escape a situation that for him is highly unpleasant (an empowerment need), it requires replacing this self-injurious action with something equally effective but more acceptable, such as asking, by word or by sign, if he can leave the situation, or do an alternative activity, or even have the pleasure of being held in a restraint. Since Durand argued these negative behaviors are communicative, it was only a short step to propose that the most desirable alternative would be a communication skill. Empirically he was able to demonstrate that when an alternative communication skill achieving the function of the challenging behavior was taught, the challenging behavior decreased. If the communication skill served a different function, however, the challenging behavior would not decrease. This was a convincing demonstration that the alternative skill was not just something else to do but another behavior that met the same needs as the negative, challenging behavior.

Every therapist for any kind of problem needs to consider and utilize this same principle. Try to discover what the function of the undesired behavior is, find out if the individual has a better alternative in his or her repertoire, and if not teach it, and then make sure this better alternative does indeed achieve the function of the one to be discouraged. If a client's voyeuristic behavior is the only way to achieve sexual satisfaction, it is very unlikely that you will have therapeutic success by introducing punitive contingencies. Psychologists generally recognize this, but think of all the interventions in which the exact function of a negative behavior has never really been analyzed or understood and yet a program has been introduced to discourage it without teaching alternatives: suspension for fighting at school, prison for pedophiles, name and shame consequences for drunk driving, and restricting access to alcohol for teenage binge drinkers, just to name a few.

Rewarding Change Directly

In other contexts or descriptions of life's journey, change is not depicted as something you have to consult a professional to achieve. Change is good. Change is inevitable. Change means you are alive and curious. The opposite of change is stagnation. Is it not equally true, however, that in life we sometimes resist change, prefer the familiar, trust the traditional, and find security in old habits? Uncertainty is aversive (Evans & Galyer, 2009). Thus we might think of change as a response class—a category of different behaviors that share a past history of being reinforced or punished and have thus become a functional class. Even in the laboratory it is possible to reinforce an organism for doing something different from what it did the last time. As already suggested, clients by definition are those people who have not been able to make changes on their own. Is it conceivable, therefore, that we can encourage specific clinical change by rewarding general life changes?

As far as I know there is no direct evidence supporting such an idea: the differential reinforcement of change. Yet it is quite commonly suggested and used by therapists, particularly behavior therapists. To encourage clients to think positively of change and the need to act differently if they wish to feel differently, behavior therapists often suggest to clients very early on in therapy that they do something different that week, something they have never done before or not for a long time. Usually the suggested action is easy to do at home or in the neighborhood, requires no resources, is likely to bring some degree of satisfaction, and is novel. At first the action might be little more than changing our environment or daily routines. Often the activity is something a little special and indulgent, designed for the client's own pleasure. After that the suggested action might be for someone else's benefit—something that brings joy, however simple, to a spouse, a child, or a friend.

These actions have no direct link to the target behaviors or the negotiated goals of treatment. It is strictly a shaping procedure. But it shows that change is possible, thus increasing hope. It permits the reinforcement of change as a response class that should generalize to the much harder changes that may need to be made as treatment progresses. And the actions themselves raise the client's overall level of material and social reward, a necessary condition for enhancing the quality of life. Behavior therapists use the spontaneous increase in overall rates of positive behaviors as a barometer for the general effectiveness of the treatment program. If you want to change you have to start acting differently.

Goal Setting

"Tell me what you want, what you really really want" demanded the Spice Girls in their song *Wannabe*. Therapists ask clients to do the same. One of the key elements of planful change is that a person has a specific goal that he or she is striving to reach and that the therapist understands it and accepts its importance. Such congruence of real wants cannot be assumed in treatment outcome trials, another way that formal treatment studies differ from practical clinical realities that require versatile understanding of change. Most life goals are implicit—"internal

representations of desired outcomes" (Karoly, 1999, p. 270). There is much, if mostly anecdotal, evidence that the deliberate setting of explicit meaningful goals increases an individual's likelihood of achieving them. A measurable goal allows for the establishment of concrete steps toward it—indicators that you are on an appropriate pathway. Achieving these steps is highly rewarding, and increases feelings of hope. This is also a common idea in cybernetic or systems models, which depend on the presence of a regulator of some kind that compares the current level of goal attainment with the level of the intended outcome. Such feedback and its resultant encouragement, has, of course, its dark side. If the goal is too distant or too hard and the steps toward it are not achieved, it is quite possible that the person will feel disappointed and lose confidence.

If the goals are not operationalized, defined in measurable terms, and agreed upon, the client does not have the incentive value arising from confirmed progress. For this reason therapists following good change principles will try to ensure that the goals that are set are attainable and realistic, as well as truly the ones desired by the client, and represented in a positive form as the things that the client will strive to achieve. To militate against the disappointment of not achieving the desired goal, therapists can prepare the client in a version of relapse prevention by reducing expectations that the goal will be reached easily and without mishap or setback. Furthermore the subgoals, the steps toward the main objective, can be set at a level that is very likely to be achieved successfully (errorless learning, behaviorists call it), as early success encourages the client. This is especially true when working with mediators such as teachers or parents who are already doubtful that change is even possible in a child with serious misbehavior or a child with very limited functional skills.

A different name for goal setting is target behavior selection. The latter concept tends to overemphasize the professional change agent as the individual who decides what the focus of treatment will be. In certain ways target selection is another name for diagnosis, or at least functional, behavioral diagnosis; again this is the assumed prerogative of the professional. Ideally target selection is always negotiated, but it is clear that in many cases persuasive therapists can ensure that the selected target fits his or her explanatory model of the nature and cause of the client's problem. There are many established guidelines for target selection. As a rule the selected target should be the most serious issue presented by the client, one that puts the client and others around him or her at the greatest risk for harm. But an equally important criterion might be the desires of the mediators as well as the client, especially if it is important to obtain a commitment from the mediators to follow through with a potentially difficult plan.

After these criteria, practical issues are next in importance—select targets that are achievable with the resources and within the time available. An additional useful criterion for establishing behavioral targets is to consider the cascade of additional benefits that might result. Later I will explain how as behaviors are always linked, selecting a "keystone" behavior might allow new skills to develop (the target is a prerequisite for something even more important to achieve, such as abandoning dietary restriction in order to interrupt the binge–purge cycle), might enhance social possibilities, and might serve to reduce stigma and discrimination that sometimes hamper efforts at social integration and rehabilitation. Although most of these criteria have been worked out with children with severe intellectual disabilities and problematic or challenging behaviors, the general principles apply equally well to all clients, particularly those especially vulnerable to social rejection and discrimination, such as people who have been in mental health services for a long period of time. But for all clients the target as a step toward something still better, rather than an end point in its own right, connects these ideas with the important recognition that change can be an ongoing process of moving closer toward a more fulfilling life. All schools of therapy espouse this ambitious objective as the ultimate therapeutic goal.

From these observations certain broad assumptions can be made about the best way in which therapists can use goal theories to enhance client motivation, both to make changes and to initiate the alternative acts that will replace the undesirable status quo. Karoly (1993) summarized them well. Therapy goals must be commensurate with the client's higher order values. They should not conflict with other life goals and daily realities of living, or with the client's temperament. (I learned this one the hard way from a dedicated mother of a very demanding child with autism. Our therapy goal of being more consistent with rewards and negative consequences clashed with her life goals of being a spontaneous, counterculture person, as well as with her daily realities of looking after three young children while unemployed. She walked out of my office with the weekly plan in her hand, but from her wry smile I knew immediately it would never be adopted.) Clients can be encouraged to think of their goals as positive, challenging states, the pursuit of which is enjoyable. Clients should be able to articulate the relevance of the treatment process to the journey implied by the treatment goals. Change goals that are ambiguous are easily overpowered by well-rehearsed negative mind-sets. As in solution-focused models, emphasis on approach and mastery-oriented goals is preferable to avoidance and focus on the past. Formal change efforts can be reduced (therapy terminated) when the change goals become an ordinary part of daily activities.

Long-Term Goals: Dreams and Aspirations

Most people would accept the common idea that a person's dreams of what he or she could do or become provides a driving force for changing behavior. These are our conscious aspirations rather than outcomes, in the sense of I dream of being a movie star, marrying a prince, or winning the Nobel Peace Prize. Having a dream about realistic goals, having aspirations, provides the incentive for performance, influencing choices and directing individual behavior. The "miracle" question elicits a vision of what life could be like if focused on solutions rather than problems. It is so important when planning change to emphasize the positive approach goals of thriving.

If behavior is dictated by context, opportunity, and past habits, however, it is interesting to question how exactly such dreams *could* influence behavior directly and thus whether they can be used in therapy to facilitate positive change. If individuals' dreams do serve as a motivational force, there are certain likely mechanisms. One of these is that the dream alters the reinforcing valence of shorter-term goals and accomplishments. If you dream of becoming an Olympic figure skater, winning a regional ice-skating competition will be a far more valued outcome than if you just skate for fun. So the dream makes the emotional valence of certain rewards more positive. Another logically plausible mechanism is that when confronted by more or less equal choices, the dream serves as an eliciting stimulus. If the choice is between lying in bed and getting an extra hour of sleep or getting up on a cold morning to get over to the ice skating rink for a practice session, it is the dream that provides the internal stimuli to evoke the latter behavior, including self-regulatory preparatory behaviors we will encounter in Chapter 9, such as setting the alarm clock to an earlier hour.

A somewhat similar mechanism whereby the dream facilitates behavior change is social. Our social networks and associations regulate our behavior. Because of your dream you associate with other people having the same dream. You read magazines about ice skating, you go on line and join competitive ice skating chat rooms, you have ice skating friends on Facebook, and you meet and socialize with other ice skaters at the rink and at the café after practice. Having the dream will change you, so making this part of planful therapeutic change means the client should be encouraged to have a dream that is potentially attainable. This is defined as something you think about, frequently, that you can fantasize achieving, that you have a sense of what that achievement would feel like as an experience, and that if you disclose your dream to your closest friends they will encourage and support it rather than scoff at it and be dismissive.

Possible Selves

An idea in social psychology that comes closest to the above account is that of "possible selves" (Markus & Nurius, 1986). "Possible selves are the mental representations of one's aspirations and fears; they are personalized goal representations of the self in desired or undesired future states" (Carroll, Shepperd, & Arkin, 2009, p. 550). In essence, the theory asserts that people, young people in particular, have some sort of idea regarding what they might become. This is not just remote aspirations, but the possible outcomes—a teenager might imagine he or she could become a teacher, a parent, a journalist, a plumber, a criminal, or an alcoholic. Children from middle-class, wealthy backgrounds are more likely to think that a possible self would be a secure professional job, whereas children from less privileged backgrounds could imagine that a possible self is being unemployed.

Unless the client is exceptionally fatalistic, these representations potentially serve as powerful deterrents of particular actions if the links to undesirable selves are known, and as incentives to mobilize and direct behavior toward their pursuit and accomplishment. Interest in this theory from the point of view of planful or therapeutic intervention arises because it might be possible to influence "possible self" concepts so as to increase motivation to strive for more positive life outcomes, particularly for young people. Similarly, certain kinds of direct experience, such as a failure experience, or certain negative emotions, such as fear, could threaten possible-selves dreams and cause their abandonment. In his study of how adolescents actually understand the psychiatric concept of "depression," Fitzgerald (2002) found that one negative experience could challenge what he called teenagers' cherished ideals of themselves. Thus failing a test at school threatened the ideal that they were scholastically very capable, or being dumped by a boyfriend or girlfriend threatened the ideal that they were lovable, eliciting depressed mood in both cases.

The experimental literature in social psychology demonstrates that threats can vary in specificity, especially when they are presented by a meaningful, authoritative person (Carroll, Shepperd, & Arkin, 2009). A therapist might imply that the academic future is bleak for an adolescent client who continues to skip school and hang with drug-using friends, or spell out in precise detail, using vivid imagery, the prospects of non-college admission, dead-end jobs, and future unemployment. From the therapy perspective, attempting to influence possible selves in a positive direction is essentially similar to motivational interviewing. Promoting and encouraging dreams has to be done with care, particularly with individuals who have strong doubts about their ability to change themselves. Almost everybody has self-doubts, which can be considered a form of anxiety. In this context there are various strategies for coping with anxiety and disappointment in a proactive way, and one of them is called bracing, which as we all know means preparing yourself for the likelihood of disappointment by lowering your expectations so that they do not excessively exceed outcomes.

It is useful for any clinician to assess a client's possible selves, however informally. But helping the client realize these dreams is fraught with complexity. Explicitly encouraging highly specific possible selves runs the obvious risk of disappointment. Past failures and disappointments serve as primes for the expectation of future failures, which the client might acknowledge; however, more probably the client will acquiesce and outwardly agree with the therapists while being inwardly doubtful and abandoning optimism to avoid further disappointment (Shepperd, Ouellette, & Fernandez, 1996). Dreams and possible self-representations are probably forged in the furnace of family aspirations, from the pessimistic "you'll never amount to anything" to the wildly unrealistic "you can be anything you want to be." People often report that their aspirations were somewhat more their parents' than their own. I had a client once, a medical student, with extreme test anxiety, who eventually admitted that becoming a doctor was his parents' dream, not something he desired and he was desperate not to disappoint them. (I'll leave the reader to make the very obvious link with his poor performance on examinations compared to all his other academic work.)

Implementation

In conclusion, dreams and aspirations provide us with a motivational mechanism that contributes to behavior change and that can therefore be deliberately activated in a therapeutic context. To help clients change they need to have a dream of what they could become, they need to have realistic and positive images of what behavior change could bring about, they need to think these outcomes are possible, and they need to have clear intentions to be different and know how to behave differently (Prochaska and DiClemente were not wrong in recognizing that some people are only contemplating change).

Those are the criteria. How does a therapist or any other change agent, including the person themselves, induce these states? Mostly we try by a combination of discourse, education, and occasionally through direct experience. Because the last of these is the least frequently used, let us consider an example first. To give someone a sense of what a possible self might be or feel like, we can give them a taste of it. If we want to change the possible self of high school students from that of a *drop-out* to a *college graduate*, we give them a taste of what the latter might be like. We arrange school visits to a university campus and we show the students the college lifestyle, taking them to the dorms, the cafeteria, and the gym. We let them sit in on an interesting lecture from a young dynamic professor and we encourage them to talk to older students from their own neighborhood about college life. The students get a sense of what college is all about and they see that it would be possible to be part of it (Beaudry, Sanders, Gibbons, & Coffey, 1995). Lots of at-risk students have no understanding of college and simply assume that it is not for them.

The same set of images, ideas, and words can be achieved through simple exposition, of course, and that is the way most therapists will be limited to when working with adult clients. The therapist provides information about possible outcomes, sometimes by giving facts and figures about how many individuals with a certain syndrome now function happily and normally in society. Then the therapist might suggest outcomes the client has never thought of, and if the therapist is lyrical and can tell a good story and weave an imaginative and rich picture of an outcome—say the joys of being a good parent—the client has new images with which to construct a possible self future. You can use structured, guided imagery, in other words simple imagination: "I want you to think of what it would be like to go to college"—let us stick with that example—"imagine being in a fancy robe at graduation with all your friends and your parents and grandparents looking on happily. Feel the glow. Think of your dad framing your diploma and hanging it in the living room. Feel your girlfriend/boyfriend kissing you and whispering 'We're all so proud of you!'"

In behavior therapy strategies such as this have been called various names: reinforcement priming, covert reinforcement, and imaginal reward. It is not a treatment per se, but it is a vehicle for behavior change. The images need to be realistic, within the client's realm of experience, and the positive feelings should be ones that are valued. The above imagery would not work that well with a highly cynical student who despises social conformity, hates his or her father, has low self-esteem, and has a grade-point average that makes him or her ineligible for college admission. Therein lies the great dilemma of group behavior change. If you take an entire class of high school students for a college campus visit and give them a taste of college life, some students will simply not like the flavor, or find it sour for other reasons, such as anxiety, social pressure from hostile friends, or financial barriers that make the possible self seem more like an impossible self. Group interventions struggle to deal with the large individual differences in how a basically good idea will be experienced by the intended clients. Individual therapy has the advantage in such situations.

Implications

I have tried consciously to keep this discussion directly relevant to planful change—as in psychotherapy—by limiting the discussion to motivation to be different, rather than motivation in general. This is due to cowardice as much as anything: motivation is a core element of psychology, central to the understanding of all behavior, and thus the source of multiple theories and explanatory constructs. Nevertheless, "motivation to change" presents a logical conundrum. Most theories of motivation accept that "all motivation is directed by aspiration—a desire to achieve some sort of positive change in the circumstances of the motivated individual" (Forbes, 2011, p. 87). Planful change is about wanting to change, and that *is* motivation.

Are there any generally accepted principles of motivation that help us understand change, rather than the other way around? A good one is suggested by Forbes, under the rubric of spheres of aspiration. He proposes three foci of aspiration. One is the pursuit of change that is directed inward—to change the way we feel about ourselves. Another is instrumental—to change the way we feel about the material world of objects. The third sphere is also outward directed—the aspiration for positive change in how we feel about our relationships with others. Forbes further assumes different levels of aspiration: being a certain way, doing certain things, and having certain outcomes. Focus and level of aspiration

Table 3.1 **Framework of Human Motivations as a Function of Focus of Aspiration Crossed by Level of Aspiration**

Level of Aspiration	Focus of Aspiration		
	Intrapsychic (Self)	*Instrumental (Material World)*	*Interpersonal (Social World)*
Enhanced expectations (Being)	Security	Empowerment	Belonging
Enhanced experiences (Doing)	Identity	Engagement	Nurturance
Enhanced outcomes (Having)	Mastery	Achievement	Esteem

Forbes, D. L. (2011). Toward a unified model of human motivation. *Review of General Psychology, 15*(2), 85–98. Copyright © 2011 by the American Psychological Association. Reproduced with permission. The use of APA information does not imply endorsement by the APA.

provide a three by three matrix with nine individual motivational domains, as shown in Table 3.1.

These nine domains have been proposed, in different ways by many different theorists, but not within one unified theory. They provide valuable categories of perhaps universal human needs and suggest important general considerations when interpreting clients seeking change. In my own work with people with significant intellectual and developmental disabilities I have long been struck by how little the profession has recognized that these basic needs explain so much of the behavior we judge pathological in highly disadvantaged individuals—especially those living in supported accommodation and institutional settings. Steven Reiss (e.g., 2004) is a notable exception. His model of 16 basic "desires" that drive behavior includes Forbes's nine, and has been useful for thinking about the limited opportunities clients with developmental disabilities often have for empowerment ("to be capable and free to act"), esteem ("to have a standing that begets respect and admiration"), belonging ("to be connected with relationships to other people in my world"), and identity ("to do things that reflect my personal taste, style, and values").

Perhaps because I have seen people with disabilities striving so hard for esteem, belonging, and identity, I am particularly sympathetic to Ward and Marshall's (2004) Good Lives Model of changing offending in people with criminal convictions. They propose that criminal behavior is designed to attain the same universal primary "goods" as desired by everyone else: personal autonomy, inner peace, mastery, and interpersonal relationships—experiences that are intrinsically gratifying and beneficial. Secondary goods, which the offender lacks for various reasons, are the instrumental ways of securing primary goods.

Treatment plans need to be specifically constructed to allow the offender's strengths and life goals, his or her own priorities, and the resources and competencies that would enable access to primary goods, as well as more effective secondary goods. Treatment goals would be *approach* goals—focused on what the client will achieve rather than what he or she will cease to do (Ward, Mann, & Gannon, 2007). This is almost identical to the philosophical principles underlying Solution-Focused Brief Therapy, which emphasize clients' strengths and past successes, on "solution building" rather than problem solving. The client's desired future is what shapes therapeutic direction.

What we need to recognize is that all human behavior is influenced by motivational forces and thus our daily planning, striving, learning, working, and playing—all of which involve change—are functions of our aspirations to meet goals and fulfill our needs. It is against that simple backdrop of ordinary activity that the need to have accelerated, targeted, planful change plays itself out. Therapists might find it useful to keep this in mind by posing the following question. Does a client's desire to be different represent a new level or focus of aspiration, or both? What appears to be a lack of motivation to change can be more clearly seen as a conflict among different motives. In the words of Billy Joe Shaver's popular Country Western song "The Devil made me do it the first time; the second time I done it on my own," we try things out in life, sometimes fortuitously, sometime opportunistically, and depending on the consequences we engage more or try to resist the next time. Because only a fraction of real life change is therapy mediated and the rest is self-regulated and socially regulated, further discussion of how people do or do not act to fulfill their own intentions must wait for a later chapter, particularly the one dedicated to self-directed change. First, however, it is constructive to examine other barriers to change, especially personality, conflict, past experiences, and current environments.

4

Individual Differences in Ability to Change

Personality and Context

There is a famous moment in B. F. Skinner's utopian novel *Walden Two* when the main character, Frazier, recalls shouting at his experimental subjects, "Behave, damn it, behave as you ought!" only to realize later that the subject was always right. Clients, too, are always right and always behave as they must, but when they show no improvement in their dysfunctional patterns of behavior or fail to implement treatment suggestions designed for their benefit and that they have agreed will be helpful, every therapist is faced with the question why? One explanation is clearly motivational—counterproductive beliefs about the new behavior or about themselves and their abilities, lack of clear goals, uncertainty regarding the costs and benefits of taking action, material rewards for the old behavior patterns—all the variables we considered in the previous chapter. But another set of explanations is more closely identified with actual, not perceived, barriers thrown up by personality traits, skill deficits, and the realities of their social and physical environment.

Individuals differ greatly in their ability to make the changes to their lives that are deliberate and designed to meet the sorts of emotional and social goals that drew them into therapy. People who are already skilled in making such changes are the least likely to seek therapy or assistance from some external source. There are, for example, striking differences in the ability of individuals to find and mobilize inner psychological resources for managing stress. Sexual abuse is always a horrifying experience, but only a few individuals are unable to cope with the trauma and seek treatment for intractable distress. In the smoking reduction literature it has often been noted that thousands of people have successfully given up cigarettes entirely on their own, using whatever strategies they could marshal. The people who come to programs to help them quit smoking are those individuals who have tried on their own but have not succeeded for long. Between one-third and two-thirds of those who go on calorie-restricting diets later regain more weight than they lost (Mann et al., 2007). People who seek treatment for depression have not been able manage their moods themselves; parents who come to parenting classes have been less successful than they had hoped in managing their children's behavior. What is it that such individuals lack?

Maybe they lack "willpower" or they did not receive a motivational interview, or they have not yet reached the correct "stage of change" and have not really made a commitment. But from a therapist's planning point of view all those concepts have limitations. What if there are significant individual differences in the ability to change and in the ability to make better use of self-regulation strategies or more natural sources of social and environmental support? If so, how can these abilities and opportunities be enhanced in clients in order to ensure quicker, greater, and more permanent alteration in behavior? To the extent that all psychotherapy is actually a specialized form of social influence, understanding a client's extant options for social rewards and how these interact with personality should be uppermost in any therapist's initial informal assessment of their client's situation. James Gibson, the great perception theorist, called environmental events and objects that permit specific behavior to occur "affordances." The complementarities of the individual's competencies and specific environmental contexts are important to understand.

In this chapter several of the possible individual difference mechanisms will be explored, and selected personality and contextual influences on change will be considered. I will examine the circumstances that make overt *behavior* change more or less difficult to accomplish, mostly because it is the topic that has received the greatest amount of theoretical and experimental attention. There is, however, a growing understanding that what characterizes people with psychological difficulties is that their *emotions* are resistant to change (Kuppens, Allen, & Sheeber, 2010). Although we often think of clients as highly reactive, having large and rapid swings in moods and feelings, this may be true for only a few, and these shifts might occur over longish periods of time. An equally common characteristic of clients is that they experience emotional inertia (Suls, Green, & Hillis, 1998). Emotional inertia can be operationalized as follows: people's emotional state at any given moment may be predicted by their state at a previous moment. Although this concept describes people who are less influenced by efforts at self-regulation and by environmental changes, it does not really explain the mechanisms. Later I will link the phenomenon to "experiential avoidance," as it seems possible that being emotionally nonreactive is a way of avoiding other complex feelings, such as disappointment, terror, or joy.

Some people have personality structures in which certain deficits or excesses seem to dominate every aspect of their individuality, especially their emotional repertoires and their social interactions. We call such patterns personality disorders. It is easy to see that if someone has a deficit in an area such as feelings of empathy and emotional understanding of others, and is incapable of feeling remorse or guilt for his or her actions, that will affect all sorts of ways in which the person interacts with his or her social world and follows conventional rules of behavior. A person such as this is described as having a psychopathic personality disorder. If such an individual were also to be involved in antisocial, criminal, or violent behavior (and obviously not all people with psychopathic tendencies are), then designing an intervention to reduce criminal behavior is going to be much more difficult than if the person had a well-developed conscience and concern for others that could serve to motivate prosocial behavior (Tyrer et al., 2010). In the popular protocol called Aggression Replacement Training for violence-prone children and youth (Goldstein, Glick, & Gibbs, 1998), a third of the curriculum relates to moral reasoning, defined as enhancing empathy and increasing a sense of fairness and concern for the needs and rights of others.

All people, not just clients, face conflict when the outcomes of certain actions are unknown, or, based on previous experience, ambiguous. There are rewards for getting emotionally close to someone, but there are risks as well, such as rejection, painful loss, and in rare cases exploitation and abuse. One of the best established principles in psychology is that when an action has the potential for both positive and negative consequences the result of this approach–avoidance conflict can be indecision. Miller (e.g., 1959) famously demonstrated that gradients for approach and avoidance differ in slope as the goal is approached. When you are at some distance from the outcome the tendency to approach is stronger; at some closer point the tendency to avoid is stronger and the gradients cross over—that is when you dither. No wonder people for whom rejection is especially distressing vacillate between engaging in an intimate relationship and avoiding one.

Barriers to Change Raised by Social/Individual Interaction

Conflicts between gain and loss, safety and risk, are everywhere. In the first chapter I introduced the impediment confronting public policy makers: most significant societal concerns are wicked problems. Policy makers have quickly come to accept that there are major obstacles to changing patterns of individual behavior. They have identified a few of the more obvious ones, listed below. Their examples come from trying to promote sustainable climate change or improve public health; I have added somewhat more clinically relevant, parallel examples: (1) Societal change may require people to give up simple pleasures (smoking, eating fatty salty food, and taking long hot showers are all *pleasurable* and thus highly rewarding; so, regrettably, are paraphilias, or self-stimulation in autism). (2) The desirable alternatives are inconvenient (waiting for the bus, drying clothes on a line, setting up a reward chart and putting stars on it for good behavior). (3) Desirable behaviors can be unpleasant or embarrassing (going for regular medical examinations, using a condom). (4) Appropriate group behavior might require challenging peers (telling friends they have had enough to drink, discouraging racist jokes at work, resisting peer pressure to participate in bullying). (5) The learning of a whole new skill is often required (adopting new farming methods, disciplining your child more consistently and positively). (6) Short-term personal gain may need to be deferred to achieve a long-term social benefit (canceling an airplane flight to reduce your carbon footprint, give up weekend time to mentor an at-risk teenager). Together these show that it is obvious that barriers to change are commonplace—the rule rather than the exception. However, in clinical therapy we are confronted with specific categories of barrier, often relating to the internal, underlying conflict between competing needs, especially between social demands and individual desires. There are three especially common clinical phenomena that emerge from such conflict: resistance, reactance, and doubts about your own capabilities.

Resistance

There is a difference between not changing and not complying with therapeutic suggestions and requirements. The term noncompliance implies a much more active, almost oppositional process to the steps toward change. The reason for this connotation is that in traditional psychoanalytic therapies there is a certain type of noncompliance called resistance. The term was used to describe intrapsychic conflict in which the client's defense mechanisms resisted terrifying thoughts from coming into consciousness. But in fact almost all therapists of all persuasions use the term to shift the blame for a common feature of the therapist–client interaction: the therapist attempts to get the client to act in some way, but the client fails to do so. More subtly, resistance is seen when the client comes late, misses sessions, refuses to talk or talks too much without thinking, forgets suggestions, engages in irrelevant intellectual debate, and perceives the therapist as the enemy—or even more subtly uncritically admires everything the therapist says.

Why does resistance happen? Clients may offer a range of excuses—they were too busy, the task was too hard, they did not quite understand what they were supposed to do, they had no opportunity that week but would do better next week, when they thought about doing it they started to think it was a bit silly, or they could not do it because it made them fearful or upset. Every one of these excuses might have validity, but the stage of change model and the traditional resistance idea essentially challenge the legitimacy of all of them, concluding that basically the client does not really want to change or is not committed to change in the first place.

Therapists who tend to be directive are perplexed by noncompliance with therapeutic suggestions. If we were to assume that the client's motivation to change is suspect, he or she might be directly challenged on this point. I have heard clinicians confront the client: "Look, we agreed that you would do this during the week and you said you understood how it would help you. Because you did not attempt these simple tasks at home, I am beginning to wonder if you are really committed to making a change?" In my experience, clients, just like your partner or your children, hate their behavior being interpreted in this way. Sometimes they will be reflective and think hard about whether they were really showing some reluctance to change, but usually they will raise barriers to performing the alternative activities that place the onus back on the therapist from the point of view of design: you made the task too hard, or not clear enough, or unrealistic knowing what was happening at home, or impractical given the client's resources or intelligence. People *do* have defensive mechanisms, particularly denial, which they use to avoid even more distressing feelings. But sometimes the clinician just has to recognize that the client had a perfectly legitimate reason for not completing a poorly designed activity or rejecting a poorly formulated cognitive reconstruction, or denying an erroneous interpretation.

Accepting responsibility for mistakes is hard for some therapists, like any of us, and resistance assumptions allow us to shift blame to the client, just as Frazier did in *Walden Two*. These blaming responses, however expressed, have the potential, according to Safran and Muran (1996), to "rupture the therapeutic alliance," and potentially increase a client's self-blame (negative self-perceptions). By accepting responsibility and discussing it, the relationship can be repaired and feelings validated, as I described in Chapter 1 when explaining "emotion talk." In a different context, but perhaps drawing on similar processes, we have found that the emotional relationship between a teacher and young children is enhanced when teachers are able to apologize for their mistakes or unwarranted moods (Evans & Harvey, 2012).

Reactance: Resistance to Control

There is a special form of resistance that is particularly pertinent to therapeutic relationships. In 1982 Sharon and Jack Brehm laid out the details of a theory they had been developing for almost 20 years. Known as "reactance theory" it addresses the consequences of people believing that their freedoms are threatened or lost. Perceived threat to individual freedom is thought to generate a negative emotional state aimed at reestablishing the lost freedom and preventing the loss of any others. More crudely, people—like Gloria—do not like being controlled and react against it in ways that will reestablish some degree of autonomy. Presumably there are individual differences in how people respond to perceived loss of freedom, hence the close connection with personality theory. For example, Beck proposed a personality concept called Autonomy for individuals who value achievement, mobility, and freedom from control (Beck, Epstein, Harrison, & Emery, 1983).

The theory of reactance has considerable empirical support, at least in very individualistic (as opposed to collectivist) cultures such as that of the United States, where personal freedom is highly valued. It has not had a great deal of impact on clinical psychology practice except in the health-related area of compliance with medical directives (Fogarty, 1997). Anyone who has tried to use coercive force to stop someone from responding the way they would like to will almost certainly have experienced reactance effects, however. Behavioral strategies attempting to control people with challenging behavior by confrontational means, including popular strategies such as time-out, often produce the exact opposite effect as the individual attempts countercontrol measures. Wrecked bedrooms, feces-smeared walls, ripped clothes, and self-injurious behavior are some of the outcomes facing nurses, teachers, and parents who have attempted to control behavior through such means. As Baumeister, Catanese, and Wallace (2002) explain, there are three essential types of possible responses to loss of freedom or choice: (1) to desire the lost option more than when it was freely available, (2) to reassert freedom by attempting to perform the restricted behavior, and (3) to aggressively attack the person or organization seen as responsible for removing or preventing the desired activity. Professionals in control of powerless people (prisoners, psychiatric patients, welfare recipients, and fostered teenagers) would do well to remember these three possibilities.

A component of the Brehm and Brehm (1981) theory is that the individual must perceive a situation as an unreasonable or unacceptable restriction on freedom. Parents who are skilled in managing the behavior of young children understand this principle very well. It is never helpful simply to order young children around or to arbitrarily thwart their desires and intentions. Instead they can be offered choices that are equally acceptable to the adult, who really does have to be in control much of the time ("Do you want to wear the red dress or the pink one?"). They can be offered a benefit (reward) for compliance ("If you get dressed quickly we will have time to stop and get an ice-cream"). And they can be persuaded that absolute choice is not optional for health, safety, or moral reasons ("I'm sorry, but you have to wear a nice warm dress when it is so cold outside").

Toddlerhood and adolescence are both developmental stages in which young people are particularly sensitive to external control as they attempt to negotiate their autonomy as a key developmental task. Smetana (2002) advanced our understanding of conflict between parents and adolescents by explaining that teenagers accept that some parental restrictions should be based on moral principles (e.g., stealing is wrong) and tacitly agree with them, some on the legitimate and fair rules and conventions set by the family (keep your room tidy; be home by 11 p.m.), some on health and safety considerations (wear a helmet when riding your bike), but some are personal (listening to hard rock music; getting a tattoo). When teenagers and parents come into conflict they are not clashing on these principles: they are disagreeing on the category into which different parental restrictions fall. Thus psychotherapy with families in conflict can be advanced by clarifying whether a disputed activity falls into the moral, prudential (health/safety), conventional, or purely personal domains (Connelly, 2001).

What is always so complex for therapy dynamics is that certain people exhibit the exact reverse of reactance. Clients may well seek treatment because they lack confidence in their ability to solve problems or make decisions without reference to some higher authority. Clients often ask therapists for direct advice, and perhaps maddeningly for them, therapists are very reluctant to proffer it. The classic irritating feature of some therapeutic approaches is to answer all questions with a question! Naturally we are reluctant to tell clients that they should get divorced, change jobs, accept a different sexual orientation, or drop out of college, even if we think strongly that such moves would be to their benefit. Instead the accepted best practice is to try to help them come to their own decision by examining the fears, lack of knowledge, and underlying motivations that might be impeding rational decision making. Nevertheless there are times when it seems simpler just to give advice, based on your own experience and professional knowledge. Clients sometimes are looking for this type of certainty from a therapist who by training, qualifications, age, clinical experience, and general wisdom seems to be better equipped than they are to know what might be best. With some clients we are looking for strategies to increase adherence; with other clients we are looking for ways to make them less needy and less dependent upon the therapist's leadership.

Doubts about Efficacy

There are three important personality dimensions that are closely linked to clients' implicit conflict between striving for autonomy and dependency on the therapist. These are the intertwined elements of self-esteem, locus of control beliefs, and self-efficacy beliefs. All three are belief systems about the nature of our personal interactions with the world and our capabilities. The earliest position, formulated by social learning theorist Rotter (1954), proposed that individuals differ in the extent to which they believe they have control over the events that affect them in life. An external locus of control is the assumption that your destiny and the things that happen in life are due to luck, chance, fate, the will of God, or any other external circumstance. An internal locus of control is the assumption that your life events are determined by your own efforts and actions. A client's attributional style—such as the belief that effort will be rewarded—makes a major difference in whether constructive behaviors will be maintained in the face of inevitable setbacks.

Albert Bandura (1977) introduced the concept of self-efficacy beliefs: a person's sense of capacity to perform particular actions. He also elaborated on Rotter's concept regarding reinforcement expectancy: the subjective probability that a given behavior will produce a rewarding outcome. Immediately you can see how relevant all this is to therapeutic compliance and helping clients make the changes in their behavior necessary to improve their lives. If clients neither believe they can perform a given behavior nor expect it to be rewarded if they do, the probability they will engage in the activity is low—what Rotter called low behavior potential. This has implications for designing effective therapy. One is that therapists should determine what their clients expect to happen before proposing a specific course of action. Another is that expectancies may be irrational and unnecessarily pessimistic, based, perhaps, on past experiences of failure, poor outcomes, or an inability to control the environment through your own efforts.

And if that sounds very much like learned helplessness, you are beginning to see the similarity with yet other concepts. The learned helplessness idea, introduced by Martin Seligman (1975), has captured the attention of clinical psychologists because it provided a plausible, experimental-based mechanism for depression. The original observations were that if an animal was exposed to inescapable shock, it was much less likely to show adaptive behavior when escape or avoidance became possible. In a sense the animal had "given up" because nothing it had tried when being subjected to painful conditions seemed to make any difference. Could this be analogous to what people diagnosed as depressed have experienced in the past? Repeated failure to rectify aversive conditions teaches the person that nothing can be done and therefore nothing is worth doing.

As a general rule therapists could try to arrange for a certain number of guaranteed success experiences in order to raise hopefulness and demonstrate to the client that positive consequences can follow. Interestingly, this exact same strategy is often recommended when designing habilitation programs for people with traumatic brain injury or developmental disabilities—introduce a few fail-proof tasks early in training and intersperse these with the more difficult ones. And because we want to encourage an internal locus of control, we can follow the advice Dweck (1999) gives to all teachers: praise children for effort, not success, so they do not attribute achievement to luck or the task being too easy. Not surprisingly, these traits (e.g., helplessness, low self-efficacy beliefs, low self-esteem) are highly intercorrelated. The conceptual overlap of these personality traits has resulted in the recognition of a possible higher-order construct called core self-evaluations (Judge & Bono, 2001). People with low core self-evaluations (i.e., a lot of clients) are not good at adapting to or creating positive change in social systems (Judge & Kammeyer-Mueller, 2010).

Although Bandura's theory of self-efficacy was rapidly accepted as a mediator of change within cognitive–behavioral therapy (indeed it was partly responsible for behavior therapy "going cognitive" in the first place), it is not without its critics. The most telling and really undeniable criticism is that the theory is so circular that it is difficult to test. If a client engages in a previously avoided behavior, such as no longer avoiding a feared object or situation, the theory goes, it is not because the fear has been extinguished but because the individual's belief has changed and the client now believes that he or she can perform the necessary approach behavior.

Specific Personality Variables Mediating Change

Although beliefs, attributions, and expectancies are all components of personality and will differ markedly across individuals, their explanatory power is limited because they are often merely other terms for the very phenomena that need to be elucidated. For example, a common clinical area in which personality traits are said to represent the individual with the syndrome is that of anorexia nervosa. Adolescents with this disorder are routinely described as perfectionists, inflexible, and rule-bound (Pryor & Wiederman, 1996), but are also high in anxiety, focused on harm avoidance, and fearful of novel stimuli (Klump, McGue, & Iacono, 2002). All of these characteristics seem little more than descriptions of the dominant features of their problem.

In this section, therefore, we will consider very briefly some aspects of personality that seem to be at a more fundamental level than simply a slightly more general description of the behavior to be explained. It has to be brief because there are so many possible personality variables. Impulsivity and risk-taking behavior, for instance, are strongly implicated in habit problems, in juvenile crime, in precocious sexuality—in fact in adolescents in general. A belief in a just world is thought to reduce empathy for victims, including yourself, since if the world is fair people get what they deserve. A favorite trait of mine is differential sensitivity to internal cues, the sensory feedback from physiological processes—the *milieu interieur*. Schachter (1968) conducted one of the classic earlier studies on insensitivity to cues signaling satiation and showed that certain individuals will eat food that is in front of them even when feeling full. The idea of sensitivity to autonomic feedback has recently reemerged as "anxiety sensitivity." Given these and many other intriguing possible facets of personality, I will begin by looking at just a few relevant traits and then will consider just one fundamental, hopefully more truly causal, mechanism.

Dispositional Resistance to Change

A novel source for our current understanding of change-relevant personality variables comes from organizational psychology, in which interest is focused on people who are resistant to changes imposed by the organization (Oreg, 2006). The relevant trait is known as dispositional resistance to change, and its components are certainly germane to clients in therapy since they are defined operationally. They are (1) routine-seeking, or the extent to which we enjoy stable environments; (2) emotional responses of stress and discomfort when change is imposed; (3) a short-term focus on the inconvenience or discomfort that might result from the change, as opposed to its longer-term benefits; and (4) cognitive rigidity, which is a stubborn unwillingness to consider alternative ideas and perspectives (Oreg, 2003; Oreg et al., 2008).

In light of the considerable cross-national support for these components of dispositional resistance to change, it appears fruitful to routinely introduce the notion in therapy. The result would be slightly different from the initial interactions with a client that occur with motivational interviewing. (1) By seeing that change is difficult for most clients, we might be more aware of the need to stress with clients the value of the constructive routines they do enjoy. (2) A therapist could also offer simple stress management techniques—not directed at the problem, but directed at the occasions in which a client tries something different. (3) Find out from the client what short-term benefits he or she enjoys from the status quo, and instead of negating them encourage the client to think about how the same (not different) benefits can accrue from change. (4) Use experiences from the client's past to suggest that the proposed new ideas may actually be ones that the client has had or experienced before.

The ability to change reflects emotional intelligence, a fairly large part of which concerns knowing how you are feeling and why. This is a form of insight, much prized in psychotherapy. In the child development literature it has been argued that the repeated experience of negative emotions may result in children focusing on their own experience rather than that of others (Eisenberg et al., 1998). Child psychologists' definitions of emerging emotion competence always include the reasoning ability of young children to predict feelings from knowledge of causes and to suggest causes from knowledge of someone's feelings, including their own. Not every child acquires that sort of emotion competence, but it can be taught (Salmon, Evans, Moskowitz, Parkes, & Miller, 2012). People also differ in their understanding of everyday strategies that might help them change unwanted behavior or increase the frequency of desired behaviors. This involves knowledge of general principles as well as knowledge of what works for them.

Flexibility versus Rigidity

As we think of the ability to change as a dimension of personality, other well-established traits come to mind. At one end are concepts such as flexible, adaptable, and ability to move with the times. At the other end we have rigid, hide-bound, fixed beliefs. In the Big Five personality model, flexibility might seem closest to the factor called Openness to Experience. However, this dimension is more concerned with appreciation for new ideas, imagination, curiosity, and adventurousness, with conservatism being at the opposite end of the dimension. Although somewhat related, this is not by itself a good description of flexibility and the ability to change. Hayes, Luoma, Bond, Masuda, and Lillis (2006) defined psychological flexibility as "the ability to contact the present moment fully as a conscious human being, and to change or persist in behavior when doing so serves valued ends" (p. 7). The second half of this definition restates what the word flexibility means in a behavioral context, although it places emphasis on values as goals. The first part is operationalized as a willingness to fully experience thoughts and feelings as they are, whether positive or negative—perhaps the opposite of being defensive?

We can turn to an idea, prevalent in cognitive psychology: cognitive flexibility, which in children refers to the ability to inhibit automatic responses and to distance themselves from the immediate situation. It is often considered a core "executive function" skill necessary for adjusting to change. More generally it is the ability to restructure knowledge in multiple ways depending on the demands of changing situations. The concept builds on constructivist theory: that people need to be able to develop their own representations of information in order to learn. It has led to computer-based exercises designed to prepare people to select, adapt, and combine knowledge and experience in new ways to deal with situations that are different from the ones they have encountered before. This "cognitive remediation therapy" has been tried with clients who seem to be particularly inflexible in their thoughts, such as young people with anorexia and people with schizophrenia (Wykes et al., 2007). Although proponents of such training believe that they are training basic brain processes, many of the tasks have a rather old-fashioned feel to them (a Stroop task, a trail-making task to encourage shifting attentional sets) compared to the sorts of fun games most young people play everyday on their iPads, such as Angry Birds and Cat Physics. And in one study of a small group of women with anorexia the subjective report by the clients was merely that the training was a pleasant diversion: it was refreshing to be focused on something other than emotion and their eating disorder (Tchanturia, Davies, & Campbell, 2007). We will encounter the potential of deliberate distraction when considering self-regulation (Chapter 9).

Personality traits are invariably dimensions with polar opposites and the opposite of flexibility is cognitive rigidity (Oreg, 2003), a concept that has been flitting in and out of psychology for the past hundred years or so, with constructs such as perseveration and reliance on fixed habits in new situations: "diminished flexibility and constrictions in the affective, cognitive, and behavioral correlates of adaptational patterns" (Overton & Horowitz, 1991, p. 3). Across an array of clinically referred individuals we find clients with a personality style that is rigid in terms of a diminished behavioral repertoire, an inability to adapt or respond effectively to changes in the environment, and being rule bound with a tendency to perseverate.

A not dissimilar concept is found in individual differences in developmental plasticity. Plasticity in biological psychology refers to the ability to adjust on the basis of experience. Belsky and Pluess (2009) have suggested that some individuals are not just affected by negative experiences (the traditional diathesis/stress model), but are easily influenced by *both* negative and positive experiences. This would mean that children with greater plasticity might benefit differentially from very positive nurturing environments in the same way that they would be seriously harmed by very negative ones. So, for example, anger proneness in toddlers (usually thought of as a negative characteristic) can result in *fewer* behavior problems than other children at the age of 5 years, if they received supportive, consistent child rearing with clear limits and instructions. Simplifying the implications somewhat, it means that some people are more likely to be influenced by experiences than others, both to their benefit and their detriment.

For these and many other personality dimensions there is a certain circularity in the argument that the client's difficulty in changing is driven by traits that greatly resemble the client's problem. If anything is to come of this topic, I think it is important to look at the more basic aspects of behavior that underlie these descriptive psychological dimensions, and I will attempt to do this in the next section.

Personality/Treatment Interface

The whole point of considering more fundamental or underlying personality dimensions is based on an extremely logical assumption that has, sadly, not as yet yielded much fruit. The assumption is that knowledge of a client's basic personality should determine the precise design of the change strategy as much as understanding the dynamics of the problem. It was really Eysenck (1967) who first made the argument, and he was able to do so because there were logical connections between his theory of personality, the implications for psychological mechanisms, and the use of these mechanisms in the design of interventions. Eysenck had first described certain personality dimensions, the best known being an emotionally Stable versus Labile dimensions ("Neuroticism"), and an Introversion/Extraversion dimension. One of the characteristics of Introverts (in the theory) is that at a resting state they are more aroused (at the cortical level), they are sensitive to stimuli, and they condition easily. People high on Neuroticism (according to theory) are likely to be emotionally reactive in threatening situations (at the limbic system level), and if they are also Introverts then fear would be readily conditioned and only slowly extinguished. There is a some evidence that this is so, but for now I do not wish to argue for the correctness of the theory, but rather to show its importance from the point of view of logic: connecting biology through personality characteristics to learning differences to psychopathology and hence to the rational design of a targeted treatment to promote change.

The New "Eysenck Theory": BAS, BIS, and FFFS

As the idea of relating basic personality processes to clinically relevant emotional behavior and its change is such an important one, it is worth taking a quick look at the modern status of Eysenck's theory in light of the most recent neuropsychological evidence. The first iteration came with the work of Jeffrey Gray, Eysenck's brilliant student who later succeeded him as Professor of Psychology at the Institute of Psychiatry. Gray (1982) reformulated Eysenck's theory according to more recent physiological, neurochemical, and anatomical advances suggesting that there are two major systems in the brain. One is responsive to reward and encourages approach activity (an example from evolutionary development might be foraging for food)—the Behavioral Activation System (BAS). The other is responsive to punishment (pain, danger, and so on), which encourages avoidance activity, escape, and hesitancy—the Behavioral Inhibition System (BIS).

Normally we would expect the two systems to be in balance as both are fundamental to survival, but it is possible to imagine that for many different reasons individual organisms differ in the degree to which one of the two systems is dominant. This immediately attracted close attention from clinicians interested in change. The concept of "reinforcement sensitivity" became popular, for example. And Carver and White (1994) developed a self-report personality questionnaire to measure BIS and BAS. Examples of BAS items are "When good things happen to me it affects me strongly" and "I'm always willing to try something new if I think it will be fun." Examples of BIS items are "Criticism or scolding hurts me a great deal" and "I worry about making mistakes." However, the BIS scale and its factor structure have been criticized; for example, it is difficult to determine whether it is a measure of fear sensitivity, punishment sensitivity, or general negative affect.

But the interest sparked in these and related topics, such as impulsivity and reward dominance (from the BAS), is nevertheless noteworthy. To give a few examples from my own laboratory (Wilson & Evans, 2002), we showed that boys described by their teachers as having conduct problems found it difficult to cease a behavior that had previously been highly rewarded and was now being penalized—this seemed like reward dominance, but also reflected the related characteristic of impulsiveness. A better example was our study of boys' and girls' judgment of what it would be like to be punished for something you did not do or not rewarded for something meritorious you did do—both of which are unfair (Evans, Galyer, & Smith, 2001). Boys, but not girls, tended to judge not getting a deserved reward as much worse than getting punished for something you did not do. This is one way to think about what is meant by being reward dominant, as it also implies being impervious to punishment.

In 2000, however, Gray and McNaughton published a substantial clarification of the original theory, better linking fear and anxiety, reinforcer sensitivity, and approach and avoidance. One reason for this was that in the earlier formulation Gray had actually divided the BIS (avoidance of threat) into a separate neurobehavioral pathway: the Flight–Fight system, which involves not just running from danger, such as a predator, but includes attack—both serving the function of escape from danger. If you do not know where the danger is coming from, however, an even better idea might be to freeze until you do, so this whole system should be called the Flight–Fright–Freeze System (FFFS). To clarify the issues of anxiety and fear, approach and avoidance, and reward sensitivity and punishment sensitivity, and relate them to personality variables that will effect change, McNaughton and Corr (2008) have produced a fourth iteration of the Eysenck/Gray theory.

First, fear, anxiety, and worry are easily distinguishable in terms of defensive direction. Fear is aroused by the appearance or perception of a threat (danger) and the autonomic arousal allows you to escape, that is to say, leave a dangerous situation (active avoidance). This could be by confrontation and attack, or you might be able to escape by freezing, especially if you are a small, not very fierce animal. If you are very fearful or if you perceive the threat as intense you might panic rather than deal with the threat in any useful way. Anxiety is aroused when there is an expectation of danger, and the autonomic arousal allows you to cautiously enter a dangerous situation or to refrain from approaching one (passive avoidance of danger). Worry, which most of us, according to Borkovec and colleagues (1983), do more often, refers to ruminative, brooding thoughts about possible dangers and threats, thus exposing us to symbolic danger via words and images. Worry predisposes us to anxiety because it fails to dispose of the threatening concern—this is one of the benefits, we would think, of teaching active problem solving (see Chapter 7).

McNaughton and Corr proposed that the FFFS is actually the system that is sensitive to punishment and relates to avoidance behavior. The BAS is sensitive to reward and to approach. The BIS is the system activated when the organism is faced with an approach–avoidance conflict; it increases attention to possible threat stimuli, increases external scanning for risks, and increases internal scanning of memory for relevant information. Personality will thus reflect attractor sensitivity (gain seeking) or repulsor sensitivity (loss avoiding). Gains and losses in this theory also relate to financial gain as well as sensitivity to other reinforcers.

Impulsivity

There is a further particularly good example of how underlying personality dispositions relate to specific behavioral difficulties clients report. The personality construct I am thinking of is impulsivity—leaping before you look, not planning ahead, and intolerance of cognitive complexity. It seems to be made up of a series of traits that are not necessarily highly correlated. As highlighted in the BAS/FFFS model, impulsivity is related to risk-taking, sensation-seeking, fearlessness (the opposite of anxiety sensitivity), poor cognitive (inner-speech) self-control, and the demand for immediate rather than delayed gratification. Despite this complexity, there is a whole raft of clinical syndromes that have poor impulse control as the underlying dynamic—road rage, opportunistic crime, intermittent explosive disorder, fire-setting, substance use, in fact just about everything we want clients to stop doing. Something that applies to too many phenomena risks being explanatory for none, and this is the question: do we gain anything in terms of helping people change by targeting the trait of impulsivity as opposed to working directly on the presenting problem? It is a very big question. Should we work on anxiety or anxiousness, obsessive-compulsive behavior or intolerance for uncertainty, criminal offending or low empathy, positive symptoms of psychosis or schizotypy (anhedonia, aberrant body schema), poor social skills in autism or theory of mind, poor academic achievement or laziness (low industriousness)?

The simple answer is that we do not precisely know, but given that, why not try both? Specific behavior problems can be targeted by specific interventions; underlying traits and dispositions can be targeted by general training strategies. The latter are very popular since they seem to correct underlying central, maybe even neuropsychological patterns, so neuroscientists like them a lot. In rehabilitation, for instance, giving people general strategies has been much less successful than teaching specific skills. In the area of intellectual disability, we have found teaching general things such as "job readiness" has always proved less successful than teaching a specific job skill, although that does not preclude some useful general skills that apply to all jobs, such as following directions or cooperating with fellow employees. *Preparing clients with a disability by teaching prerequisite skills led to the well-known complaint in special education: "Pre means never." This is a significance topic, relating to target behavior selection, setting therapeutic goals, pivotal and keynote skills, generalization, long-term outcome expectancies, changing one behavior in order to change another, and many other themes we have been looking at. My own, bias, perhaps obvious by now, is to recommend a greater emphasis on the targeted behavior: gambling not impulsivity or domestic violence not callousness. But when clear hierarchical connections between a problem and the underlying trait exist, personality change will potentially yield the broadest and longest term benefits.

Context Determines Behavior

In his landmark book on personality, Walter Mischel (1968) made the case that people behave differently in different contexts. Traits are not consistently expressed or revealed across different environments. His convincing treatise provoked a storm of controversy and changed forever the shape of personality research as investigators struggled to determine what aspects of personality could be considered fixed. Mischel's book was actually about assessment, which makes the whole concept of consistency of behavior particularly relevant to the understanding of change. Good assessment should determine what factors are influencing behavior—change those factors and the behavior changes.

Because of Mischel we also know that neuropsychological and personality constructs do not function in isolation from environmental conditions. And so the other important part of barriers to change can be found in contextual variables. We now need to consider influences on behavior completely different from explanations based on traits and personality dynamics: socioecological influences (Oishi & Graham, 2010). This is not because there is a conflict between the importance of personality and the importance of context. Far from it; the two sources of influence are not only equally important but also closely intertwined.

The Fundamental Attribution Error

As important as Mischel's demonstration that personality characteristics were not consistent across different situations was Lee Ross' articulation of what he called the "fundamental attribution error" (Ross, 1977). This is our tendency, when explaining behavior, to overvalue personality-based or dispositional explanations and to undervalue situational explanations. An interesting twist to the fundamental attribution error is that when explaining our own behavior we are more likely to justify it on situational grounds, whereas when it is someone else's behavior we tend to blame the way they are rather than the situation they are in. This difference is known as the actor–observer bias. Therapists are especially prone.

Gilbert and Malone (1995) elaborated on the fundamental attribution error, calling it, in less memorable terms, the correspondence bias. They defined this as "the tendency to draw inferences about a person's unique and enduring dispositions from behaviors than can be entirely explained by the situations in which they occur" (p. 21). One of the features of everyday understanding about behavior is the importance we place on why it occurs. These judgments have a very strong influence on how we respond to the behavior of others. If a parent attributes a child's misbehavior to an internal disposition ("he's naughty") or to a negative motive ("he's trying to provoke me"), the child is more likely to be punished than if the attribution is more forgiving ("it was an accident" or "he's too young to know any better") (Azar, Nix, & Makin-Byrd, 2005). Such attributions not only influence the way a child will be treated by the parent or teacher, but will also shape therapeutic treatment in exactly the same way. Your intervention plan, perhaps unknowingly to you as a practitioner, will be largely determined not by the scientific data on the validity of a treatment method but by the causal attributions you make for the problem being addressed—think back to the arguments made in Chapter 1 about the causes of a person's weight or a child's activity level.

One way Gilbert and Malone proposed to mitigate the correspondence bias is to help an observer understand that he or she may not be seeing the situation in the same way as the other individual is. There are numerous social psychology experiments that indicate that we have difficulty separating our assumptions from the construals of another. If you knew that a situation was dangerous it is harder to accept that someone else assumed it was safe and thus acted—in your view—recklessly or thoughtlessly. How often have you made that judgment about your teenager? Because of the work on "theory of mind" we now presume that this limitation in understanding another person's understanding is a feature, maybe even an explanation, of autism (Baron-Cohen, Leslie, & Frith, 1985). But actually we all show it to some extent. There are numerous versions of cognitive therapy in which the attempt is to encourage the client to recognize that their egocentric reading of another meaningful person's behavior may be entirely different from that person's own construal.

A second possible way to reduce correspondence bias is to encourage people to reserve making a dispositional judgment until there have been more extended opportunities to observe behavior in different situations. Gilbert and Malone presented considerable evidence that people tend to make these dispositional judgments first. A teacher who has already decided that a pupil is a "trouble maker," "holy terror," "conduct disordered," or "hyperactive" is much less likely to consider situational influences such as domestic discord at home, the structure of the classroom rules, or coming to school hungry. Helping trainee clinicians start with functional analyses of behavior and seek contextual influences (including socioeconomic, cultural, and lifestyle; Evans, Herbert, Fitzgerald, & Harvey, 2010) can reduce correspondence bias. We should repeatedly point out to trainees that in most cases they have seen the client in only one somewhat unusual setting (Swann, 1984).

Types of Environmental Influence

Environments control behavior in extremely complex ways. One source of influence is simply the behaviors that are physically possible. Snow permits skiing and tropical beaches permit snorkeling; these affordances ensure that the activities are not interchangeable. When driving a car in traffic, most forms of direct physical aggression are unfeasible; rude gestures, swearing, and revenge fantasies are eminently possible. If the client is in a prison cell, sexual assault on a female partner cannot occur. Children eat more junk food if there is a fast food restaurant near their school (Currie, DellaVigna, Moretti, & Pathania, 2009), as do truckers when fast food is all that is available at truck stops. In many settings behaviors are physically possible but strongly proscribed by the rules of the setting. You are capable of making or receiving a cell phone call in a movie theatre, but the behavior is rare because it is socially sanctioned.

Other environments regulate behavior because the role of the agent in the setting is learned through implicit rules and modeling. The university professor can deliver a lecture in a wide variety of ways but there are limits on the general categories of behavior called teaching—there is an explicit role that is very different when the same person is watching his or her favorite team play a game of soccer. Even anticipated future environments influence behavior through motivation. Once you have made the commitment to run in a marathon, a demanding training and exercise regime becomes more probable.

Physical conditions such as climate have strong influences on behavior and mood. In the United States, violent crime rates are higher in cities with high average temperatures (Anderson, 2001). Because of the general public's fascination with Seasonal Affective Disorder, most ordinary people are well aware of the influence of cold dark weather conditions on mood and depression (negative affect), even without knowing the scientific evidence (e.g., Young, Meaden, Fogg, Cherin, & Eastman, 1997). Anyone who has recently had a vacation in a pleasant sunny resort will tell you how beneficial it was for enhancing motivation, positive mood, and general well-being. What psychotherapists often forget is that many of their clients, especially those in the public mental health system, never or rarely experience relaxing holidays and the renewal from significant if temporary changes of environment.

A further type of contextual influence is the availability of resources and opportunities. In Wilson's study of nonrecidivist men with psychopathic traits who had spent time in prison for violent offences, most were living in more remote rural areas with limited access to the social and environmental conditions that allow criminal behavior—bars, liquor stores, drug dealers, gang members, and so on. Stimuli of hunger elicit food seeking or foraging behavior, but eating—the consumption of food—can occur only if there is food available. Rozin and colleagues (Rozin, Kabnick, Pete, Fischler, & Shields, 2003) showed that food portion sizes in French supermarkets, restaurants, and cook books were smaller than in the United States and suggested that this contributed to differences between the two countries in terms of average body weight. Not surprisingly, portion control is a major therapeutic recommendation to people hoping to eat more healthily. Even satiated rats will eat a second whole meal again if presented with a contextual stimulus that has in the past been paired with food (Weingarten, 1983).

Environmental restrictions thus restrain and facilitate behavior, but fortunately we can often control environments. If you want to learn to snorkel in the middle of winter you have to find a heated swimming pool, or if you want to go skating in the middle of summer you need to find an indoor ice skating rink. Thus it may well be that the degree to which people are able to influence and regulate their own behavior is not just a function of something like flexibility, but the extent of their knowledge of contextual influences and their access to environmental resources that sustain or elicit desirable patterns of behavior. One of the best established "big picture" concepts in psychology is that environments and behaviors interact in order to determine current functioning. Let us consider this a little more closely.

Personality/Situation Interactions

Ironically, Mischel, having set the proverbial cat among the personality trait pigeons, relented later and proposed that there *were* stable individual difference variables that interact with features of the environment (Mischel & Shoda, 1995). These, he suggested, were at the level of cognitive-affective mediators: encoding strategies (what you pay attention to and the meanings you attach to them), expectancies (what you expect to happen if you do something), subjective values (your personal values determine what is rewarding to you), and self-regulatory systems and plans (figuring out how to achieve your long-term, desired goals). Self-identity must be one of the most important mediators of person/environment interaction, especially if we differentiate between *verification strivings* (the desire to know ourselves) and *positivity strivings* (the desire to feel good about ourselves) (Pinel & Constantino, 2003). People's cognitive-affective dispositions in all these areas will affect how they deal with the world and the world with them—crucial principles for all behavior change, as will be asserted again in Chapter 8.

From a more behavioral perspective Staats (1975) had already developed a rather neat way of conceptualizing personality/situation interactions in a model particularly suited to planful behavior change. He argued that some environments are essentially deficit environments—they do not offer the choices and the opportunities that permit complex learning to take place. Similarly, some personality repertoires are deficit repertoires—individuals have not acquired a sufficient range of keystone or pivotal skills (see Chapter 7) that allows new learning to build hierarchically on the old. The classic example of this might be the child who comes to kindergarten without having had the benefit of a rich home environment in which useful preschool skills have been acquired: counting, recognizing letters, enjoying a story, following instructions, waiting your turn, and sharing. If this child comes to an early education program that is well designed so his level of learning is understood by teachers who can form a caring relationship, then he will probably acquire the necessary basic skills and do fine. Conversely, if a child comes to preschool with lots of early stimulation, where creativity is encouraged, reading is loved, and emotional competence is high, but where the educational program is limited, rigid, or chaotic, then his or her skills will most likely not counteract that environmental deficit.

What is objectively the same educational environment for two different children will shape and control behavior in completely different ways. A teacher uses praise and negative consequences, gives instructions, and offers help in pretty much the same way to all children. But the boy who has come from an abusive home in which physical discipline is harsh may be very hesitant to approach a new adult teacher and so gradually he has fewer and fewer opportunities for social interaction with this teacher and becomes less favored and possibly less liked. He soon learns that other children are treated more positively despite the teacher's efforts to be fair to all. Differential treatment leads to resentment and hostility and from there to conduct problems. Classroom conduct disorders in children provide a perfect example of how trying to change behavior without changing the general environment is extremely difficult. Classroom environments have a distinctive atmosphere and this can either promote positive behavior in the majority of children or create a climate in which negative behaviors predominate (Evans & Harvey, 2012).

It is with changing the inappropriate or excessive actions of people with intellectual and developmental disabilities that the concept of stimulus antecedents and how they need to be changed has come to center stage as a tactic for changing behavior. Very specific stimuli have been shown to trigger challenging behavior, sometimes physical, such as a fluorescent light, and sometimes social, such as a verbal reprimand. These eliciting stimuli are just like the specific cues that evoke a fear reaction in an adult client with a phobia or cues that evoke anger-related aggression in violent individuals. Where possible, we gain considerable therapeutic advantage by simply removing these stimuli from the client's environment. Even if these eliciting stimuli are difficult to eliminate from everyday environments, their temporary removal affords a treatment program the chance to develop alternative behaviors.

It is also possible to teach discrimination so that the individual responds to a much narrower and more realistic range of cues. To give a simple example using fears, if a child is afraid of dogs we can, according to the above ecological principle, reduce the overall expression of fear by keeping all dogs away. But what a child needs to do in real life is learn to be cautious around fierce, unleashed, aggressive dogs, and to be perfectly relaxed around tail-wagging, face-licking, friendly dogs—a discrimination task. Thus, we would teach children to approach and maybe pat friendly dogs and to be wary of, by standing still or avoiding, fierce dogs. Operant conditioning theorists prefer to talk about discriminative stimuli as setting the stage or the occasion for the event that it signals and so they talk about it as a setting event.

Ecology and Change

I have been focusing on specific triggering or eliciting stimuli as they provide a very elaborate set of possible strategies for facilitating at least short-term behavior change. If an undesirable behavior typically occurs in a given context or situation, change the situation, at least temporarily, and the behavior will change. People with very explicit fears know this—if you are afraid of heights or elevators do not look for an apartment in a high-rise condominium building. Some people will tend to eat snacks because they are in front of them not because they are hungry, and so if you are trying to reduce your unhealthy intake of salt and cholesterol, do not stock your pantry with your favorite corn chips. As will be shown in Chapter 9, many people learn to manage their behavior through exercising control of their physical environment. But situations are usually made up of hundreds of possible stimuli occurring in hundreds of different possible combinations, and there are many situations that cannot be avoided. Work environments, including classrooms, can be dull, repetitive, or frustrating. Unlike leisure activities, work is done for someone else, who usually dictates the terms and makes the performance demands. Clients with poor communication skills (often true of people with disabilities), or limited power (also true), often have little opportunity to decline to do tasks, to set their own pace, or to carry out a task in their preferred way. Often work and classroom situations can be quite negative, responding to none of the nine motivational needs introduced in the previous chapter. Negative situations evoke challenging behavior (Meyer & Evans, 1989).

Let us break this down a little more carefully. Challenging behavior might be an indication of frustration or general unhappiness. Or it might be more explicitly serving the function of getting out of a disliked task, or communicating that you wish to do something else entirely. Either way, if you can explain that to your manager or supervisor, which most of us can, then usually some sort of accommodation or compromise can be arranged. But when you do not have those skills you have a tantrum, throw things around, break stuff, and generally act like a frustrated 2 year old. In certain settings you might have those communicative skills but have so little power that they do not allow the objectionable conditions to change in any way. Someone in prison might fit this circumstance, especially as the environment tends to be generally unpleasant, and, in particular, tends to be very controlling, thus increasing the likelihood of reactance.

In any of these situations, the antidote to disruptive behavior is to be less controlling, offer more choices, and modify the available activities so that they are more interesting or engaging. There are hundreds of published examples of the success of this general strategy for people with intellectual and developmental disabilities (Harvey, Boer, Meyer, & Evans, 2009), but somewhat fewer for people in other restricted circumstances. If the primary trigger here is that the programs are monotonous and unpleasant, making them more interesting is sufficient. If the reactance comes about because in addition to being boring the programs are being dictated by an authority figure, then offering more choices and lowering the demands for success would be the modification required.

There are, however, other triggers in this situation. For example, if the activities are interesting but difficult, then the person will experience fewer successes and more failures. If the challenging behavior (remember this is aggression, disruption, noncompliance, and self-injury) is triggered by failure experiences, then the changes that need to be made are to match the level of difficulty to the client's capability and ensure higher levels of success and fewer failures. In classroom situations good teachers do this automatically—adjusting the demands of the tasks to the competence of the students. Many therapeutic situations require clients to perform new and perhaps difficult tasks—social approach for clients who are very shy, or negotiating conflict in married couples, or functional daily skill training for someone who has had a traumatic brain injury. The competent therapist gauges the difficulty of such tasks for the client and suggests initial activities or tasks that are very likely to be successful and thus rewarded. If no simple levels of difficulty can be found, then difficult tasks can be interspersed with highly familiar ones that are certain to bring success.

Implications

If I am right and clients differ in their affordances for change, either because of trait characteristics or ecological conditions or their interaction, it follows that therapists have to try to manage the likelihood of changing (changeability) as well as the specific therapeutic strategy to bring it about. Perhaps this aspect of intervention design represents the true "nonspecifics" of therapy. The therapeutic alliance (Chapter 10) would thus be simply a small subcomponent of enabling change.

Not all therapy is about getting people to do things, but much of it is, especially if we expand the meaning of that to getting people to think about things in new ways. But if we begin to imagine the likely impediments to change we can share responsibility with the client for managing suggestions for action that will not encounter major obstacles. To do this requires some understanding of barriers. There are barriers due to attitude and belief and barriers due to lack of knowledge and understanding. There are barriers due to never really making the commitment in the first place but being too unassertive or shy to say so. There are practical barriers such as cost, opportunity, available time, and appropriate location. There are barriers due to the fact that the actions are not easily performed or make you feel uncomfortable when doing so—something very common in clients with anxiety disorders. There are barriers due to a lack of energy and difficulty in making the effort—something that is very common in clients who are depressed. There are barriers caused by conflicting goals, seeking rewarding versus avoiding punishment. All of these barriers are related to personality/environment interaction. They are all proportionate to the feeling of urgency to change and the belief that these actions will assist in the change process. In other words, clients have self-efficacy beliefs (and doubts) for the actions that might lead to clinical improvement in some other, targeted behavior.

Interactional concepts, now often referred to as constructivist theory (Kahn, 1999), alert us to the fundamental principle that people are not passive recipients of environmental influences: they are agents, not objects. Clinicians need to be constantly mindful of that fact since we typically see clients in only one setting, the clinic. Behavior is also situationally determined, which is a closely related fact that needs to be born in mind because it is such good news. Situations are going to be so much easier to tweak than personality dispositions. Situations create opportunities, but they also throw up barricades. Clients make fundamental attribution errors just like any other observer of behavior. When they do so, they may attribute their problems to their own limitations, producing feelings of low self-esteem. Or they may attribute their problems to fate or superior mystical forces, resulting in feelings of helplessness.

Of all the long-standing environmentalist traditions in psychology it is probably Urie Bronfenbrenner's (1977) ecological model with its different levels of influence that will be most familiar to contemporary psychotherapists. But does this perspective convey a full appreciation of the importance of social ecology (physical, social, and interpersonal environments) in helping clients change (Oishi & Graham, 2010)? Kurt Lewin, in the 1930s, drew an analogy between psychology and the history of physics, reminding us that Aristotle believed objects' tendencies to directional movement resided in the bodies themselves. Galileo, on the other hand, although conceding that the properties of an object were important, saw that these properties had a crucial relationship to the object's environment. Lewin (1931) urged psychologists to get out of the Aristotelian mode and think more like Galileans. Psychological dispositions may be genetically determined and tied closely to neurological systems, but if they can at least partially be attributed to learning experiences, then learning experiences should be able to change them. I will now look at how these might be planned.

5

Conditioning

Changing the Meaning and Value of Events

Pavlov told good stories. One of his best was how his laboratory was inundated during the 1924 Leningrad floods, and he and his assistants had to rescue the dogs from their submerged cages in the basement. Because the kennel doors were low and the water was high, the dogs had to be dragged under water before being helped to safety. Later, however, when back in their little harnesses to perform the standard experiments on conditioned salivation, the dogs' previous learning was disrupted and they continued to show strong emotional signs of being quite traumatized (Todes, 2000). I've got a good dog story too. When I moved with my family to a 100-acre dairy farm in upstate New York, our suburbanite dog made the fatal mistake of putting his wet nose against the electrified fence. He proved that learning can take place in one trial and he never went near a piece of wire again; he would even shy away from wire clothes-hangers.

In these two examples we see the full range of associational experiences that change behavior. When the stimulus is discrete and somewhat familiar, such as a strand of wire, and the associated event is unambiguous, such as pain, the effects are tightly focused. When the situation is novel, complex, and volatile and the associated ordeal is diffuse, life threatening, prolonged, and unpredictable (floods, combat, rape) the effects are pervasive and destabilizing. Pavlov's interest in "experimental neurosis" brings us to the very core of understanding behavior change that has the kind of intransience that must be achieved in therapy if therapy is to have any merit at all. Permanent change is neither plausible nor even always desirable, but there does need to be some carry-over from the therapeutic experience to meaningful change in behavior as it affects day-to-day living and lifestyle.

The integrating idea is quite simple: people benefit from therapy to the extent that they learn two things: (1) to reevaluate and respond differently to events and situations—both present and remembered—that previously caused distress (what this chapter is mostly about); and (2) to acquire and use new desired habits and skills and unlearn interfering, unwanted ones (the topic of the next chapter). This includes learning new "habits of the mind"—highly automatic and stylized thoughts. Learning and unlearning are the essence of planful change. You have a client who is unable to swallow solid food for fear of choking, another who cannot stop gambling despite heavy financial losses, or a child who is too anxious to go to school. Even though you may not fully understand how these patterns of behavior originally developed, or even if you understand the origins but cannot expunge them, one thing seems certain: change for the client will require some sort of new learning, however that is achieved.

Learning in this context does not mean what we call in everyday parlance book learning, such as being able to recite *Ode to a Nightingale* or remembering Boyle's Law. There are occasions, clinically, when clients may need simple, clear verbal information and factual knowledge about things that are otherwise mysterious, confusing, or misleading, and these will be mentioned later in the chapter on cognitive change (Chapter 8). In the present context learning also excludes motor skill acquisition, such as learning to dance the Highland Fling. Neither does it include perceptual learning, such as recognizing a face you have seen only once before. The learning that is relevant to unwanted habits, emotional reactions, and maladaptive thoughts is the learning often referred to as conditioning: classical and instrumental. In the next two chapters I am going to explore conditioning, as we understand it in modern psychology, and try to show that it is an essential element of how and why people change.

Approach and Withdrawal (Avoidance)

Before doing so, however, I want to propose a simple framework for linking together the previous discussions of motivation and personality with the topic of learning, especially emotion learning, and the concepts of reward and punishment. This is a theme that has pervaded psychology from the start. The notion is that human behavior (actually the behavior of all organisms) can be divided into approach and withdrawal (often a bit misleadingly called avoidance). For humans, with our vast symbolic capabilities and vivid imaginations, this does not have to be a physical movement in space toward or away from a desirable or threatening situation. Sending a romantic Tweet to a lover is approach, as is watching an opera or peeling an orange (assuming you plan to eat it rather than throw it). Writing a "Dear John" letter is withdrawal, as is walking out of the opera in the middle of an aria or spitting out a red hot chili pepper. We approach or plan to approach things we like and enjoy and that are familiar (the stimuli are appetitive, they give pleasure), so these things also serve as rewards, and we escape or avoid things that we dislike or that are unusual (the stimuli are aversive, they cause pain), so these serve as punishments. I have already explained in Chapter 4 that three different neural pathways independently regulate these two essentials of adaptive functioning.

Particular emotions and attitudes are associated with approach and withdrawal, as has been hinted at by the use of words such as liking and disliking. Signals of impending pleasure will themselves become positive, and signals of potential pain are likely to become aversive in their own right. Signals informing you of the likelihood of a positive or negative consequence create expectations. Expectation of reward is synonymous with the emotion hope; expectation of punishment (pain, injury, loss) is roughly synonymous with anxiety, which facilitates avoidance. (The actual appearance of danger evokes fear, which facilitates escape.) If we approach with a positive expectation and fail to get a reward, the emotion is disappointment (if the goal attainment is blocked, the emotion may be frustration or anger). If we escape an aversive situation or actively avoid and fail to receive an expected punishment, the emotion is relief. Thus, approach and withdrawal both have the potential to elicit positive feelings (the behavior was successful) as well as the potential to elicit negative feelings (the behavior was a failure). There are nuances to this basic outline we will have to acknowledge. Approach, being a more active form of conduct, yields energizing sorts of feelings: positive emotions such as elation and excitement and negative emotions such as anger and guilt (guilt should motivate you to make amends). Avoidance, tending to be more passive (yes, sometimes we run for cover, but often we hide or freeze on the spot—Roelofs, Hagenaars, & Stins, 2010), yields more quiescent emotions: positive emotions such as contentment and serenity and negative emotions such as shame (shame makes you want to hide, to cover your face, to wish the ground would swallow you up).

In human experience there are typically costs related to simple approach or simple avoidance. Most situations require elements of both: although hot, the chili pepper might make your burrito taste really delicious; the amorous Tweet to your lover might be misconstrued and result in rejection; sitting through the opera without complaint might have pleased your partner. So, as everyone knows, the majority of human endeavor consists of conflict between approach and avoidance, balancing the desires to maximize pleasure and to minimize pain, remembering that these are not necessarily material or physical outcomes.

Classical Conditioning

One of the triumphs of experimental psychology during the first half of the twentieth century was to reveal many principles of basic learning. In the broad field of learning theory there are two indisputable universal forms: instrumental conditioning (operant learning) and classical conditioning (respondent conditioning). These may turn out to be simply different experimental preparations rather than reflecting fundamentally different principles, and perhaps all learning requires the same underlying brain mechanisms involving associative processes, synaptic connections, consolidation of memory traces, and the recall and use of information. However, the difference between behavior changing (1) as a function of its consequences (contingency), and (2) as a function of the pairing of stimuli (contiguity), is a useful one that has served psychology well.

At one time Skinner (1938) thought that only overt actions that physically change the environment could be modified by their consequences (their effect on the environment), and only involuntary "respondents," or automatic reflexes, could be modified by pairing stimuli contingent on each other but not contingent on what the organism does. There are numerous examples demonstrating that this is a false distinction (Pear & Eldridge, 1984), but the essence of the idea is important for therapy. If a boy is described as school phobic, his reluctantly walking to school or refusing to climb onto the school bus is an instrumental behavior by which he controls his environment. His screaming, trembling, and vomiting at the sight of the school or the school bus are reflexive reactions of the autonomic nervous system (emotional respondents) that are primarily controlled by environmental cues. The child's emotional (respondent) reaction will have an effect on his social environment; if this effect is something desirable, then the respondent behavior can become an operant. The child can use emotional reactions to obtain desired outcomes—attention, comfort, treats, exemptions, whatever. Nevertheless, there is a useful difference between behavior that is controlled by the stimuli that elicit it and behavior that is controlled by the stimuli that are its consequence, blurry as the distinction can become.

In this chapter the focus is on classical, or Pavlovian conditioning, which relates to changing the meaning, value, and significance of stimuli rather than responses. Everyone knows about Pavlov's salivating dogs. Understanding them is not quite so easy, and it is arguable that today we do not know much more than Pavlov did (Bitterman, 2006). If you ask undergraduates, after explaining the basic phenomena, why the dog salivates at the sound of the bell (ticking metronome, or whatever the conditioned stimulus, CS, might be), they quite reasonably say things like "well, the bell reminds them of the food" (the unconditioned stimulus, UCS) or "when they hear the bell they expect to be fed." Most students are right up there with Tolman and the "cognitive revolution" in psychology—it all concerns information: learning *about* what leads to what. Students are typically expectancy theorists.

But the simplistic cognitive explanation, if not downright wrong, is certainly tautological. After explaining the basic phenomenon of extinction (the conditioned response, CR, decreases when the CS is presented repeatedly without the UCS), you can again ask students why this effect happens. The answer usually is "Oh, I guess the dog doesn't drool anymore because now it realizes that it will not get fed after all; now the bell signals 'no food.'" So then you tell them about spontaneous recovery and ask them why that occurs, and then they have to say "OK, after a little while, the dog reckons that maybe things have changed and that now the bell might mean the food is coming after all, and"—they add in triumph—"that is why the salivation response in spontaneous recovery isn't usually quite as strong as at the end of acquisition, because the dog isn't really sure that food will come now."

These mentalistic explanations may have some legitimacy; certainly modern conditioning theory has played around with probabilities. Rescorla (1988) argued that conditioning occurs only when the UCS is more probable in the presence of the CS than when the CS is absent. The CS has to mathematically predict the UCS, even though the CS and UCS are often paired or the UCS might also occur without any CS warning. There are theories suggesting that the CS comes to represent the UCS, perhaps by evoking a memory or representational image of the UCS (Holland, 2008). The best demonstration of this likelihood is revaluing the UCS after conditioning. This can be done, for example if the UCS is an alcoholic beverage, by pairing the drink with a noxious substance. After that, the previously positive CSs that signaled alcohol, such as the sight of the bottle or the smell of the whiskey, are no longer positive and do not elicit the urge to drink, even though they themselves were never paired directly with the unpleasant substance. The CS often comes to have the same hedonic value as the UCS. That makes a great deal of sense to us humans: words obviously acquire their hedonic properties through association. Words such as "bacon" and "pancakes" elicit salivation; words such as "square" and "edge" do not (Staats & Hammond, 1972). The specific words will depend on your culture, religion, and upbringing, but the principle is universal.

Fortunately for a unifying approach to clinical therapy, we do not need to understand fully the mechanisms of classical conditioning; all we need to do is apply the known principles correctly. Thus, if we have a child client—like those described by Friedman and her colleagues—who has been receiving chemotherapy for cancer, and that child vomits when seeing the hospital, we can reasonably say that that is an instance of Pavlovian conditioning (conditioned nausea, with the radiation or drug treatment being the UCS) (Okifuji & Friedman, 1992). If we wish to prevent such a reaction what we need to do is create the conditions for extinction (amelioration) or for conditioned inhibition (prevention). Examples of clinicians using overshadowing (presenting a novel, highly salient taste cue between food and the chemotherapy) to prevent taste aversion to normal food represents an elegant example of the relevance of conditioning principles to planful change (Brodberg & Bernstein, 1987).

Analyzing smoking and alcohol abuse provides a further way that conditioning principles offer a valuable element to broader treatment. For a regular smoker, the cigarette pack, the taste and smell of the cigarette, and the situation in which the smoker regularly smokes become conditioned stimuli (the effects of nicotine on the central nervous system are the UCS/UCR) and the CR is the urge or craving to smoke (Lazev, Herzog, & Brandon, 1999). This is equally true with the sight, taste, and smell of alcoholic drinks, especially in the right context, such as a bar. Repeated drug use over time means that the positive valence of the various drug-related and contextual cues increases—an effect known as increased (sensitized) incentive salience. This increases the positive valence of other associated rewards, such as peer acceptance by other smokers. Repeated exposure without nicotine to smoking-related stimuli (i.e., extinction, CS alone) can reduce cravings and urges (Bevins & Palmatier, 2004).

Classical Conditioning as Explanation

Understanding and using the principles of classical conditioning were of profound significance for the development of behavior therapy, the first psychological therapy to be based on principles derived from experimental psychology. There has been a long and productive link between classical conditioning and behavior therapy, starting with the infamous demonstration by John B. Watson and Rosalie Rayner (1920) that fear of a previously neutral-ish object (a white rat) could be induced in a 9-month-old infant (little Albert B.) by a procedure resembling the Pavlovian paradigm. Anyone who has worked with a child who has had an intensely aversive but ultimately harmless experience has hands-on knowledge of similar events. A toddler I know who was barked at and chased (UCS) by a friendly but misguided sheepdog (CS) is now fearful of all unleashed dogs (stimulus generalization), even many years later.

Early behavior therapists reasoned that if simple phobias for rodents, insects, dogs, heights, flying in planes, or swimming are acquired through a mechanism resembling classical conditioning, then maybe they could be eliminated through similar mechanisms. We do not actually know why little Peter, described by Mary Cover Jones (1924), was frightened of rabbits, but slowly bringing the rabbit closer and closer to him, while he was eating, was a systematic desensitization therapy, very similar to the Pavlovian extinction procedure. So perhaps "extinction" is a valid explanation for Peter's reduced fear. Behavior therapy built very successfully on these parallels, despite the fact that the Watson and Rayner (1920) study has never been convincingly replicated in the laboratory: legends are powerful. Conditioning can be thought of either as a casual mechanism—exposure to a feared stimulus *is* Pavlovian extinction—or as an analogy (it looks like Pavlovian extinction in terms of procedure).

Controversy arises when evidence is presented that people can have highly aversive even life-threatening experiences and not acquire a phobia. You can fall off a ladder, be bitten by a dog, burn yourself at a barbecue, or get an electric shock plugging in an appliance without becoming phobic of heights, dogs, hamburgers, or toasters. Similarly, you can be fearful of heights or dogs without ever having had a fall yourself or a bite that you can remember. This is the gist of a long and rather pointless debate in the field; it is pointless because the two confirmed phenomena (trauma without phobia and phobia without trauma) do not prove that traumatic experiences resembling classical conditioning are not, in certain circumstances, the origin of irrational fear (fear of a relatively harmless object). We also know that even after the UCS has been devalued (perhaps through repeated exposure so that it no longer elicits fear or distress), the fear conditioned to the CS during the original conditioning will continue to be elicited by that CS (Laborda & Miller, 2011).

Incubation and Inhibition

Many years ago Eysenck recounted an experiment conducted in Russia in which the experimental subject, an unfortunate dog, was, unlike mine with the electric fence, deliberately given one classical conditioning trial with a very intense, traumatic experience as the UCS. After a short delay the CS was presented alone, without the UCS, which should have resulted in some decrease in the dog's conditioned autonomic response (CR, fear). That is the usual extinction effect. Instead the autonomic indices of fear—heart rate, for example—increased. After a further delay the CS was presented again and the CR increased still further. Eysenck (1968) called this incubation. He explained it on the grounds that the conditioned fear response was in itself so aversive that when it was elicited it essentially represented another aversive conditioning trial: the CS-alone presentation was not a neutral event at all.

Today we identify clinically that people can fear their own fear responses, especially the fear of having a panic attack. The phenomenon goes by various names such as fear of fear or anxiety sensitivity. I have suggested that in many clinical examples the secondary distress actually arises because the elicited or anticipated fear or anxiety directly interferes with skilled performance in a socially embarrassing way (Evans, 1972). Male sexual impotence is the classic example of anticipatory anxiety interfering with penile tumescence. I had a slightly less dramatic example of a client who was so anxious about her hand shaking when signing a check in front of the bank teller that the muscle tension that was part of her anxiety response made her hand tremor so much she could not sign the check. After choking on food and nearly dying, clients can become so tense about eating in public that they have difficulty swallowing (Evans & Pechtel, 2010).

In other situations the conditioned fear response does not inhibit performance directly but makes the individual especially wary of situations that are not objectively dangerous. A client of mine who slipped on wet concrete while walking next to a swimming pool illustrates this process quite well. She fell backward with no bodily support at all and the back of her head slammed against the concrete. She was very severely concussed and some months after the accident was referred to me by her neurologist who felt that the extent of her traumatic brain injury could not explain her unsteady gait and reluctance to walk without a cane. Not surprisingly, I soon discovered that she was most hesitant to walk outside on wet days when there might be puddles of water and wet sidewalks. Her conditioned fear of slipping made her tense, interfered with normal walking, made her constantly seek out physical supports and solid objects she could hold on to, carry her cane in case it rained, and worry about the soles of her shoes. These secondary "safety-seeking" behaviors obviously maintained her excessively cautious behavior that had originated in classical fear conditioning. We quite often see similar behavioral dynamics in people with much more severe anxieties, such as panic or agoraphobia.

The original neobehavioral theories of Hull and Spence struggled to maintain the concept that what was associated in any contiguous (in time and space) pairing of events was a stimulus–response (S-R) connection (Spence, 1950). However, there is now evidence from many different sources that in addition to S-R associations, stimulus–stimulus connections are what underlie many different phenomena of classical conditioning and that these associations are equivalent to simple associative memory (Holland, 2008). The animal that has been sequenced through both acquisition and extinction procedures with the same CS has two memories: the bell means food and the bell means no food (Capaldi, Martins, & Altman, 2009; Comstock, Hammer, Strentzsch, Cannon, Parsons, & Salazar, 2008). The second memory does not cause the first to be forgotten. If you start the procedure by presenting the stimulus alone (it signals nothing) and then use it as a CS, acquisition is delayed (inhibited). As a CS this stimulus is not neutral; the animal has heard it before and at that time it signaled no food. We also know that if you first pair stimuli A and B, and then subsequently you condition fear to B, by pairing it with nasty event C, stimulus A, never paired with anything threatening, will now evoke fear (classical conditioners call it "sensory preconditioning"). Operant conditioners later discovered this same phenomenon and called it "stimulus equivalence" (Zettle, 2011).

Evaluative Conditioning

The best way to appreciate the significance of classical conditioning for planful behavior change is to realize the most important feature we are talking about is changing the emotional meaning of stimuli, their valence. A very effective way to change people is to change their patterns of likes and dislikes. We approach what we like and avoid what we dislike. Make lattes popular and desirable and suddenly everyone is sitting in Starbucks with their laptop computers. Pair the taste of a frozen banana daiquiri with the taste of our own vomit and that cocktail will seem repulsive and be avoided, often for long periods—even the thought of it will make you nauseated. In light of the evolutionary importance of learning to avoid harmful and contaminated foods that would make you ill, the emotion of disgust can very readily be conditioned to the taste and smell of relevant, ingestible substances.

Clinical experiments on clients with addictions and paraphilias carried out in the 1960s and 1970s provided countless demonstrations that the positive valence of inappropriately desired objects (pictures of naked children, highly unhealthy foods, cigarettes, alcohol) could be deliberately changed through association procedures that looked very much like the pairings arranged in classical aversive conditioning experiments. There may be other ways that stimuli change their hedonic value either up or down, but this way, at least, is known to be effective and is called evaluative conditioning (Martin & Levey, 1978).

A long time ago in my laboratory at the University of Hawaii we wondered if we could change the likeability of liquids of different colors and tastes by pairing them, in a Pavlovian procedure, with a foul odor—pyridine gas (Busch & Evans, 1977). Pyridine is harmless in the minute concentrations that we puffed into participants' noses, but it has a particularly unpleasant, disgusting smell. The experiments were designed to test an evolutionary notion, novel at the time, that organisms were "biologically prepared" to associate tastes and smells with chemically harmful stimuli, such as poison. Thus, so the argument went, you could not condition aversion (dislike) of alcohol by pairing it with electric shock, but you might be able to do so when pairing it with a nauseous substance. We were certainly able to change people's preferences, but the precise evolutionary fit between the CS and the UCS was not so clearly demonstrated.

Happily we moved off chemical aversion and tried a few related experiments with just words as the UCS. Words have highly emotive properties—their connotative meaning. Staats (1968) had demonstrated that positive and negative words could serve as a UCS and make neutral words paired with them more positive or negative. Essentially he proposed that through hundreds of early conditioning experiences that was how words acquired their emotional significance. Words, whether spoken or just thought, are very powerful emotionally. Just thinking about our own death if triggered by the word "funeral" causes little unconscious pangs of fear, resulting in us seeking reassurance by, for example, expressing more pronationalistic beliefs, which creates a sense of security. This well-replicated phenomenon—called "terror management theory"—has been demonstrated in many different ways (Pyszczynski, Greenberg, Solomon, & Maxfield, 2006).

So what we asked in a laboratory demonstration was whether a simple association with emotive words could be used to influence desirability. We paired words such as CHOCOLATE with relevant unpleasant words such as PIMPLES or CAVATIES, or irrelevant unpleasant words such as CANCER or POVERTY. Both procedures changed liking for actual chocolate as measured by a behavioral test: in a pseudopreference task, in which participants thought they were tasting and rating different candies for a marketing campaign, those participants who had had aversive verbal conditioning ate less of the chocolate, particularly when the UCS words were relevant. Because words have denotative meaning as well as emotional valences, it is likely that certain forms of association will occur more easily because of semantic relevance. Behavior therapists have used this fact as a self-control strategy. Someone who is trying to reduce carbs and eat less chocolate can be encouraged, when tempted by the sight of a chocolate bar, to generate semantically relevant associations that help to alter preferences through counterconditioning. Saying to yourself "chocolate will give me pimples" or "chocolate causes cavities" sounds a bit simplistic, but it should reduce the positive valence of the chocolate (De Houwer, Thomas, & Baeyens, 2001).

Wonderful, Wonderful Two-Factor Theory

Instances of basic conditioning actually involve both instrumental and classical contingencies. That is to say there is always a relationship between the individual's behavior and its consequences (instrumental relationship) and there is a relationship between the context (the setting, discriminative cues for the reward) and the consequences (classical relationship). There is one heavily researched paradigm in which this dual relationship seems to be especially important, and that is the experimental procedure known as active avoidance learning.

This arrangement in the laboratory is one in which an aversive, painful event (such as an electric shock) is signaled by an auditory tone or a light. The animal can escape the shock by performing some action, typically jumping over a small barrier into a safe compartment where there is no shock. It is easy to see that the cessation of shock (and its painful effects) serves as a reward for the instrumental actions of escape. This is called negative reinforcement. But after a few learning trials, the animal does not wait around for the shock—as soon as it hears the warning tone it leaps to safety, thus avoiding the shock entirely. This pattern becomes quite persistent, and the animal will avoid the shock for trial after trial. Well and good, except for one thing. If the jumping behavior was reinforced by cessation of the shock, what is reinforcing the avoidance jumping, since no shock is now forthcoming? For all the animal "knows," the shock has been turned off, and in fact it sometimes has, particularly if you want to extinguish the avoidance (barrier jumping) behavior.

Why in this experimental paradigm is the animal's avoidance behavior so persistent? First Mowrer (1939) and then Miller (1948) suggested a simple answer. During the escape trials jumping led to cessation of shock and was thus instrumentally rewarded (factor one), but there was a pairing of the warning tone and the shock, so that through classical conditioning fear would be conditioned to the warning signal (factor two). When the animal starts to avoid, the warning signal is turned off, thus resulting in an immediate cessation of fear. Reduction of fear is reinforcing, Miller reasoned, and that is what is maintaining the active avoidance behavior. You should be saying to yourself, why doesn't the *fear* extinguish once active avoidance is taking place? The answer is that because the animal jumps so quickly and the warning tone is turned off so fast, not much of an extinction trial is really being offered. If the animal were to experience the tone without the shock (classical extinction) in a more prolonged situation in which avoidance was not possible, the fear should extinguish. Then, when avoidance is again possible, the animals should fail to make the avoidance response, since the tone now signals nothing or maybe even "no shock." And that is exactly what happens.

The potential relevance to human behavioral dynamics should be obvious. Even though the shock is turned off, so to speak, we try to avoid situations that make us fearful or uncomfortable and because we avoid them we are not exposed to simple extinction trials that would show that they are not objectively dangerous. I have put that deliberately in a sort of layperson's common sense, cognitive interpretation because there are many objections to the details of two-factor theory and conditioning interpretations in general. But the one overarching idea, which seems so crucial to many forms of intervention, is that we do things not to avoid the objective harm that we think might result, but to avoid unpleasant emotional feelings. If we engage in a behavior that seems inappropriate or maladaptive, but it is one that results in the termination of pain, anxiety, fear, shame, stress, tension, or any other negative feeling, then that behavior will persist through negative reinforcement. We actively do things to turn off unpleasant experiences and to escape or avoid negative feelings, regardless of how those feelings originally came about. To change that behavior we need to change, or learn to tolerate, the unpleasant feeling.

In recent years, any deliberate strategy that allows us to minimize or avoid negative experiences, whether unpleasant thoughts or feelings, has come to be called experiential avoidance (Hayes, Strosahl, & Wilson, 1999). The new insight from this renaming is that people may differ in the degree to which they can tolerate these unpleasant private experiences. We might label this "anxiety sensitivity" (or depression sensitivity, or guilt sensitivity, or overreactive Flight–Fright–Freeze System, FFFS). If that is so, it could explain why feelings such as anxiety or depression are so often struggled against by clients. Conceivably, therefore, the struggle is their problem, rather than the negative experience per se. Alternatively, if someone has been severely stressed—for example, by the trauma of sexual abuse or assault—the strategy used to reduce or avoid those feelings (we often call it coping) might be quite successful for a while but then end up resulting in further negative outcomes (Pechtel, Evans, & Podd, 2011). Common examples seen clinically of ineffectual "coping" are strategies such as abusing drugs or alcohol, suppressing all feelings (numbing or experiential avoidance), or resisting positive, romantic sexual encounters. Individuals who are emotionally traumatized as young children experience early-onset anxiety, which contributes to substance abuse, in turn stressful life events, less social support, and thus more severe symptoms of psychopathology in adulthood (Kendler, Gardner, & Prescott, 2001).

Psychotherapists accept that there must be many different ways in which unpleasant feelings about situations that others find neutral can come about. I personally think that classical conditioning is one of them. Yes, it may be true that most people who fear heights have never fallen off a cliff or a ladder, and people who have fallen off a ladder do not necessarily develop a conditioned fear.

But if you wanted to create a fear of heights in someone (and why you would I don't know) then arranging for them to fall and hurt themselves seems like a sure way to achieve it. After an earthquake collapses a large portion of your house around you (UCS for terror), aftershocks that merely shake the ground (CS) elicit intense, if momentary, fear (CR). I worked with a child client who had a strong fear of traffic and of crossing busy streets. He had been knocked down by a car outside his school and his ankle was pinned under the wheel of the car for many minutes before he could be freed. Cognitively he knew that cars were generally not arbitrarily dangerous as long as he stayed on the sidewalk, but when he saw moving traffic he panicked and froze.

The clinical task was to extinguish this little boy's fear. I can think of many ways of doing this. The first thing is to make sure—speaking analogously—that the shock has been turned off and there is no true threat. That is problem number one right there—cars *are* dangerous. The shock is not off, it is just not likely to occur. The second thing is to encourage approach rather than avoidance, to allow extinction to take place. In what is problem number two, encourage is the operative word, since forcing him to be exposed to moving traffic is likely to produce intense avoidance reactions. We also want approach to be more rewarding than avoidance, which is problem number three: before the fear is extinguished, the negative reinforcement of avoidance by fear reduction (experiential avoidance) continues to be quite powerful. Finally, problem number four, if exposure to traffic could be arranged, we do not want the fear response to be so intense that some sort of "incubation" process is going to occur. Parents know this only too well. They push the child to confront something he or she is afraid of; however, the fear reaction is so strong that the parents panic and remove the child from the situation, thus resulting in escape behavior being reinforced (by fear reduction). The fear is now even stronger.

Telling children that dogs are not dangerous and that there are no monsters under their bed is a fine thing to do—reassurance never hurts—but it will generally not extinguish severe anxiety. To achieve this, new learning, based on actual experience, is required. Meaningful therapy is about new learning, and learning comes from doing, from experiences. People feel anxious when they perceive a threat (both physical and psychological). If the threat is realistic then the anxiety is highly adaptive and will motivate caution in the form of avoidance or looking for ways of staying safe. When you tell your child that playing with matches is dangerous (verbal conditioning) you do not expect or want them to become *phobic* about lighting a match. You want them to do so in a safe way—exercise caution. If the threat is unrealistic, however, we might expect the anxiety to be reduced over time. But with people experiencing intense anxiety, like a panic attack, there is a realistic threat—paradoxically it is that they will panic or feel intense anxiety and perhaps lose control and be publicly embarrassed. Situations (stimuli) that cause anxiety or distress in general *are* aversive because they cause anxiety and distress. Worrying about worry, thinking it is uncontrollable, and being concerned about its consequences for mental and physical health (lack of sleep or the harm of hypertension) is a phenomenon dubbed "meta-worry" by Wells (1999) and is hypothesized by cognitive theorists to be the underlying dynamic for generalized anxiety problems.

I worked once with an airline pilot who had become extremely fearful of flying (I will not mention the airline he worked for). He was not anxious about crashing or causing harm to himself or his passengers, essentially because he did not foresee that as very likely. What he was terrified of was that in an emergency, even one he had been trained to handle easily, he would have an anxiety attack and lose control so that the co-pilot would have to take over the plane. Any little warning signal in the cockpit triggered anxiety, which triggered more intense anxiety, mediated by thoughts of loss of control. You can call this incubation, or fear of fear, but the dynamics are that the threat is real, not imagined, and very easily remembered. You cannot change the valence of the situation by arguing. The client knows objectively that it is not dangerous, but that does not make it less threatening psychologically.

Emotional Memories

Simple conditioning principles seem very relevant to planned behavior change, either in terms of setting up experiences that would allow an unwanted or maladaptive conditioned response to extinguish, or setting up experiences that would create new associations and allow the meaning of stimuli to change. However, learned and unlearned associations are laid down in memory, and once we have to bring memory into our explanatory picture, mechanisms become more complex again. If we experience a terrifying or otherwise highly aversive event—something like food poisoning, or witnessing someone being injured, or undergoing an unpleasant medical procedure—we rarely come away from such experiences with one emotional response conditioned to one stimulus. Instead we are much more likely to have what memory researchers call episodic memories of the experience—a quite complex recollection of the context, what we were doing at the time, and what we felt, including both the physiological changes and the interpretation we placed on those feelings (Reisberg & Hertel, 2004). These emotional memories may depend on how the experience was encoded and then how it was stored, or consolidated, so that all the contextual and emotional elements will be remembered, often for a very long time (Smith & DeCoster, 2000).

In therapy, as in life, we encourage clients to recall upsetting, traumatic, incidents and to talk about them. What we want to happen is that although the facts of the incident will be remembered, the strong affect associated with it will fade. We want the conditioned emotion to extinguish, but not the overall memory of the events. For one thing, remembering a highly threatening or dangerous situation might make us more cautious about getting into the same situation again.

If someone has had a bad car accident we do not expect or want the memory of that to completely disappear. We want people to recognize dangerous situations on the road, to wear their seat belt, to slow down, and not to talk on their cell phone while driving. But we do want the intense emotion elicited at the time to be reduced sufficiently that the person does not develop such a strong, unfading phobic reaction that they cannot drive in a car without feeling panicked. If, on the other hand, the person carefully avoids the recall of the details of the traumatic incident, these emotions have little chance of ever being extinguished.

This is basically how Levis (Levis & Malloy, 1982) explained the persistence of negative affect following traumatic experiences—if you do not recall them, do not think about them, and do not talk about them, the associated affect cannot extinguish. You are turning off the warning bell before you can experience an extinction trial. Thoughts and memories as visualized and verbalized are events with powerful stimulus properties that elicit negative emotions and cue even more negative thoughts in a chain reaction. It is a profound recognition by Levis that such an arrangement will lead to active, if mental, avoidance of such memories. Because we will not engage in those painful thoughts the negative affect associated with them remains unextinguished. Another feature of that model is that one reason we would not want to recall, think about, and talk about an experience is because initially, when doing so, the associated affect is extremely unpleasant. Therapy has to find ways of encouraging the necessary recall of the memories, including picturing the situation in our mind's eye and talking about events in considerable detail.

Cognitive theorists tend to refer to thinking about a negative experience such as a social interaction for someone with social anxiety, or a failure experience for someone with depression, as event "processing" (Dannahy & Stopa, 2007). Truly, reflective people always evaluate their performance, reevaluate it, rationalize it, and through repeated recall redefine the experience so that it is stored in memory for later recollection as positive, neutral, or negative, relevant or not to self and the future. That this process of rumination and reevaluation takes place between therapy sessions as well as within exposure treatment suggests a further way in which the therapeutic encounter (within the formal session or when talking with friends) affects everyday functioning, so that mood and other self-reported aspects of experience fluctuate completely independently of the therapeutic "dose." Nebulous as these concepts are, they support the broad idea that what a client goes away and thinks about or experiences between sessions interacts with the specific experiences of the session itself as well as with the homework recommended and other assigned tasks. In such a dynamic interaction between therapy experiences and subsequent life experiences it is no wonder that change during treatment is not—as I emphasized in Chapter 2—a smooth linear process. The standard session-opening therapist's question "How was your week?" might be better posed as "What were you thinking and feeling this week about what you learned last session?"

Many circumstances enable stimulus revaluation—a safe therapeutic setting and a calming therapist who instills trust, or prior training in strategies to manage emotion (such as relaxation, or controlled breathing), or requiring recall of the traumatic event little by little by following a hierarchy, or offering additional hypothesized cues to probe for the recall of the memories despite the negative affect (that is what happens in Levis's implosion therapy). But the one thing that would be counterproductive is allowing clients to escape the memory and not think about it just because thinking about it makes them feel bad (experiential avoidance).

Physiological Sensations as Aversive Stimuli

Many bodily sensations, especially those associated with fear, anxiety, and anger, are highly unpleasant. That is why we seek to avoid or escape them. So if someone is particularly averse to such feelings we might anticipate a strange paradox—that negative feelings give them negative feelings. Classical conditioning is about the conditioning of very basic, automatic, physiological responses—the pit in your stomach before an examination or the dry mouth before a speech, the hot flush of embarrassment, the heart palpitations when about you are to be attacked, and the muscle tension of anger when disrespected.

If a person has poor emotional control (regulation ability), the early sensations of negative affect often precede a more intense, prolonged episode of emotion, identified as a panic attack. Panic involves incapacitation and is particularly unpleasant. If bodily changes provide exteroceptive cues prior to panic, then these milder bodily sensations become CSs for conditioning further physiological change. A possible way to alter this incubation-like affect is to expose the client to cues while at the same time providing some combination of reassurance, support, and emotional control strategies. Creating these milder, safer sensations in order to desensitize a client to them is not terribly difficult—heavy rapid breathing, for example, gives rise to hyperventilation, or being spun around in a chair causes feelings of dizziness

The key thing about any autonomic physiological responses, apart from their aversiveness, is that although easily elicited they are not easily controlled by voluntary means (Unger, Evans, Rourke, & Levis, 2003). It is possible to control the motor behavior these autonomic nervous system reactions usually give rise to: just because your mouth is dry and your palms are sweating you do not have to run off the podium in the middle of your speech. But the actual sympathetic and parasympathetic responses themselves are very hard to stop at will. Words and thoughts having the opposite emotional value is one way of regulating them. This is why in systematic desensitization we say to the client "think now of a PEACEFUL, PLEASANT scene." This allows the physiological response to be muted when the fear-arousing, phobic stimulus is presented, either in reality or in imagination. Hopefully we then get extinction rather than incubation.

You cannot, however, simply alter feelings by telling people that things are safe (don't be fearful), are not likely to eventuate (don't be anxious), and are not their fault (don't feel guilty).

Implications

Why, out of all the important phenomena studied in psychology, did I select classical conditioning for special attention? The reasons are partly historical. Behavior therapy began with the direct application of classical conditioning principles. This in turn led to a rich and intense relationship between psychological theory and clinical practice. But in contemporary behaviorally inspired treatment protocols there are few that really resemble the classical Pavlovian paradigm and as therapists we would only very rarely use laboratory-like conditioning procedures with clients. What classical conditioning really represents is not a method to be followed literally, but a parable—a tale about how the value attributable to stimuli can be increased or decreased and made appetitive or aversive. In other words, classical conditioning is an explanatory paradigm that has great utility when used at the level of analogy, or of a model, rather than confirming underlying mechanisms.

There is one particularly intriguing thing about this position clinically. When a client has a fear reaction that appears to have been acquired in a traumatic incident, such as a fear of swallowing arising from an incident of near death from choking, there is little point in telling the client that it is unlikely to happen again. His or her fear is not based on lack of knowledge of probabilities. The fear response is automatic and is not under voluntary or cognitive control. It might be in some clients. Fear of eating a raw egg might be based on erroneous information that there is a salmonella epidemic; if you have evidence to the contrary that should allay their fear. But telling children that dogs are not dangerous after they have been bitten by one seems to be the wrong approach, when conditioning principles are understood.

To say that classical conditioning is about the valence of stimuli certainly broadens the topic far beyond what an experimental psychologist would recognize as the classical conditioning *procedure*. In June 2011, after an outbreak in Europe of a deadly strain of *E. coli* bacteria, German public health officials blamed cucumbers from Spain. Spanish cucumbers were no longer popular, no one would buy them, and thousands of tons had to be destroyed. This is not exactly classical conditioning but it is associative learning using words. People in Europe did not fear cucumbers. What they feared was getting sick and possibly dying. As Levis (1991) clarified, people do not literally fear heights, they fear getting injured or maimed; they do not fear swimming, they fear drowning.

The most obvious difference between the laboratory study of classical conditioning and real life influences producing change is that the stimuli used in the laboratory are all always pretty well meaningless to the subject. But in human experience with the overwhelming exposure we all have to words, pictures, and other images, the stimuli in our lives are laden with layers of emotional significance and associations with other symbols rich in emotion. Americans will respond emotionally to the Stars and Stripes; in one study simply exposing people to a picture of the American flag made them react more conservatively and patriotically up to 8 months later (Carter, Ferguson, & Hassin, 2011). Millions of people around the world feel hope, fervor, and joy at the symbol of the Christian cross. These are learned associations—you were not born feeling arousal to the blue Star of David or disgust for the red and black Swastika the same way you have inbuilt startle reflexes to loud noise or leg jerks to a blow on the patellar tendon.

Classical conditioning is about changing the valence of stimuli (including words, thoughts, and other symbols)—the input side of an organism's interaction with the environment. In the next chapter we will examine the output side of the equation by considering the other major paradigm for studying learning, instrumental conditioning, or what happens after the organism responds. Classical conditioning is about the rules concerning the relationship among events, regardless of the individual's responding; instrumental conditioning is about the rules concerning the relationship between responding and the consequent events.

6

Contingencies
Reward and Punishment in Therapeutic Change

> If you faithfully obey the commands I am giving you today... then I will send rain on your land in its season, both autumn and spring rains, so that you may gather in your grain, new wine and olive oil. I will provide grass in the fields for your cattle, and you will eat and be satisfied... [But if not, I] will shut up the heavens so that it will not rain and the ground will yield no produce, and you will soon perish from the good land.
> (Deuteronomy 11:13–17, New International Version, 1984)

Reward and punishment are the cornerstones of human and divine justice. In psychology, one of the best established principles is that an organism's behavior is controlled by external contingencies. Deliberately changing behavior by managing rewarding and punitive consequences is one the great technical success stories of psychology. Thorndike's Law of Effect essentially stated if an action is rewarded it will tend to be repeated; it will become more probable in the future. Reward "strengthens" a stimulus–response association, Thorndike (1932) argued, which is where the term "reinforcement" comes from. Skinner's version of what is basically the same law was that behavior is a function of its consequences. This allowed him to avoid the tricky circular problem of knowing what is rewarding without first claiming it is anything that strengthens behavior. In fact, Skinner was not fond of the term reward for the same reasons, and many operant conditioning researchers today continue to prefer the seemingly more neutral term reinforcement, although I will use them interchangeably. Thorndike's rewards were pieces of salmon; Skinner originally used cut up pieces of dry spaghetti—a far cry from "grain, new wine and olive oil," but seemingly serving the same function.

Note that I am already using a variety of terms for the same phenomenon (changed behavioral outcomes): "strengthening," "more probable," and "repeated." So let me emphasize that these changes in probability are not absolute, they are not context free. The increase in probability is true only for certain conditions, usually the stimulus conditions present before the behavior was rewarded, or those that signaled the likely availability of the reward. Thus, the strengthening idea does not really mean that the behavior literally becomes stronger, but that the connection or *association* between the contextual cue and the behavior is strengthened: in the presence of that cue a given behavior becomes more likely: in Thorndike's words "the animal had formed a perfect association between the sense-impression of the interior of that box and the impulse leading to the successful movement" (1898, p. 10).

The alternative words and the concepts they signify are not just instances of pedantry. These words carry considerable meaning, sometimes precise and sometimes surplus, especially for clinical contexts. If we say a school child's studying behavior has increased as a result of a reward contingency being imposed, what exactly do we mean? Does it mean the child will study harder or longer, or in the presence of homework cues (textbook in his backpack) will be more likely to engage in study than in an alternative activity? If these are optional alternative characteristics of behavior, which is the one we want to see more of? That is a question taking us back to an earlier discussion of "be still, be quiet, be docile": what behavior change is actually desired in clinical practice? We can also see it is not really likely that the behavior of studying is itself an entirely new skill. (In some circumstances a child does not study because he or she does not know how to—a skill deficit we will come to presently.) What we are actually trying to do is to make studying behavior fill a greater percentage of the child's time when the homework cues (situational demands) are present. We do not want the child to be doing homework during family times when it is not desirable to be studying. Modifying the duration or intensity of study behavior could be thought of as a motivational influence rather than a learning one.

The difference between learning a new skill and performing a previously acquired one is a distinction that has been confusing the learning field for a long time. Thorndike's cats did not literally learn *how* to get out of the puzzle box he constructed, nor did they work out the solution to the puzzle; they learned to step on a paddle that opened the door of the cage, which then let them out to get food. Although the response was not exactly new, its probability changed from low to high. Probability was measured by response latency: the time between being put in the puzzle box and depressing the little paddle. This time parameter steadily decreased over trials ("trial" always means "learning opportunity") until eventually the response occurred almost immediately after being placed back in the box and the latency reached asymptotic levels—it could not be performed much quicker. This steady decrease in latency could be plotted against trials and the resultant function was an operational definition of learning—the learning curve. It is common in everyday vernacular to hear people talking about being exposed to some new experience and saying that they were on a "steep learning curve," meaning, of course, that they had to learn new habits very fast.

These niceties aside, it is very clear that many properties of behavior are shaped by their consequences. It is true that when a rat—the usual reluctant participant in instrumental conditioning studies, since cats rarely adhere to any behavioral principles—is taught to press a lever in the Skinner chamber the original act of depressing the lever is largely accidental, often caused by the rat leaning on the lever with its forepaws while stretching up and exploring its new environment. The lever makes a distinctive click (later this will serve as a secondary reinforcer) and a pellet of food drops into the feeding trough where it might or might not be found by the animal. If it is not found and consumed right away, the lever press response is not strengthened—consequences, or their symbolic representations, need to be immediate in order to provide feedback as to the specific response that is earning the reward.

To encourage lever pressing a researcher is likely to "bait" the lever by smearing a small amount of food over it and thus causing the rat to spend more time nosing around it. Key pecking by pigeons (the experimental subjects Skinner preferred—the "key" here being a little round plastic disc set in the wall of the chamber) is slightly less iffy because pigeons tend to peck at things, anything, in the presence of food. Pecking around is part of its natural foraging behavior, unlike lever pressing by the rat. Watch a pigeon walking about on the ground next time you are at a park and you will see what I mean. As a result of these differences it takes a while for the rat's depression of the lever to become a simple, minimal-effort, one paw action, but once it does the subsequent changes produced by the reward contingency are largely with respect to the pattern of repetition of the response and not the shape or form of the behavior. Rats end up depressing the lever in their own idiosyncratic ways; the researcher does not care, because the action is defined mechanically as enough force on the lever to activate the electronic mechanism that records a press. The most common dependent variable in operant conditioning research is the frequency of the response plotted against time—its rate.

However, many other properties of the response *can* be developed by differential contingencies; for example, it is possible to make only harder, more effortful depressions of the lever earn the reward, so that industriousness in humans is easily shaped (Eisenberger, 1992). Generating infrequent responding by ensuring only low rates get rewarded is often useful clinically when a child's targeted problem is that he or she does something too often. It is also possible to make the animal depress the lever in different ways, such as with both paws rather than one, or with its nose rather than its paw. If the animal is a dolphin being trained for a marine mammal entertainment show, then leaping out of the water higher and higher can be consequated. Pretty much any behavior the animal is physically capable of performing can be differentially rewarded and thus shaped into a distinctive pattern by rewarding successive approximations of the desired end behavior

Species-specific behaviors that occur naturally in the wild or as a result of selective breeding (if your dog is a Golden Retriever it can easily be taught to fetch your morning paper), are more readily shaped than totally novel behaviors, such as getting a circus dog to ride a trick bicycle. With humans, depending on the contingency operating, we can produce effortful, graceful, even flawless responding. Often, however, it is necessary to get only the basic task done. If the contingencies require task completion, a student will whip off a B– assignment the night before it is due; if the contingencies demand excellence, the student will put much more time and effort into writing a good essay. Because in education the contingencies are often ambiguous, individual differences in motivation, such as competitiveness, fear of failure, desire to please the teacher, and perfectionism, may be stronger determinants of quality of performance than are unspecified reward contingencies.

Hedonistic Principles

I have already mentioned that Skinner (and thus behavior analysts today) was always careful to define reinforcement not as something the individual likes or enjoys or even needs, but as something that serves to make an action more probable. This strict emphasis on operational definition was considered necessary since the only way to judge whether a stimulus is liked is by seeing if it will strengthen behavior. But that is not strictly true. With people we can find out what sorts of things someone likes by asking them, or, if they are nonverbal (an infant, or someone with a significant disability), by giving them choices and seeing which one is selected or by measuring how much time is spent looking at one stimulus rather than another. In practical terms a reinforcement survey is extremely useful to any psychotherapist—you can find out ahead of time what things (including people and activities, not just material objects) a client really desires. There are many such surveys available, such as the Reinforcement Survey Schedule (Cautela, 1977), or for children the Reinforcement Inventory published by Integrated Behavioral Solutions, 2000 (see Corcoran & Fischer, 2000).

Other learning theorists had no problem with defining rewards in terms of their hedonistic value—how much they were enjoyed. Clark Hull (1943), for instance, hypothesized that reinforcers worked through a mechanism of reducing basic biological drives, or secondary, conditioned drives (incentive motivation). We tend to think of an event, or an outcome, as the reward—a drink when you are thirsty. But it may be the pleasure you get from slaking your thirst that is reinforcing, just as an action that removes a barrier to goal attainment is reinforced by anger reduction. Although food is a necessity of life and serves to reduce hunger drive, foods of different tastes are not equally enjoyable—Skinner's rats had to be very hungry before they would work for dry spaghetti. There is an incentive value even for those things essential to survival. Many studies have shown that primates will work for variety (suggesting a "curiosity drive"), thirsty rats prefer sweet-tasting liquids to plain water, and children and other humans can be strongly reinforced by information that stimulus events are going to be certain, rather than unpredictable. Knowing you are going to get punished sometimes seems preferable to being uncertain you will get rewarded. Getting immediate feedback that your responding is correct is highly rewarding—look at the intensity and persistent of young people playing electronic games on their computers, iPads, or cell phones.

One of the complex challenges when understanding reward is that although it is true that reward determines behavior, it also seems that behavior affects how pleasurable are its outcomes. The obvious example of this is familiarity. Although novelty can be highly rewarding, considerable degrees of pleasure can be derived from engaging in actions or having experiences that are very familiar. It seems likely that this is a potential barrier to change. If we enjoy doing the things we are used to doing, it may be necessary to help clients concentrate on those familiar patterns that are not maladaptive or destructive in some way, so that the simple pleasures of familiar settings and activities can be sustained. Asking clients to change everything is not a sensible way to help them change anything.

A different way in which the desirability of a reward can be influenced is by the degree of effort required to obtain it. As a general rule an outcome is more highly valued when greater effort is required to obtain it. There are many possible explanations for this effect. One is that if there is a discrepancy between your beliefs and your actions, this creates an uncomfortable feeling, or dissonance. One way to reduce this discomfort is to change the belief so it is now more in keeping with your behavior. Working hard for a small reward could generate these dissonance feelings, which are then alleviated by now valuing the reward more than you did originally. This well-known phenomenon of cognitive dissonance (Festinger, 1957) has widespread corroboration. However, animals show the same effect and it is hard to imagine that rats and pigeons "need to justify their behavior to themselves or others" (Zentall, 2010, p. 296). It is likely that there are complex contrasts effects at work, Zentall has argued. Oversimplifying somewhat, if you work harder or longer but fail to get a reward for it, you will get frustrated. When the reward finally comes you not only get the reward you also get relief from the aversive frustration and so the reward has greater value.

Incentives and Rule-Governed Behavior

Rewards have such a dramatic influence on behavior it is always surprising—to those of us who remember that Skinner (1958) taught a pigeon ten-pin bowling—that they are not used more widely in a formal way in treatment programs or as the foundational principle of any systematic program of behavior change. True, in the early years of behavior therapy, especially "behavior modification," there were literally hundreds of published demonstrations of the therapeutic benefits when desirable behavior was rewarded. With contracts (specifying performance/reward relationships), point-earning systems, star-charts, treats to be earned for good behavior, stock options or other bonus systems, and all the other variants, the rule—if you do this you will get that—really seems to serve as an incentive system and is thus closely tied, operationally, to the topic of motivation already discussed.

Because language can specify relationships and events that have not been experienced directly, most human reinforcement contingencies are specified ahead of time by verbally stated relationships: "if you put your toys away, you can watch a DVD" we tell the 5-year-old child. Although this is called "rule-governed behavior" that phrase is slightly misleading. The rule in the previous example was more a restriction than a promise—"you may not watch a DVD until your room is tidy"—and was only a rule if permanently in place and agreed to by both parties. Rules that are consistently enforced and promises that are reliably kept probably serve the same function. But the main point is that the parent does not need to wait until some sign of room tidying has occurred and then rush in with a reward, the way we have to wait for the cat to accidentally press the paddle. We simply tell the child what the contingency is, and, assuming parental approval is both desirable and probable, that serves as an incentive to perform the action. Nevertheless, spontaneous reward is equally powerful—praising or otherwise recognizing the desired behavior of an employee is such a potent method of ensuring more of the preferred behavior that effective organizations use the old parental principle of "catch them when they are being good." Verbal information can also convey the standard with which the action is to be performed, as well as what will happen if it is not performed. The client beliefs that therapists describe as irrational are verbal rules people have imposed on themselves, with untested expectations regarding consequences of interpersonal behavior.

Note that many "if A, then B" relationships are conditional—"only in the presence of C." In the animal laboratory the implicit basic rule might be "if you press this lever, you will get a pellet of food." If this is true only under a certain condition—"when a blue light is on"—the blue light is called a discriminative stimulus and it eventually controls behavior (no point wasting your energy pressing the lever when the blue light is off, because you will not get fed). If this same conditional relationship is expressed verbally, the conditional context is sometimes called a frame: "if you are very quiet *during the sermon*, we'll go to Kentucky Fried Chicken after church." What is called Relational Frame Theory (Hayes, Barnes-Holmes, & Roche, 2001) confirms that verbal rules are almost always context specific and thus context always influences behavior. Often people know the response/reward relational rule ("if I publish lots of papers I'll get promoted"), but do not fully appreciate the implicit contextual frame that is operating conditionally ("as long as the promotions committee respects those journals").

And so it is that when the promise of rewards is translated into treatment programs there are subtleties that require common sense as well as psychology. Take, for example, the use of a voucher-based incentive system for reducing substance abuse (e.g., Higgins, Alessi, & Dantona, 2002). Cocaine-dependent outpatients earn points worth about a quarter for each drug-free specimen, with bonuses for consecutive negative test results. In a typical trial people can potentially earn almost $1000. But they do not get the money. They exchange their vouchers for retail purchases made for them by the clinic staff. Like almost all token reward programs over the years, there is a "response cost" contingency embedded in the agreement: the value of the voucher is reset to 25 cents if a specimen is positive or is not provided. That contingency does not work well in classroom settings. If a child loses all or most of his or her points and cannot earn them back that day there is a natural "what the heck" reaction; the child might as well enjoy the freedom of being bad, as there is nothing left to lose.

In any event, classrooms are poor environments for imposing artificial rewards. If only one child's inappropriate behavior is targeted, then rewarding that child for what is expected of others is judged unfair. If the contingency applies to the group, the child who is the spoiler and loses the reward for the class is vilified. Generally speaking, when it comes to rewards, children are more like dolphins than rats or pigeons. Sometimes dolphins would rather play than earn rewards.

Caveat

The power of reinforcement as a principle does not translate into proof that clients or any other humans are driven only by materialistic rewards or the satisfaction of biological needs, although a few will be. The medical scientist is undoubtedly reinforced altruistically by the contribution that many hours of laboratory work will make to the health of others. However, the pleasure of seeing an experiment turn out as predicted, having your name printed in a leading journal, attaining the the praise and admiration of your peers, or reaping the benefits of salary and promotion are all reinforcements sustaining research and scholarship, even when it is mostly conducted for its own sake. It is not a stain on the human condition that we do things that bring us pleasure. What is remarkable is that through socialization, perpetuated by genetic history, so many altruistic, artistic, spiritual, and intellectual experiences can bring us as much if not more pleasure than the reduction of primary drives.

There are, however, functional differences between intrinsic and extrinsic rewards. Lepper, Greene, and Nisbett (1973) published the evocative experiment that was the first to demonstrate that if children who had intrinsic interest in an activity were given an external reward for engaging in it, when that external reward was withdrawn they would show less interest (engage less in the activity) than they did originally. The effect has been replicated many times and the implications spelled out in a slightly alarmist book entitled *Punished by Rewards* (Kohn, 1993). Kohn pointed to the aversiveness of not receiving an expected reward, which, as mentioned earlier, children see as especially unfair. He highlighted the negative effects on cooperation in organizations and promoting competitiveness at school, with students focused on the reward and not the task.

Like any controversy there are counterarguments. One of the strongest is that the issue demonstrates that the term rewards should not be used interchangeably with reinforcement; reinforcements are always defined in terms of their function. However, the implication to consider is to be cautious with external reward contingencies as you may get what you wish for.

Irrespective of the true mechanisms and complexities of reinforcement there is one fundamental principle that should be recognized if your goal is promoting new behaviors rather than desisting from old ones. Behavioral variation is essential for new behaviors to be established. Just as spontaneous variation in the members of species makes natural selection possible in evolution, so variability in responding permits the shaping of new forms of behavior. This is well accepted in clinical assessment—the functional analysis—when we focus attention not only on the occasions when, say, a person reports a headache, expresses anxiety, or craves a cigarette, but also on the times the client does not. In terms of intervention planning the same principle holds. We can consequate a desirable behavior (even an approximation to one) only if it occurs. It is very difficult to change behavior clinically if clients cannot be persuaded to try something new and overcome their behavioral inertia. I mean no disrespect to clients by drawing a parallel with children who are fussy eaters. "Try it, you'll like it" we say to our children, "just have a taste, you don't have to eat the whole thing. Look, mommy likes it. Mmm, yum, yum. Have just one bite and then you can have some ice-cream"—persuasion, modeling, reinforcement sampling, successive approximations, conditioned reward. The similarity to strategies used with many clients should be apparent.

Secondary or Conditioned Reward

If you were trying to shape the behavior of a dolphin to jump out of the water and through a hoop, it would be a little hard to give the dolphin a fish reward at the very moment it goes through the hoop. Catching that moment is important, because one of the known principles of reinforcement is that it is most effective when it comes shortly after the response to be strengthened. This might be due partially to the informational value of the reward (it is a signal: "Yes, that's what I want; you got it right"). Either way, immediacy is important—"clean up your room and I'll get you an ice-cream next Thursday" is not likely to result in a tidy room. So what does the dolphin trainer and the wise parent do? He or she associates a previously neutral symbol with the reward; the signal indicates with some certainty that the reward is or will be forthcoming and thus obtains its own rewarding properties. This is called a secondary or conditioned reward. In dolphin training it is usually a blast on a whistle—if the dolphin goes through the hoop the whistle is blown; the animal receives a symbolic reward and sometime later will get the sardine when the whistle is sounded again. The whistle becomes a sort of substitute sardine. For a child it might be a smile, a "good girl," a little hug, or a star on a star chart—Kohn notwithstanding. Of course, in most human situations all our primary needs are taken care of: we get our sardines regardless. Thus, although the social approval may signal the probability of other good things, in reality these rewards become highly valued in their own right, often more so than the material rewards available.

Could the mechanism for secondary reward be the conditioning of positive affect, originally elicited by the primary reward and now equally elicited by the secondary one? Put rather simply, the whistle becomes pleasant for the dolphin, eliciting hope, and possibly signaling the end of hunger. The sight of a bottle of alcohol can calm a heavy drinker long before the physiological effect of the alcohol has been experienced. Staats suggested a simple model for thinking about these interrelationships. A stimulus predicting reward has a cue function—it comes to control the behavior, it is a discriminative stimulus. It also acquires a rewarding function for other behaviors. And because through association it comes to elicit a positive emotion, the stimulus itself becomes liked or desirable. He called this the A-R-D (Attitude-Reinforcement-Discriminative Stimulus) function of any stimulus, particularly verbal and symbolic stimuli, associated with reward—it will have a positive attitudinal valence, serve as a reinforcer, and have a discriminative stimulus function, regulating behavior. Each of these processes is well-known and has been shown to be valid in many diverse research studies, but putting them together this way was a useful model. It also indicates further that in a learning situation there are instrumental relationships between response and reward, but there are also associations between stimuli (both external and internal) and affect. All learning situations involving rewards and punishments have classical contingencies (associations) embedded within them.

Practice Makes Perfect (Sometimes)

It is slightly embarrassing that after a hundred years of learning research we are still citing Thorndike for important principles. However, Thorndike articulated two very basic laws of learning that have really stood the test of time. In addition to the Law of Effect, which as we have just seen is all about reinforcement, he proposed the Law of Exercise, which states, essentially, that when behavior is repeated it becomes stronger; it is "stamped in." We know this to be true from countless everyday observations, but we also know that mere repetition does not really improve performance very much without some sort of feedback. Thorndike (1932) recognized this and revised the Law of Exercise to include that proviso.

Nevertheless, the sheer repetition of an action seems to strengthen it, especially when we are dealing with simple habits, such as picking, hair pulling, thumb sucking, or daily routines. Repetition of behavior always occurs in a context, and as such salient cues in that context often evoke the behavior. Lots of people who smoke light up a cigarette after a meal or with a cup of coffee. The cues present in that context become powerful triggers for the behavior of lighting the cigarette, and the related desire to smoke, especially if the action is thwarted, is interpreted as an urge. Stimulus control of behavior is one of the most important things to assess when designing an intervention—what cues are likely to elicit the behavior we hope to reduce or suppress? Remember too that most activities we wish to increase or decrease consist of long complicated chains of specific actions. Each response in the chain produces its own internal stimuli (interoception and proprioception) and these play a role in regulating the next action in the sequence. You will know this if you have ever had an injury that prevents a specific response from occurring—suddenly your usual smooth routine of taking a shower or getting dressed is interfered with because the cue complex guiding this motor pattern is disrupted.

Analyzing and understanding the formation of habits is a venerable topic in psychology. William James (1890) devoted an entire chapter of his textbook on psychology to it. My Kindergarten teacher wrote in my report card "Ian must remember that habits begin as cobwebs and end as steel chains." I do not recall what nefarious habit she had identified—sucking my thumb or biting my nails or twisting my hair around my finger all seem likely candidates. In any event she was simply repeating Thorndike's Law of Exercise. But it was Guthrie (1935) who emphasized that in addition to repetitive practice, it was the stimulus context in which responses were repeated that came to have such a powerful influence over behavior, and Dunlap (1932) who provided a number of clinical examples. Clinically there is more emphasis on strengthening the behaviors newly acquired in therapy and less on breaking the old habits, but they are essentially two sides of the same coin.

As change requires that new behaviors (including cognitions) become more probable, clients have to practice their new found skills. They can practice these in the clinical setting, in the presence of the therapist, but the consulting room is usually the wrong cue complex. It is much more useful to practice these skills in the settings in which they will be used or when confronted with stimuli likely to trigger the old, unwanted, behavior pattern. For a long time now in cognitive-behavioral therapy, this sort of extratherapy practice has been called "homework," but essentially it is practice in a meaningful context.

There is a great deal of data supporting the value of client engagement in homework exercises prescribed by the therapist (Kazantzis, Deane, Ronan, & L'Abate, 2005). Practice involves two components—rehearsing the skill itself, such as sitting at home and carrying out your meditation exercises, and implementing the skill when it is needed, such as doing a brief relaxation exercise before doing a stressful task, or preparing a small healthy snack instead of bingeing on yesterday's leftovers. The designation of these practice sessions as "homework," analogous to what children are required to do at home after school, is slightly unfortunate. Most people have negative connotations about homework and so when cognitive–behavioral therapists introduce the concept they usually have to do so with a little proviso, or off-hand joke, that it is "nothing like homework during school days!" It might be simpler just to give up the term homework and describe the task for what it is: practice of the new skills or habits in a relevant context. Clients seem to benefit from being told that for change to become established the onus is on them to practice. They know the old adage about practice making perfect.

What cognitive therapists often refer to as "automatic thoughts" can be conceived of as habits—a fixed idea or knee-jerk verbal response that has been overlearned and practiced so that it is now reliably evoked in certain situations or possibly triggered by other thoughts. Cognitive restructuring has as its goal the outcome that in the same situations other, less negative, emotive, or irrational thoughts will be more likely to occur. Because the undesirable thoughts are cognitive habits (occur with high probability), they cannot really be changed by argument and disputation from the therapist. So the idea of homework practice was introduced to encourage the client to rehearse the new thought repeatedly.

If co-workers in the office are giggling to each other, the automatic thought "They're laughing at me" is probably erroneous, but makes the person feel bad. It also functions to promote self-monitoring ("What silly thing might I have done?") and avoid embarrassment (saying "Hi guys! What's the joke?" when it might be you). Practicing the more rational alternative ("They must be sharing a little joke among themselves") can easily be stated to yourself, but can just as easily be pushed aside by the dominant, habitual thought ("But maybe they are laughing at me"). Because of this, more sophisticated forms of cognitive therapy try to replace irrational or false habits of mind (beliefs) with more correct, adaptive ones, through a range of other techniques. These might include approaches such as stating a more general rehearsed self-statement: "But my thoughts are not reality—I've actually no idea what they are laughing at." The purpose here is to create a distance between the thought and the action or feeling that it might otherwise (erroneously) trigger, which is not that different from any other habit-breaking technique.

Punishment

The thorny topic of punishment in psychology is part of instrumental conditioning, but gets its own section because it contains some tricky issues for planful behavior change. The other side of the Law of Effect is that if a behavior is followed by a noxious (unpleasant, aversive, painful) stimulus it will be *less* likely to be repeated in the future. If reward is seen as something that strengthens behavior, then punishment could presumably be thought of as something that weakens behavior. But that raises an immediate problem. It is often the case that after a response's probability of occurrence has been reduced by contingent negative stimuli, when those stimuli are removed the response reoccurs very rapidly rather than remaining gone from the individual's repertoire. Because of this, various theorists, including Skinner himself, suggested that the punished activity is "suppressed," but not eliminated. The individual is no longer producing the response while under a punishment contingency, but that does not mean the response has been extinguished—or forgotten.

A reason punishment is difficult to study experimentally is that we need a reliable behavior to punish in order to investigate its effects. Usually in the laboratory that behavior is one that has already been shaped by a reward contingency; thus punishment often involves introducing a conflict between potential rewards and potential punishments. To add yet another wrinkle, it is possible to think of acquisition of an instrumental response not purely as the increase in probability of that response, but as a decrease in the probability of all other relevant responses. Thus, punishment is not a decrease in the probability of the punished response but an increase in the probability of other (incompatible) responses in that situation. We also know that if an operant behavior is followed by an aversive event (a painful shock) and then followed by food, the animal will keep responding—endure the pain or starve is Hobson's choice. But, and this is the lesson for parents who punish and then cuddle children, the animal will soon continue to respond only when the shock is present. Punishment becomes a discriminative stimulus for approach.

There is a further feature of the experimental conditions used to study the effects of punishment (and reward) and it relates closely to practical applications: the responses *elicited* by punishment or reward play a role in what happens next. Defensive systems are activated when threatened with danger and pain, and defensive responses can be quite varied, usually fleeing or freezing, but counterattack if escape is not possible. If these responses elicited by punishment are different from the behavior being consequated, then they will facilitate behavior reduction, but if they are similar they interfere with the contingency effect. In appetitive behavior the opposite is true. What happens after a rat has pressed a lever and gets a pellet of food? Obviously it eats it. Because this involves the use of its paws, the consummatory response is incompatible with lever pressing for a short period of time. In a pigeon study, things are different—when the little grains of corn are dispensed, the pigeon pecks at them. Pecking is the very behavior being consequated. As a result, we have a phenomenon known as autoshaping. If you dispense corn randomly (noncontingently) into the pigeon's Skinner apparatus, rates of pecking, including the crucial one of pecking at the disc, go up. You can increase the operant by noncontingent reward when the behavior evoked by the reward is similar to the behavior being shaped. I can think of numerous clinical occasions in which I have been encouraging parents to reinforce their children with praise (which often elicits social approach), only to have them come back and say it did not work. When the active, boisterous child was engaged, as the parent wanted, in a quiet, solitary activity in the house, and the parent delivered fulsome praise, the child stopped what he or she was doing and ran over to the parent. For the parents, this proved that behavioral principles did not work. I knew that it proved the exact opposite—they work only too well.

This relationship between the behavior being consequated and the behavior elicited by that consequating event is particularly evident with punishment procedures. What laboratory behaviors are elicited by aversive stimuli such as electric shock? Often, but not always, it is some sort of freezing behavior. This phenomenon is used to estimate the level of fear an animal has. If the animal is thirsty and is lapping at a water spout, that lapping stops when a stimulus is presented that has been paired with shock in the past. This preparation is known as conditioned suppression. So if punishment is designed to cause nonresponding, punishing events eliciting freezing will be especially effective. But certain aversive stimuli cause the exact opposite—they elicit fleeing, not freezing. If a rat or a mouse can see a cat coming toward it, it will run. If it hears or smells the cat but cannot determine where it is, it will freeze. Getting shocked in the back legs will make a rat run (in an activity wheel, for instance); getting shocked in the front legs will make it stop—you would do the same if the threat was in front of you rather than behind. If receiving a punishment makes the child cry and have a tantrum, then being punished for crying and having a tantrum is utterly pointless. If pain elicits aggression in children, then causing them pain for being aggressive seems equally futile once basic principles of behavior change are understood.

Further Stipulations

The contingency known as negative reinforcement is one in which there is an ongoing unpleasant condition that is terminated by a given action. The cessation of the unpleasant stimulus condition reinforces the behavior that made it stop. The classic practical example is when a very harried and stressed parent is dealing with bothersome, fighting, arguing, noisy children and loses patience and yells at the children or, worse yet, spanks them. When the upsetting child behavior ceases, as it will at least for a while, the parent's harsh disciplinary practice is reinforced, even though the cessation of the unpleasant condition is only temporary. If the child also stops the unpleasant behavior briefly because of the negative consequences (yelling or spanking), he or she has not learned any preferable alternatives. Thus, in the words of Gerald Patterson (1982), who first described this important pattern, the child and the parent are caught in a "coercive trap," each one controlling the other by aversive means.

As explained in the previous chapter, if you can produce a behavior that relieves you of pain or anxiety, albeit only briefly, the behavior is likely to be strongly reinforced and thus become habitual. If the behavior that reduces an intensely negative feeling also produces negative consequences that only occur later, then this individual is also caught in his or her own coercive trap. For example, when a teenager deliberately cuts himself or herself, the immediate physical pain may be much less than the intense psychological distress the young person is feeling. The action of cutting is thought to reduce these negative feelings, perhaps by distraction or by creating pain that is under your control. Pain you inflict on yourself often seems more tolerable than lesser pain that is inflicted unpredictably from an outside source. Binge eating or gorging on fattening food may have negative consequences for the individual later, but the immediate effect is to reduce the feelings of anger, anxiety, or self-loathing that the client with a serious eating problem may be experiencing.

If rewards work hedonistically by generating pleasurable emotions that are then connected to the actions themselves, it is plausible that punishment—especially verbal reprimand and criticism—works by generating unpleasant emotions (fear, anxiety, sadness) and that these are then associated with the action that resulted in punishment. We have a large amount of evidence suggesting that punishment conditions unpleasant feelings to the punished action. What do we call such feelings in everyday parlance? Guilt. If you perform an act that has been punished in the past, even if there are no external negative consequences currently, you will probably feel some small degree of discomfort. This would appear to be conditioned anxiety. I am not suggesting that this is the only mechanisms whereby a conscience is developed—fear of consequences for certain behaviors can be induced in many ways, especially through symbolic means such as pictures and verbal statements, as every religion has used since time began to control the behavior of its adherents. But the conditioning mechanism is an interesting one because it relates to the possibility that if children do not condition readily, or if the punishment occurs too long after the transgression, then they will be less likely to develop a conscience and less likely to confirm to societal rules for moral and ethical conduct (Aronfreed, 1968).

When punishments are severe enough to elicit fear it seems highly likely that fear will be conditioned not to the punished behavior, which might have occurred sometime in the past, but to the agent of punishment. The likelihood of children becoming fearful of the adult who punishes them too severely is very high. Quite apart from its effect on otherwise important positive relationships, it is very obvious that when the punishing agent is no longer around the child need not fear the consequences and can engage in the proscribed behavior with impunity. Because we can never monitor children and youth all the time, if prosocial behavior is controlled only by fear of the consequences of transgressions, socially desired behavior will occur only in very circumscribed conditions. Anyone working with delinquent youth who have not internalized the desire to behavior appropriately will know that is exactly what happens. Punishment certainly controls behavior, no doubt about it, but not in the ways we want.

Punishment generates emotional responses just like reward does, except these responses are negative and undesirable. If a punishment contingency is in place the best way to avoid getting that noxious experience is to refrain from performing the behavior. In other words, a punishment contingency can be thought of very much like avoidance, but passive avoidance, not active avoidance. Naturally this similarity has led theorists into recognizing that if nonoccurrence of the response (the passive avoidance) is sustained and no punishment is delivered, the reinforcement for that could be a reduction in negative affect. Fear will have been conditioned to the context in which punishment stimuli are delivered, as well as to the proprioceptive feedback from the punished response. The organism manages negative affect by not responding, and if it is conditioned to the stimulus complex of the behavior in context, then it cannot easily extinguish.

This is the same argument as the two-factory theory of active avoidance. It might help explain the unexpected results of punishment, since a change in cue complex would mean lessened fear. The most obvious change is when the punishing agent (some authority figure) is not present, or the setting is altered (now being outside the institution, say). So it is not surprising that the suppression of even harshly consequated behaviors in real life does not generalize well. And humans, needless to say, can simply calculate cognitively the chances of being punished (being caught, being observed): people who have not internalized social responsibility speed on the roads when they are fairly certain that no police, radar, or traffic cameras are around. If we add to this mix the well-established finding that some people are insensitive to punishment (not to the pain, but to the emotional contingencies), then relying on punishment to benefit clients seems to be a forlorn, but ever-present societal hope.

Some Implications for Practice

Whatever the mechanism, the reality is that when actions result in highly aversive consequences, the individual will tend not to repeat them, for a while, that is. Punishment, therefore, has been used by parents (and sometimes teachers, and certainly social institutions of reform) for generations to try to regulate the behavior of children. It is only quite recently that modern societies have raised the question of the appropriateness of child-rearing practices inflicting pain or inducing fear in children: corporal punishment such as spanking or striking a child. Alternative forms of negative consequences seem more suitable, such as loss of privileges, verbal reprimands, and "time-out." Because corporal punishment is now regarded as unacceptable in many cultural groups, spanking children is often associated with poor parenting strategies in general. Despite this confound, the evidence is very clear that spanking is harmful to children's development (Briesmeister & Schaefer, 2007).

Behavior analysts, impressed with the reality of the principle of punishment, tended to explain this failed relationship as one arising from misuse of the principles of punishment. For example, parents who hit their children might not do so clearly contingent upon specific, defined behavior, might be inconsistent in their use of punishment, and might use a lenient intensity, and research shows that delayed latency of punishing events make them less influential. But because it seemed like punishment principles could be implemented in proper professional contexts, these arguments gave rise to the suggestion that punishment had a clear-cut role in expertly designed programs to eliminate highly undesirable excess behaviors in children and other clients. Ethically, the justification for causing a client pain came from the much greater harm that the challenging behavior was causing, both to the clients themselves and to others. All in all it seemed as if we had a certain technical understanding of the best ways to make punishment successful, so there was considerable justification for using punishment to change intractable, illegal, dangerous, self-harming behaviors. And so applied behavior analysts did just that.

I will not go into a full history of the use of punishments in the management of challenging behavior in children and adults with severe developmental disabilities—what became known as the aversives controversy. However, the controversy is a fascinating illustration of a number of central contentions of this book: (1) that a limited set of principles of behavior change does not provide a sound basis for the development of meaningful and effective treatments; (2) that validation trials may show a treatment produces change, but cannot show that another one might not have performed even better; (3) that unless being carefully monitored, negative outcomes (iatrogenic effects) are usually not revealed in conventional treatment trials; (4) the translation of a change principle into a treatment method often distorts the principle because of hidden biases and unrecognized cultural assumptions in the clinicians using the principles; and finally (5) because a treatment approach is possible does not mean that it is ethical (or humane, and respectful of clients' rights). I will give a brief synopsis of the controversy to illustrate each of these points.

Principles are limited. Unlike the experimental procedures whereby punishment has been studied behaviorally, the challenging behaviors exhibited by children with developmental disabilities, such as self-injury (head banging, skin picking, self-biting), aggression (hitting others), self-stimulation (pica, rocking, flicking objects), and destructiveness (breaking property, throwing objects, ripping clothes), all serve some sort of function (Carr, 1994). As they are being maintained by other contingencies, these would need to be well assessed and understood before attempting to change the behavior using an added punishment contingency. Also, aversive stimuli selected for punishment would be capable of conditioning fear in the child to the situation, including the clinician administering the punishment.

Other methods might be as good or better. Single case studies showed that punishment procedures resulted in a reduction of challenging behavior (Cataldo, 1991). But could a positive approach have produced a comparable result or one that is more stable and longer lasting? By conducting a meta-analysis of the reported treatment studies (none of which was a direct comparison), my colleagues and

I were able to show that nonaversive, positive interventions could produce a result just as effective, and possibly more so, as aversives (Scotti, Evans, Meyer, & Walker, 1991). Part of the problem with the treatment outcome literature on aversives was that it was not possible to determine if there were side-effects, either good or bad, since few studies reported them formally, despite sometimes commenting that they were common.

Principles were badly translated. If a child is engaging in an inappropriate behavior "for attention" (gaining attention is the function; social reaction is the reinforcement maintaining the behavior), it is a reasonable intervention strategy to try to ignore it. But a few children, particularly those with developmental disabilities, do not get much positive social attention, and because that is pretty well universally rewarding, we would need to find other positive behaviors for carers to attend to, rather than simply remove the one thing the child is trying to obtain. This should shift the clinical emphasis firmly to skill development. Similarly, if the behavior is punished, it is done socially, and so the attention it entails, even if negative, could really be a reward rather than a punishment.

"Time-out" was originally conceived as time out from the availability of reinforcers, especially social ones—a kind of extinction procedure. But as it can be aversive to be placed in a small locked area, the event is usually that of punishment. If the behavior that is being punished has the function of controlling the environment, the time-out period permits controlling actions to continue, so children often do things like physically resist and when finally forced into time-out will break windows, yell, scream, and pound on the door, or smear feces on the walls. When that happens, the time-out period is usually extended and so the entire pattern is repeated.

Time-out as a clinical procedure, therefore, does not fit the punishment principle of behavior change nor the extinction principle. Time-out can be used somewhat more constructively with young children. The child is told to leave a conflictual or noncompliant situation and to go off by themselves, say to a bedroom [or what Supernanny (Frost, 2006) calls "the naughty stool"], to calm down and to think about the situation, and, when back in control of their arousal, to return and maybe apologize as specifically as possible for the transgression. This strategy does represent a mild punishment, insofar as the child does not like the experience and feels the parental disapproval as aversive, but is really an opportunity to be able to exercise some self-control skills. If the child lacks those skills completely, the time-out procedure will not work.

Ethical concerns. There are very basic ethical principles when conducting any psychological treatment. One of these is informed consent. The clients with intellectual disabilities who were subjected to aversive procedures in the past were never asked to give their consent. Consent cannot be given by a primary caregiver as the parent of a child with a severe challenging behavior has an obvious conflict of interest. When various advocacy groups started to protest the use of aversives in these treatment programs, those clinicians who actively promoted these methods argued that clients had a "right to effective treatment" (Van Houten et al., 1988). But as there were other effective treatments available that did not involve aversives, clients' rights are really for "the most effective, least stigmatizing treatment with the fewest negative side-effects." The proaversive proponents also asserted that nonscientific arguments were being used in clinical judgment. However, the whole point of having and using professional ethics is based on the inevitability that all clinical judgment involves decisions and considerations that are related to humanistic and practical concerns (Léduc, Dumais, & Evans, 1990). Just because it is possible to introduce a certain type of intervention does not mean that it is desirable to do so (Lovett, 1996). Fortunately, it is now widely accepted that teaching alternative skill sets is the appropriate strategy for changing a wide range of socially undesirable behaviors.

Skill Development

We talk a great deal about teaching skills in therapy, especially in the behavioral tradition. Assertiveness was among the first of such skills to be considered therapeutically, to be quickly followed by social skills (especially for children with disabilities and people with schizophrenia—Bellack, Mueser, Gingerich, & Agresta, 2004), communication skills (in marital therapy), parenting skills, and then problem-solving and coping skills. In all of these cases skills are loosely thought of in much the same way as any other complex behavior sequence, whether a sporting skill, an artistic talent such as drawing, or a complex performance such as a circus act. Skills require a great deal of practice, with the desired competence modeled or explained in some way, timely feedback has to be available, and usually there has to be some sort of pay-off or reward to sustain the drive for constant improvement.

When the skill being taught is a basic life competence, such as simple cooking, knowing how to operate a computer, taking care of personal hygiene, getting yourself dressed, or finding your way around the neighborhood, a simple task analysis usually suffices for identifying the components of the skill sequence. These are the everyday things that are often taught to people with intellectual disabilities or to people in rehabilitation programs who have lost skills as a result of a traumatic brain injury or other cause of brain damage. A task analysis is a very useful way of breaking up the activity into its essential components and ensuring that clients have these components and can emit them in the correct order in a fluid way.

Much complexity arises, however, when significant cognitive elements are involved in the skill in the form of judgments, decision processes, choice-making, and so on. Safely crossing a road in busy traffic is a skill that young children in urban areas need to learn. But what is the critical component that many children are missing that makes them unsafe? Is it that they cannot control impulsive acts, or are there other deficits in judgment? Recent research using simulation suggests that some young children judge safety in street crossing only on the basis of the distance of the approaching car, and do not factor into their judgment the speed of the vehicle and the time it will take them to walk across the road (Congiu et al., 2008). Once that is known as the skill deficit, training programs can be geared directly to remedy it. In fact, for some so-called skill areas, these are the only important elements, such as in problem solving.

The idea that clients often lack skills rather than being unable to use them or refusing to use them for some reason is an important one for any formal behavior change effort. Today we hear a great deal in the popular media, echoed in all seriousness by many psychologists, that teenagers behave in erratic, irresponsible, and risky ways because of the way their "brains are wired" and the fact that they have not reached appropriate levels of maturity in neural development. However, seriously problematic behavior of the kind that concerns adult society is exhibited by only a small fraction of the adolescent population, especially across different cultural and ethnic groups. It is far more plausible to assume that some adolescents have not had the effective learning opportunities that foster anticipation of consequences, judgments regarding alternatives, concern and empathy for others, and other self-regulation skills that will be discussed in Chapter 9.

Implications

Instrumental conditioning principles appear much less controversial than classical conditioning. There is little opposition in contemporary treatment approaches such as cognitive–behavioral therapy to the general idea of the importance and effectiveness of reinforcement contingencies for changing behavior. At one level that seems like a correct inference—the value of rewards for changing and sustaining behavior is really indisputable. However, we have seen that at a different level, things are not quite so simple and straightforward. Human behavior cannot be explained as a series of operants controlled by their consequences. Reinforcements have incentive value; rewards can be anticipated. Rewards might be fair and delivered as promised and yet still not meet a person's expectations. Rewards have strong symbolic value—the treat given by a parent for a task well done may really serve as a signal for a far more valuable commodity, parental approval. Rewards may be delivered to just one or two members of a group for behavior that is better than that of the others. Does that shape high performance standards in the rewarded individuals or does it shape competitive behavior? If effortful or difficult tasks are strongly reinforced, does this promote a whole class of behaviors that might be called something like industriousness?

A long time ago Tinklepaugh (1928) reported a finding that has become a classic, because it is a good story. Hungry monkeys are quite willing to perform an operant task for lettuce as a reward. However, if given a choice they prefer fruit—so would most of us primates. If monkeys who have been working for fruit are switched to a lettuce reward, they refuse to eat the lettuce. In fact, they show fairly strong signs of displeasure. Reinforcement contingencies are powerful means of behavior change, but not always in the expected direction. When used therapeutically, these many properties of reinforcement do need to be understood.

Be wary of highly artificial reinforcement schedules. It should come as no surprise that if a child is reading a book because the child expects to get cash from his or her father (a promised material reward is maintaining the activity), we run the risk of reducing reading behavior once the material reward is no longer forthcoming. Worse still, it is possible that the level of reading outputs will drop below the previous baseline. Surely it is obvious that the reward for reading is intrinsic to the activity: enjoying the story, getting excited, and wanting to know how the book ends, and social—being able to tell others about the book and share your enjoyment of it. (Think about why we have book clubs. Reading would appear to be a solitary activity, but like language, it has implications for sustaining social interactions as one of its implicit rewards.) No sensible clinician would suggest a material reward to encourage reading behavior in a child; a better approach is to make sure that the books available are easily read but a little bit challenging, are exciting, are related to many other interests the child has, and get discussed with friends, teachers, or parents after the book is finished. This is what we call encouraging children to read. It might need a bit of priming, just like we have to smear a little food on the lever to get the rat to start nosing around it. The stimulus of *a book* needs to be a positive attitudinal one, however that is arranged. And we have to make sure that there are few competing activities—playing with X-Box or watching TV and videos provide stiff competition for something initially more effortful, such as reading.

Most behaviors we want to change have intrinsic material and psychological consequences, which, because these are not as noble as the enjoyment of reading great literature, give them an apparently compulsive quality. Pathological lying in children, for example, often results in material gains but also satisfies implicit emotional needs by gaining sympathy, admiration, and avoiding punishment. In planning change, when the goal is to reduce or eliminate undesirable behavior, one of the most important diagnostic questions is to ascertain its function. What is the person getting from performing this behavior? Well-rehearsed activities produce action tendencies when foiled—the urge to perform the blocked behavior. And if they are also satisfying a need or achieving a positive outcome in some other way, simply removing the consequences (extinction) or adding conflict by introducing an additional negative outcome (punishment) will further preclude the desired change. Equally functional, emotionally effectual alternatives need to be found. All of which leads us nicely into another major domain of behavior change: no behavior exists in a vacuum, and, furthermore, emotional responses regulate overt actions and provide a potent motivational force for approach and avoidance. We thus need to examine much more closely the fact that all behavior occurs as part of a dynamic system—behaviors are all interrelated.

7

Response Relationships

The Dynamics of Behavioral Regulation

There is a movie called *The Ruling Class* (1972) in which Peter O'Toole plays a British aristocrat who has the delusion that he is Jesus Christ. He goes about harmlessly mad, doing little harm. He then gets treatment—psychotherapy and electroconvulsive therapy—and the delusion disappears. But by the end of the movie he has now become a violent hater of women, believing he is Jack the Ripper. In the early days of behavior therapy, one of the criticisms leveled against it, especially by psychoanalysts, was that as it seemed to be focused on the symptoms rather than the underlying causes of distress, removal of one symptom would merely result in the appearance of another. This presumed phenomenon was known as symptom substitution.

Behaviorists scoffed at this suggestion, arguing that there was no evidence to support it. But because both behaviorists and psychoanalysts saw human functioning, especially psychopathology, in dynamic terms (analogous to physics, forces drive behavior change; Galbicka, 1992), before long behavior therapists had to accept that the concern was valid. Simply put, the issue was this. If a behavior had a certain function (served a psychological purpose; was under the control of a contingency), removing that behavior without addressing the emotional (pleasure, or pain reduction) or motivational (drive reduction) needs it achieved could well result in some other behavior taking its place. The likely cause of symptom substitution was not quite what the psychoanalysts proposed, but there were well-accepted and obvious psychological mechanisms that could account for why changing one problem might inadvertently facilitate another.

Some of the evidence for such substitution came from a somewhat humbler source than the exciting world of dynamic forces at work in adult psychoneuroses. Meyer (Voeltz) and I were conducting research on undesirable, challenging behaviors in young children with severe developmental disabilities (Voeltz & Evans, 1982). When looking carefully at our own clients, and also reading similar research reported in the literature, we noticed that it was *not* uncommon to find that as one problematic behavior was reduced, a second might appear or at least increase in frequency (Evans, Meyer, Kurkjian, & Kishi, 1988). We soon realized that far from being an exception, this behavioral substitution was the norm in treatment studies and clinical case reports. The good news was that the new behaviors were not inevitably undesirable. Side effects could be good as well as bad. These "collateral effects" could be positive as well as negative. If training one response leads to improvements in others—what I identified earlier as response generalization when the others are all part of a response class—then positive collateral effects can be said to have occurred.

Regardless of whether these collateral effects were clinically desirable or unwanted, what was rather interesting from the literature was that although the researchers would mention them in the discussion section of their published articles, they rarely planned for them, monitored them, or measured them in any formal way (Scotti, Evans, Meyer, & Walker, 1991). This was clearly a result of the tradition in behavior analysis of studying only one selected operant at a time. Selecting one target behavior in this way ignored the obvious fact that behaviors were likely to be interrelated within any individual's repertoire.

There were many other authorities making the same general point. In fact, within personality theory the notion that people have complex repertoires of interrelated behaviors is the fundamental idea. Staats (1975) had made the strong case that behaviors are often independent variables for the emergence of other behaviors. Many responses, he reasoned, are arranged in cumulative, hierarchical patterns, such that the presence of one behavior or set of skills, reading for example, is a prerequisite for another set of skills, learning second grade social studies. The child that comes to Kindergarten *without* simple skills in manual motor dexterity (cutting, pasting, drawing) or in social behavior (sharing, waiting your turn, following the teacher's directives) is at a serious disadvantage for further learning.

The way behaviors are organized within individual repertoires and the influence of one set of responses upon another are therefore critical ingredients of treatment planning, outcome evaluation, and the facilitation of long-term therapeutic change. The construct of personality has been sneaking in and out of this whole discourse in various ways. We have asked if there are individual differences in people's ability to change, and we have looked at personality/treatment interfaces in which there may be individual differences in conditionability, or sensitivity to reward versus punishment. In Chapter 2 I briefly raised the issue that individuals diagnosed with a psychotic disorder may long for a life more normal and fulfilling than simply a reduction in symptoms. If we were to improve the quality of life and reduce overall stress, would the distressing clinical symptoms of psychosis be reduced as a consequence? Or, conversely, if we reduced the more unusual elements of hallucinations, delusions, and thought disorder, would this increase the chances of making friends, returning to work, and feeling useful and needed? Clearly the answer to such questions will lie in our understanding of response relationships within individual repertoires—what contributes to what?

Constructs Operationally Defined

There is a perennial confusion in psychology with regard to understanding response relationships when we cross from one mode of responding to another (Cone, 1979). Nowhere has this been more clearly seen than in the long struggle to operationalize an emotional state, for example, anxiety. There are basically three ways in which anxiety is manifest—physiological (somatovisceral) changes such as an increase in heart rate that produce strong negative sensations, verbal statements of anxiety (e.g., "I'm scared," which is not quite the same as self-report of those physiological changes, e.g., "My heart's pounding"), and the act of avoiding or escaping specific objects or situations (Lang, 1968). We could say that these represent physiological, cognitive, and overt behavioral aspects of anxiety, but the question is whether they are equivalent, substitutable signs of an underlying state, or whether they are different channels of expression of the state we call anxiety. It is certainly clear that they generally cooccur. If you have social anxiety your palms sweat, you express discomfort, you say you feel unsafe and people are judging you, and you avoid or get away from social gatherings as quickly as you can. But it is also possible that these three channels do not always cooccur: despite being tense, having a pounding heart and sweaty palms, and reporting that you feel anxious, you might still stay in the social situation. Numerous experimental studies in which the three channels are simultaneously monitored confirm that these three manifestations of anxiety do not always cooccur (Evans, 1986).

There are many good reasons for this, some of which are well illustrated by our social anxiety example. Socially anxious people in the public domain have learned to mask their physiological reactivity so that they appear outwardly calm. Sometimes there are benefits for staying in a social situation despite feeling intense discomfort. And there are often strong social pressures on people not to verbally express anxious feelings and to rationalize their avoidance behavior in other ways. All these examples represent situations in which the individual has managed to gain control over some facet of emotional manifestation, suggesting that these are truly separable components of an emotional state. But a more fundamental issue is whether in general these three components work together because they have causal interconnections. Because you heart is pounding you feel and express the negative emotion you call anxiety. Because the intense physiological changes called anxiety are so aversive you avoid or escape a situation so that the negative affect will diminish—the important idea underlying two-factor theory. Or because you are about to run away, your heart beats faster and you get a knot in your stomach as your digestive processes slow down.

The idea that there are three ways in which emotions are manifest—the "triple response" concept—has not gone unchallenged, particularly from those who argue that the function of anxiety is to access and process information: focus attention on the threat, judge its severity, and recall and compare previous protective strategies (Zinbarg, 1998). These are the sorts of processes, as we have seen, that are hypothesized to be managed by the Behavioral Inhibition System (BIS) neural system (Chapter 4). Eifert and Wilson (1991) pointed out that there has been confusion between the content and the method of measurement. They also projected that it is possible to distinguish between subjective feelings (affect) and processing information, reflecting more of a judgment about anxiety-provoking situations, such as the rapid recognition of potential threats or making assumptions about other people's reactions. Although this revised model of the components of anxiety and the different ways they can be measured is undoubtedly more precise, it does not take away from the important conclusion that emotional states, such as anxiety, are both manifest and measurable in a number of different channels, and these may not be alternative measures of a single construct, but potentially independent expressions of the hypothetical construct called anxiety. The debate remains as to whether any one of these three (or four) components has causal superiority within the cluster. Do you interpret people's reactions to you negatively because you are tense and sweating; or do you label your pounding heart as anxiety not excitement because you want desperately to run away from the social situation?

Constructs as Response Classes: Shared Functions

In the above example I am suggesting anxiety is a general construct (a psychological state) that can be operationalized by virtue of the different elements of which it is typically made up. The same can be said of clinical depression, which is made up of symptoms (e.g., insomnia), anhedonia, and melancholy thoughts. Many overt behavioral categories are also constructs that subsume different behaviors all having properties in common. Childhood aggression is a good example. Different behaviors are labeled aggressive if they have certain properties in common: they are designed to coerce others, they often cause pain or harm to others, and they are usually triggered by blocked goals (frustration/anger) or threats to safety (fear). A child might be judged aggressive if he or she kicks and bites peers, pulls hair and spits, is cruel to animals, is verbally abusive, or sends unkind text messages. Obviously several children do all of these things at a rate or frequency, or with a greater lack of provocation, than would be expected from the norm. Thus, we think of these actions as symptoms of aggressiveness, not just as a series of discrete and totally unrelated behaviors. And indeed they are highly substitutable. Clinically we would not try to change a child's biting behavior and ignore hitting, spitting, and hair pulling. Or if we did, we could reasonable expect these alternative forms of the problem to increase or even emerge newly as collateral behaviors. This is because these activities are interrelated since they are different forms or behavior sharing a common function. They represent a class of behaviors, different components of a socially constructed category, that are more or less interchangeable.

A response class (a series of different activities that share controlling properties) can be generated through the exercise of a contingency rule. This is logically similar to concept formation, in which the rule might be "anything edible with a pit that grows on a tree," thus forming a construct that includes olives, peaches, and avocados. A rule such as "do what I say" if followed by a reward generates the response class of compliance. A response rule such as "do whatever I do," shaped through differential reward, allows children with disabilities to acquire the general skill of imitation. It is, unfortunately, a bit harder to teach them when to imitate the trainer's actions and when not, but in principle at least it is a useful response class to inculcate. Children's play is a response class having many different forms but only one function: it is partly defined by having intrinsically pleasurable consequences and partly by being not directed by or demanded by an adult.

Behaviors within a response class have different probabilities of occurrence. In the early days of classic learning theory it was argued that in any given situation a number of substitutable responses are possible, based on past learning history. The one that occurs will be the one with the highest associative strength for that stimulus context—"habit strength" (Hull, 1943). If that response is blocked or prevented in some way, then the response with the next highest level of associative strength will occur. Within any individual repertoire a range of responses capable of satisfying a need exists, each with different probabilities of occurrence. There are countless clinical situations in which this simple idea has relevance. For example, we might want to encourage a child to eat healthier foods. Ordering a hamburger instead of a salad is simply a more probable response, due to differences in incentive value (taste), speed of reduction in hunger cravings, and lots of others, but both choices do serve the same function. To make choosing the salad a more probable response, we might want to make it tastier, easier to prepare, more accessible (cheaper, less waiting time), and so on. I am not designing a healthy nutritional program for children, merely emphasizing that if there are a number of potential responses all serving the same function within a repertoire, fostering the healthier alternative requires increasing the attraction of the currently less likely one.

Another childhood example can be found when parents complain that their children are spending too much watching television and not getting outside and having adventurous activities the way they used to do when *they* were children. But all children have a repertoire of highly substitutable activities each of which serves the function of being entertaining and fun. There would be little point trying to substitute doing homework for watching TV, as these activities serve completely different functions. To reduce TV watching and replace it with a currently lower probability interesting and potentially more cognitively beneficial activity, it is necessary to facilitate accessible, safe but adventurous, reasonably high habit strength alternative play activities *before* limiting or restricting the child's access to TV (blocking the most probable response in the leisure time repertoire). Again, I am not designing a complete program to increase children's activity levels (desirable a public health goal though it may be—witness Michelle Obama's "Let's Move" initiative), but merely emphasizing that by understanding this organizational structure of response interrelationships we can facilitate planned behavior change.

When social service agencies try to facilitate such alternatives for detached youth engaged in antisocial behaviors—drug experimentation, drinking, carrying a weapon, tagging, irresponsible sexual behavior, petty larceny, and truancy from school—they may try to introduce a range of alternatives, including nonleisure, unexciting, or low habit-strength activities such as job coaching. However, it is important when designing interventions to keep the function of the undesirable behavior you are trying to reduce clearly in focus. In Blandy's (1971) interesting book *Harvest from Rotten Apples*, he explained how clubs set up for youth in economically deprived areas in Britain had a new ping-pong table installed, but as none of the young people ever played table tennis on them, after a while they stopped attending the youth center altogether. Children with autism also often lack leisure skills, especially social play, but even more so lack effective communication. Clients with expressive language deficits are more likely to engage in self-injurious behavior (McClintock, Hall, & Oliver, 2003). Carr and Durand (1985) showed that intervention plans were successful only when the alternative behavior being encouraged had precisely the same communicative function as the undesirable one they were trying to reduce.

Some response classes are purely arbitrary, created by social conventions and legal requirements. The response class of "safe driving" is made up of different behaviors such as driving at the speed limit, not using a cell phone, coming to a complete halt at a stop sign, and glancing regularly in the rear view mirror. Driving researchers have recorded that in the presence of a police car or traffic officer all of these behaviors become more probable (Ludwig, 2002). They have also noted that drivers tend to sit up straighter. There is no law against slouching, so presumably this added component is somehow part of a pattern of actions controlled by the stimulus "proving I am a safe driver." In other words, previous training creates a response class of somewhat arbitrarily linked behaviors. When individuals move from one structured environment to another, such as moving to a new classroom with a new teacher or moving to a new marriage with a new partner, only some of the collection of behaviors within the class of "these things make this person happy" may be appropriate in the new environment.

Other Organizational Structures

There are, in addition to response classes defined by a common function, many other possible structural relationships defining how behaviors might be interrelated within a repertoire. In simple behavioral chains, as would be found in many well-rehearsed routines, the performance of one response becomes the cue for the next one in the sequence. Each link in the chain sets the occasion for the next. More complex structures are hierarchical, as already mentioned: one action or skill is a prerequisite to the subsequent acquisition of others. In education we are well aware of the importance of such chains. If you do not know that numerals represent numbers of objects it is hard to learn how to add and subtract using numerical symbols; if you cannot first float and hold your breath under water it is hard to learn to swim. In clinical contexts such sequences are equally important. If you cannot listen to your partner's point of view, you cannot communicate effectively, and if you cannot communicate you cannot solve problems equitably, and if you cannot negotiate problems you cannot spend mutually enjoyable time, and if you cannot do that you cannot share intimacy and you will not be happy in your relationship. Marital therapists can give much more specific detail to such chains, but generally agree that there are these cause–effect sequences that have to be recognized if the goal is to change a dysfunctional marriage (Jacobson & Christensen, 1996).

There is an additional basic structure that deserves mention. This is the idea not of a chain, a hierarchy, or a sequence of behaviors, but of a keystone behavior on which a great many other behaviors depend. In some contexts these keystone behaviors seem to be prerequisites for many otherwise unrelated behaviors. In childhood learning, for example, observing the behavior of others and imitating it (modeling) are fundamental to learning a great many other skills. Understanding language, or having at least a rudimentary communication system, is critical for learning not just one sequence of skills, but is the keystone to learning many discrete, unrelated competencies.

In remedial settings these keystone behaviors are often called pivotal skills, especially when they are missing in the repertoire and need to be developed for widespread benefit (Koegel & Koegel, 2006). You can see right away that for a child with a deficit repertoire of learning competencies, such as a child with an intellectual disability, it would make a great deal of sense to focus your instructional efforts on these pivotal skills such as imitation (see Chapter 11) or language comprehension, because once the child has these abilities other things will be learned naturally and, incidentally, not just those competencies that are taught directly. Following the gaze direction of others or being directed to a target by pointing is something most infants do from about 6 months of age. Children with autism are less likely to show these emerging skills; if they can be taught them it has widespread benefits for learning other things. Children with autism can also be taught to self-initiate: by learning to approach others in a socially acceptable way, to join a group, or to gain entry into a game, many new opportunities for social interaction become available.

Various actions have the effect of creating many new opportunities to *access* far-reaching response-reinforcement contingencies. In behavior analysis these have been called "cusp" behaviors (Rosales-Ruiz & Baer, 1997). Every parent who has seen his or her infant go from sitting to crawling will know of the new opportunities for behavioral consequences (both positive and harmful) afforded by the emergence of that specific skill. For adults, activities such as going to college or foreign travel result in major new opportunities for reinforcing experiences. The cusp concept was originally proposed by Bijou (1968), who strongly disputed developmental principles such as stages and milestones. Cusp behaviors are neither prerequisite skills nor universal milestones. Hitting a tennis ball with a racquet when you are 3 years old is not a pivotal skill like curiosity or play. But when you go on to win a tennis tournament at the age of 4½, as Serena Williams did, life-changing new opportunities present themselves. Buy your child a puppy and it generates performance demands for training and exercising the pet. It might require your child to make sure the dog is fed and in return generates skills of caring, empathy, and the pleasure of receiving affection and loyalty.

It has to be admitted that the search for keystone behaviors, particularly those that prop up a whole repertoire of undesirable behaviors, has not proved particularly easy. What might be the one keystone that supports and sustains all of the antisocial behaviors of delinquent youth? Is it undue peer influence and the inability to resist peer pressure? Is it impulsivity and poor self-control? Is it hostility toward parental rules or authority in general? Any or all of these might be plausible keystone behaviors and there is little definitive research to identify the right one. Very often the causal variable is the absence of a pivotal skill, for example, not having (or not having access to) socially sanctioned leisure skills (playing soccer, reading alone for pleasure, hiking, playing in a band in the garage). Young people who spend significant time in such activities spend less time in antisocial, criminally nuisance activities.

Nevertheless, the idea of the pivotal skill or the keystone behavior represents another of the many structural arrangements whereby elements within individual repertoires might be causally related, and this is encouraging for planned behavior change, particularly prevention. Putting it absolutely simply, in order to change one behavior you have to change a behavioral precursor. Being aware of this is very useful for planning behavior change because it is often so difficult to get at the targeted behaviors directly—they might be secretive, private, occur rarely, be hidden in some other way, or unlikely to emerge until future opportunities present themselves. How do we begin to change the sexualized behavior of a child who occasionally molests other younger children in secret, or the relatively infrequent behavior of fire setting, or a distressing paraphilia in an adult client, such as exhibitionism or voyeurism?

One important way in which pivotal skills lead to broadly beneficial change is through mechanisms relevant to prevention. Teach a toddler "hands are not for hitting" and you prevent aggressive, disruptive behavior in elementary school. Increasing young children's emotion knowledge results in improved prosocial behavior, because giving children the language tools for identifying emotions in themselves and others enhances all aspects of emotion competence, such as knowing of strategies that can be used to self-sooth and control your feelings. I have already explained how emotion talk that increases emotion knowledge has widespread social benefits. Formal cognitive skills in problem solving have been successfully taught to school children with beneficial results in preventing school behavior problems (e.g., Guerra & Bradshaw, 2008). Some of these pivotal skills are taught in a formal elementary school curriculum, emphasizing friendship skills, self-control, social problem solving, and the emotion competence mentioned earlier (Greenberg & Kusché, 2006).

There is plenty of evidence from the educational field of the benefit of teaching people to learn from new experiences. This is sometimes called learning to learn and it helps place the individual client on a learning trajectory. "Future learning frequently requires 'letting go' of previous ideas, beliefs and assumptions. Effective learners resist 'easy interpretations' by simply assimilating new information to their existing schema; they critically evaluate new information and change their views (accommodate) when necessary" (Bransford & Schwartz, 1999, p. 93). That "letting go" ability is doubtless one of those many individual difference variables that relate to differences in a client's potential to change, analyzed in Chapter 4.

Problem Solving as Therapy

A pivotal skill that has been quite extensively researched within psychological therapy for both adults and children is that of problem solving. It is the psychotherapeutic equivalent of the old adage: give a man to fish and you feed him for a day; teach him to fish and you feed him for the rest of his life. Within the cognitive–behavioral therapy (CBT) tradition, the concept was originally introduced by D'Zurilla and Goldfried (1971). However, it has been most vigorously championed and developed in recent years by Arthur Nezu. He and his colleagues and students have extensively evaluated its application in both health psychology contexts (coping with diabetes or cancer, for example) and mental health areas (depression and anxiety) (Nezu, Nezu, & D'Zurilla, 2007). They call it "problem-solving *therapy*" for the reasons discussed at the beginning of this book—our field likes to think of discrete treatments rather than principles of change. Nevertheless, the essence of the approach is to provide the client with a set of generalizable, meta-cognitive, pivotal skills—how to go about solving problems—and only the solutions that emerge are likely to be specific to a particular kind of syndrome, personal distress, or emotional challenge.

It is not really possible to do justice to the approach within a few paragraphs. Yet the basics are actually quite simple and straightforward. Nezu divides problem solving into (1) social problem solving and (2) a relational/problem-solving model of stress. The former essentially refers to the challenges and vicissitudes of everyday life and how we resolve them; these may be major events, such as job loss, or relatively minor events, such as forgetting an appointment. The latter division is somewhat more closely tied to Lazarus and Folkman's (1984) hugely influential ideas about stress and coping, where the problems are specifically likely to overwhelm the individual emotionally. Usually, effective coping in such situations is "problem-focused" coping, hence the close connection between problem-solving therapy and models of coping. However, Nezu explains that "emotion-focused" coping in which clients are taught to reduce or modify negative feelings can be just as useful in some contexts. Stressful life events need to be thought of as "problems to be solved" rather than overwhelming disasters. Note that when trying to manage major problem situations, daily challenges and hassles can derail constructive solution generation, so problem-solving skills need to be applied at many different levels of significance.

The actual components of problem solving are fairly standard. First, this "therapy" really resembles teaching in which the strategies are explained, modeled, and rehearsed, feedback is provided, and finally practice is extended and implemented. Many of the components are almost identical to elements emphasized in Acceptance and Commitment Therapy (ACT): seeing emotions as not undesirable in themselves but signaling that a problem exists; using metaphors such as a red traffic light to encourage the client to "stop and think"; and normalizing problems as part of the rich panoply of living. Clients are taught not 12 but five problem-solving steps, mnemonically represented by the word ADAPT: have an attitude that is positive, define the problem, alternative solutions need to be generated, predict the outcomes of each one, and try the best one out.

Sometimes good problem-solving strategies are known to clients but are just not being implemented; clients complain that if they could sit down and think rationally and calmly about their problem, they would, but they feel too overwhelmed to do so. Nezu's partial answer to this is to assess by questionnaire what the client's current (probably dysfunctional) problem-solving style and barriers are (such as being impulsive or avoidant), thus allowing the teaching of the skills to be tailored to individual needs. Also, the underlying mechanism of change might be more than acquiring new strategies. The exercises provide a structure allowing the causes of clients' distress to be isolated from the cognitive and emotional experiences that have, in a sense, become the problem. Anxiety and depression are not the problem; they are the result of wrestling—unsuccessfully—with the problem. It is in this way that giving clients a way of distancing themselves from the struggle of the problem is not dissimilar to the principles of ACT. What I find so beneficial about this whole approach is that it recognizes that so much of the emotional distress we label as psychiatric symptoms can be traced to stressful life events, both daily crises and more major calamities, including chronic and life-threatening illnesses (Read, Mosher, & Bentall, 2005).

People can be taught general problem-solving skills as alternatives that are incompatible with ineffectual worry, avoidance, or giving up.

Problem Solving as a Pivotal Skill for Children

Like all skill development described in the previous chapter, problem solving requires dividing the task requirements into components. The early work on interpersonal problem solving for very young children by Shure and Spivack (1982), which became immensely popular, required a fairly rigid formula to be followed: generate possible solutions (without censoring any of them), thinking through the pros and cons of each one, and then selecting the strategy with the greatest likelihood of success. Children's ability to think through the possible consequences of different actions was assessed by a What Happens Next Game in which hypothetical actions were described to children and they had to predict the most likely events that would happen next. In Shure and Spivack's well-conducted randomized controlled trial of their "I Can Problem Solve" protocol with preschool children, the results of the training showed not only improvement in the cognitive components being taught but also in improved behavior. A longitudinal evaluation showed benefits into the fourth grade.

Some of my own doctoral students conducted a number of studies on highrisk children in our region at the time (e.g., Mdaka, 1994). Our general conclusion was that children of all ages could indeed learn the formal processes that they were taught: brainstorming solutions, predicting the consequences of their actions, and understanding cause–effect relationships in interpersonal situations. However actually using these strategies in the heat of real life situations was another matter entirely. Like so many other topics in changing behavior, we have come to recognize that both context and individual differences contribute greatly to successful use of problem-solving skills. Take the example of self-managing behavior in the context of a chronic illness such as diabetes. In addition to requiring general problem-solving skills, to be successful the child needs specific knowledge about the disease, the ability to transfer past experiences, and attitudes or self-efficacy beliefs regarding the potential of problem-solving strategies (Hill-Briggs, 2003).

Compatible and Incompatible Behaviors: Behavioral Economies

A crucial principle of behavioral organization is that some behaviors are incompatible with others. This could be based on physiological polarity (you cannot be calm and anxious at the same time) or on temporal incompatibility (when you are doing one thing you cannot be doing something else). This is less true for feelings and thoughts, and certain automatic overt activities, which is one reason why emotional expression, cognition, and simple habitual behavior can be thought of as separate categories of human conduct. Nevertheless, emotional responses often disrupt smooth motor behavior; in clinical contexts the physiological activity we call emotion interferes directly with skilled performance.

As far as complex overt behavior patterns are concerned, if you are playing soccer or practicing the guitar you are not tagging other people's property. Despite many teens' belief to the contrary, you cannot be texting a friend and doing homework at the same time. A number of behaviors interfere with each other because they rely on equivalent control mechanisms, such as attention. This is why talking on a cell phone and driving is now prohibited in many jurisdictions. All behavior has its opposites, sometimes the polar opposite, or reverse of the action, and sometimes just the nonoccurrence of the action. The nonoccurrence of wetting the bed is being dry at night; the polar opposite (and the behavior we want to see in children who are enuretic) is waking up and going to the toilet in the middle of the night if you need to.

A person cannot literally be doing nothing. Of course your partner may interpret your lying in a hammock with a mai tai instead of mowing the lawn as doing nothing, but it is equally an activity that fills the available time. Any behavior perceived as meaningful (has a purpose and is recognized) is more actively pursued (Ariely, Kamenica, & Prelac, 2008).The idea that behaviors fill available time means that we have a fixed sum "economy" of possible activities. This is why behavioral interventions that focused only on reducing an excess behavior (by using punishment contingencies or extinction tactics) were doomed to failure. The undesirable behavior (acting as Jesus Christ) might decrease, but another one (acting as Jack the Ripper) might increase. It seems plausible that if we focus on adaptive, appropriate alternative behaviors to the one we wish to see reduced or eliminated, we will have greater success in doing so if the new behavior is not only an alternative but is also *incompatible* with the undesirable behavior. One type of incompatibility is physical—the two behaviors cannot occur within the same ecological space. So extinction of lever pressing can be aided by switching the reinforcement contingency to wheel running. In fact, extinction can be seen not as the decrease in frequency or probability of one behavior, but the increase in frequency or probability of other, incompatible behaviors.

When you have clients with emotional disorders to modify, rather than when you are training rats, the situation is a whole lot more complicated, but the principle is still useful. Imagine that you are trying to extinguish the compulsive hand-washing behavior of a client with obsessive–compulsive patterns. Have you defined what you expect the client to do instead? After the client has touched something he or she believes is contaminated, our usual instruction is something like "now try *not* to go and wash your hands." In the therapy room we might encourage touching a "contaminated" object and then ask the client just to sit there—this is exposure (to the feared stimulus) with response prevention.

That is a basic CBT treatment strategy. What happens is that at first the client sits there getting increasingly anxious but eventually that anxiety dissipates and is extinguished. We might consider enhancing the response prevention by filling the time with something incompatible with hand washing. Possible things to do other than hand washing are briefly using a hand sanitizer (socially acceptable form of cleaning), taking your lunch out and starting to eat a sandwich, typing an e-mail to a friend on your Blackberry, putting the contamination item in the garbage, and loading the dishwasher or folding clothes.

Behavioral Interrelationships Are Context Dependent

Much of our purposeful behavior is made up of sequences of responses that unfold with regularity once certain cues trigger an action or environmental supports are put in place. The young person who steals a few spray cans of acrylic paint is initiating a tagging sequence, even if it occurs days later. These contexts constrain behavior and allow very complex (well-defined) sequences of behavior to occur. Once these constraints are in place, the appropriate sequence is more probable, and it does not have to be a well-rehearsed routine, it can be an entirely novel sequence.

Imagine you have been invited to deliver a talk or an academic paper, or had a poster presentation accepted at a conference for the first time, perhaps in a foreign country, sometime in the future. Once the commitment is made, it requires a whole sequence of routines and subroutines to be enacted: applying for funding or leave, making the relevant airline and hotel reservations, converting the presentation to PowerPoint, working out how you will kennel the dog while you are away, and many others, right down to setting the alarm clock the night before an early flight. For some this planning may be all last minute and done in a rush, but the necessary routines do fill time and make the next step possible. Many people who are clients of mental health services may have similar long-term goals and dreams of foreign travel and having new adventures. But without the structure imposed on their lives of having formalized commitments and arrangements supported by their employment, their daily routines can be quite nebulous, subject to random events, and focused on immediate needs and self-interest. When helping clients change it may be very important to know whether their daily lives are planned and purposeful, or lack specific direction, and thus are likely to be influenced by unpredictable circumstances.

Planning, which involves knowing and anticipating the behavioral routines required to fulfill future goals, ensures that behavior change is focused, but does not necessarily ensure that it is constructive and positive. You can plan to rob a bank as well as plan to go to college. But planning, like problem solving, is one of those categories or classes of behavior that facilitate transition to new environments—they enhance generalization and transfer, topics we first encountered in Chapter 2. It is important in therapy, when hoping to leave a client with a

Dynamic Interrelationships

I have asserted that overt behaviors are negatively reinforced by the reduction of highly unpleasant affect. This important insight is illustrated clinically when a person engages in checking behavior resulting in an immediate decrease of anxiety that the door might not have been locked or the gas fire turned off; checking is so powerfully reinforced we call it a compulsion. If someone is feeling depressed, angry, or rejected, binge eating can inhibit these unpleasant feelings, and bingeing becomes an ingrained pattern. It is not surprising that any careful reading of the works of Mowrer (1960) and Miller (1948), who between them developed two-factor theory, shows that they were very much influenced by dynamic models, including classical psychoanalysis. Miller was also well aware of how some of the symptoms of traumatized soldiers who had experienced combat, particularly amnesia and emotional numbing, could be explained as ways of avoiding the devastating painful memories and experiences of warfare. In his explanation of positive psychology, Seligman (2002) likens coping mechanisms to scabs over a physical wound. It is best not to pick at them if healing is to occur.

We have all experienced this at one level or another. We may be angry at someone else's behavior, which serves to mask our own feeling of guilt for a share in responsibility for a bad situation. Behavior therapy, like dynamic psychoanalysis and unlike cognitive therapy, has always assumed that a given feeling can mask another. One of the most compelling examples of this is the argument put forward by Stampfl and Levis (1976) that removing defensive types of feeling does not eliminate the more basic and more devastating underlying feeling—these are left to fester and to motivate other behaviors in the future.

Experiential Avoidance and Acceptance

Behaviors that reduce highly aversive feelings are strongly reinforced and persistent, even though these behaviors might themselves result in punitive outcomes. To the outside world, these acts appear irrational, or inappropriate, or maladaptive, but the short-term relief is greater than the longer-term disadvantages. But what if we could find ways of decreasing the negative emotion motivating all these maladaptive behaviors? Could part of the problem be that the person is simply overly sensitive to unpleasant emotional feelings? Perhaps the client has intense avoidance of negative experiences because of a personality characteristic: excessive sensitivity to anxiety and other unpleasant feelings, or low tolerance of distress?

Part of this sensitivity could be not just to distressing feelings but to perceived threats from the environment. These threats might be social, such as fear of embarrassment from fainting or vomiting in public, or they might be the threat of further pain and distress, such as fear of getting deep vein thrombosis on a long airplane flight. When such threats are present, the individual will focus on the situations that allow for avoidance or escape from them. Although this proposition sounds a lot like two-factor avoidance theory, it has been give a different name and is usually called "safety seeking" behavior (Salkovskis, 1996). This is a very apt description. For example, people who have panic attacks or fear open busy places will be focused on what they need to do to stay safe, such as sitting at the movie theatre at the end of the row so they can get out quickly, or planning where they could sit quietly in the shopping mall if they felt dizzy. The reason this is so interesting from the point of view of helping people change is that it seems likely that these are the very behaviors that although motivated by allowing people to feel a little relief from anxiety, actually maintain the anxiety because they are continually thinking about possible catastrophes, and perhaps are closely monitoring their feelings to sense if an attack is coming on that they need to do something about. Thus, treatment, paradoxically, might focus on ways of discouraging these safety-seeking behaviors: stopping in some way the "experiential avoidance."

Two strategies to achieve this have been developed that have gained a degree of empirical support—that is, they seem to work at least for some. The first of these is to try to reduce the perception of threat. Although clients seek "safety" the reality is that they are not usually in much danger. The threats are often social, such as being embarrassed or losing your dignity by having an intense emotional reaction in a situation most people take in their stride. Thus the client might be asked to specify more precisely what the worst thing that could happen might be and then to reappraise both the threat level of such an event and its probability of occurrence. Reduce the perception of threat and you reduce the safety-seeking behaviors. Reduce them and the anxiety will extinguish in the absence of any further distress.

The second strategy consists of trying to reduce the experiential avoidance by increasing the client's tolerance for negative affect, especially fear and anxiety. This can be approached through verbal persuasion, redefining negative feelings as information, safe, valuable components of life experience, that subside of their own accord, and other reconstructions, all of which fall under the rubric of increasing acceptance. Raising tolerance can also be attempted, through graduated exposure, which is useful if the negative affect is itself feared because of worse outcomes such as a full-blown panic attack. If bodily sensations are aversive because of what they might signal (conditioned stimuli), classical extinction techniques, as already explained, are possible.

Does (or Should) Personality Change with Treatment?

Personality constructs, particularly traits, are really response classes. Personality repertoires consist of interconnected patterns of responding. Take the example raised in Chapter 4, impulsivity. If a child who typically darts across the road without looking for cars exhibits other behaviors such as suddenly starting a new game or grabbing food before anyone else, he or she will be judged as impulsive. This trait means that children will respond rapidly to changing stimuli without first appraising the situation or thinking about what should be done. We have to be careful not to explain their dashing across the road *because* they have the trait of impulsiveness, but by understanding the trait we can better understand why they act in these ways, and better articulate what we need to alter in their repertoire to make them safer when walking down the street. So the question remains. If treatment consists in changing the basic behavioral repertoire, does that mean we are changing personality? Or could we teach a child good road safety without trying to alter his or her basic impulsive personality style?

To answer the question, it would be useful to consider anxiety again. Clients who experience chronic social anxiety often describe themselves as "worriers." In the absence of a stimulus or specific situation the client might report generalized anxiety, accompanied by feelings of dread or vague concerns about negative outcomes (Hofmann, 2007). These anxious thoughts and feelings can be addressed therapeutically a number of ways, but what if the client has a significant predisposition to anxiety? People have been described as having marked individual differences on the trait of Neuroticism (Eysenck), Neuroticism versus Emotional Stability (one of the Big Five dimensions of personality), or a dominant Flight–Fright–Freeze System (FFFS) (Corr & McNaughton, 2008). The latter two characteristics represent distinct neurophysiological pathways and patterns of brain activity. When anxiety is treated clinically do we expect to have a labile, neurotic, defensive person who is no longer anxious about certain things, or do we expect, in Neil McNaughton's nice turn of phrase (2010, personal communication), to have "reset her/his personality"?

A very common argument in recent therapy approaches, especially that of ACT, is that a viable treatment of anxiety will not immediately make the client less anxious but will ensure that these anxious feelings do not inhibit or prevent the individual from engaging in desired goal-directed activities (Hayes, 1989). The client may continue to be socially anxious but goes to the party anyway and has a reasonably enjoyable time. If you have not altered the client's perception of the threat but have ensured that he or she will not act defensively (flee) in the face of the threat, you have at least begun the process of "resetting" personality. That would appear to be the preferred outcome, although perhaps not from the client's perspective. Clients want to be free of anxiety and worries, not functioning despite them. (The therapist's hope, it should be made clear, is that once the defensive, avoidant behavior is reduced, the unpleasant feelings of anxiety will subside.) It would clearly be best if we can change the mechanisms underlying the chronic and persistent anxiety without modifying the adaptive and valuable features of anxiety as the barometer for impending dangers.

Personality Itself as the Target for Change

The question takes on a different hue when clients' problems are judged as reflecting something wrong with their whole personality, and not just some features of their day-to-day coping with stress or managing conflict, dealing with threats, and avoiding danger. Clients for whom the entire individual repertoire seems overly interconnected are judged to have a "personality disorder." What this means is that a very basic mechanism within their individual repertoire uniquely and consistently influences their behavioral responses across a wide range of situations. And not all situations, of course. The contexts relevant to personality disorders are the *social–emotional relationships* we have with others (e.g., antisocial, dependent) or within ourselves (e.g., narcissistic, schizotypal). For example, if *any* and *all* forms of intimate social relationship elicit anxiety or distress in a person, that individual's entire repertoire of social contacts, friendships, romantic relationships, or closeness with workmates, for example, will be *avoidant*. If the person also fears rejection and abandonment, then avoiding intimate relationships is not a workable strategy. Clearly, a person with both sets of needs is likely to be in even more extreme conflict and to behave erratically across a range of social contexts, constantly testing them.

A different example, touched on already, is the personality characteristic labeled psychopathy. In this case the individual is said to lack a well-developed conscience and to have little empathy for the feelings of others. People labeled with this personality profile are said to have callous, unemotional disregard for others. If such individuals also exhibit criminal behaviors (and not all do) or are part of an antisocial group then we could predict that they are likely to be violent as well as unconcerned with the rights, feelings, or needs of others (Harris & Rice, 1997). Such feelings partially help nonpsychopathic people to care about others and thus be more prosocial. To bring about change, therefore, should the personality deficits (lack of empathy, lack of conscience) be what are targeted, or should we be trying to find a way of curtailing criminal behavior regardless of these underlying deficits? The former seems logical but difficult; the latter would have to rely heavily on external factors, such as in the case of the men described by Wilson.

Implications

Response relationships, chains, and hierarchies affect our evaluation of treatment outcomes. In Chapter 2 I questioned what exactly *is* therapeutic change, if the direct effects of treatment are merely the behavioral means to psychologically meaningful ends? This is not an inconsequential clarification. Consider, for example, Casey and Berman's (1985) meta-analysis of psychotherapy outcomes for children. These authors differentiated between "reactive" outcomes—those things directly taught or targeted in therapy—and the more general, longer-term clinical outcomes that are presumably the objectives for the psychological treatment of children in the first place. Only if these reactive measures are included in the analysis are the effect sizes yielded by cognitive–behavioral treatments significantly greater than for nonbehavioral therapies (Weisz, Weiss, Alicke, & Klotz, 1987). If treatment-reactive outcomes really promote, in a cumulative-hierarchical chaining fashion, the outcomes we desire, then their achievement is valuable. If not, we may once again be confronted with the problem of observable but clinically and socially rather meaningless change.

What has hopefully been demonstrated in this chapter is that one response often facilitates another, either because it serves a cue function or because it is a necessary component of the second activity. But because all responses interact with the environment, which we cannot always control, firm prediction about which specific behavior will influence another cannot be made with certainty. The person with the diagnosis of psychosis, who has learned to test reality and no longer treats other people with suspicion, might still have difficulty making a friend unless likely companions are available and in some cases are tolerant of other possible oddities in the person's behavior, such as their speech, or social skills, or even appearance. Whether improving one behavior reliably improves another is not easily predicted in advance.

There are, however, various basic behavioral elements that seem to underlie a whole raft of more specific responses. We know enough about social situations to be able to state with some assurance that a child who is capable of using language to ask for things will have much greater success in regulating the environment than a child who has no communication system. Teaching communication skills should be a priority for children who lack them. If a child does not actively attend to the things going on around him or her, it is very difficult to respond appropriately to social cues or to teachers' instructions. In trying to improve the adaptive behavior of a child with autism, therefore, teaching a skill such as active attending or one such as the ability to imitate observed actions represents potential enhancement of pivotal skills that have many beneficial consequences.

Emotional expression can be represented in three different ways, but to make clinical life complicated, these three aspects do not always agree with each other—measures of the three types of reaction do not inevitably correlate. In real life this lack of concordance is highly adaptive, however. If, as a person with a psychotic disorder, one of your "symptoms" is extreme social phobia, the fact that it is possible to approach people despite that fear, and that it is also possible to engage in a social interaction without showing too much fear in your facial expression, is very fortunate. Because once you have made the social contact (approach) it is likely that your fear will subside, assuming that the social context is not a hostile one and that you are able to objectively judge it as safe. So to encourage social contact and potential friendships in a client with psychosis, I am not going to wait until I have tried to extinguish social anxiety as manifest in all three components. I would want to encourage approach despite fear (acceptance), in contexts likely to be safe and reciprocating, teaching the client to mask his or her anxiety to the greatest extent possible, and to have reduced the client's suspicion or paranoia sufficiently that he or she can accurately judge whether the social interaction is accepting and positive. Understanding the dynamics of response interrelationships creates endless rich therapeutic possibilities.

It has also been shown that cognitive processes under our control can cause an emotional response. Everyone knows how to become sexually aroused—all you need to do is to think of a past erotic experience, to imagine an erotic scene visually, and perhaps to say certain words to yourself that have been associated with past sexual satisfaction. Cognitions have this effect because they function as stimuli that are as good—or almost as good—as the real thing (and sometimes even better if your fantasy life is rich enough). Cognitions in the form of inner speech can also direct our behavior as readily as a direct instruction from someone else. Cognitions are not as bounded by physical space and time as overt behavior. They can and do cooccur, sometimes with completely unrelated activities, such as daydreaming. Therefore the relationship between cognition and other aspects of behavior presents a very special case of response interrelationships. This will be scrutinized next.

8

Cognition

Changing Thoughts and Fantasies

If anyone were to doubt the emotional effect of words or the manner in which a vision of a possible future can change the present, let them read again, or listen to, the speech of Martin Luther King Jr. delivered on August 28, 1963, at the Lincoln Memorial in Washington, DC. And mental imagery being what it is, I imagine that few people, certainly few Americans, cannot, as they read this, hear in their own minds the precise timbres of the words "I have a dream that one day this nation will rise up and live out the true meaning of its creed," or the crescendo of the very final words from the old spiritual: "Thank God Almighty, we are free at last!" Our minds are laden with remembered words and images, fragments of songs and tunes, some dim and some vivid, but all capable of evoking intense affect.

In earlier chapters I have repeatedly articulated the separation between cognitive events and overt behaviors and emotional reactions (thoughts, actions, and feelings)—an artificial way of dividing up psychological life but still useful from a planful change point of view. Think for a moment of Nezu's strategy of helping clients manage their feelings of despair when trying to cope with life's stresses by teaching them systematic problem-solving skills. These skills are cognitive, involving verbal analysis of situations, constructing possible solutions, making choices, and so on. Only when the chosen solution becomes an action plan that is implemented does the cognitive analysis result in trying out new patterns of overt behavior. Or think of Ajzen's theory of planned behavior: only when the individual has beliefs in the value of the action (attitude), in the normative social acceptability of the action, and in the perceived controllability of the action, will the intention lead to its performance. These beliefs are cognitions. In this chapter we are going to examine cognition as its own phenomenon, able to influence emotions and actions.

Cognition often refers to a parallel "stream of consciousness" running alongside and frequently independent of other ongoing actions. When someone is sitting on the bus, taking a long walk in the woods, laying bricks, attending a lecture, or lying in bed hoping to go to sleep, he or she is able to think (carry on considerable internal dialogue as well as nonverbal daydreaming), sometimes completely unrelated to the activity, but possibly closely related to their mood. If you are hiking in the woods and you are thinking of the blister on your heel, the weight of your pack, wishing you had not eaten your last chocolate bar because now you are thirsty as well as hungry, and wondering if it will rain before you get back to your campsite, your negative cognitions are only partly controlled by the external sensory features of the experience. Conversely, if, in the identical situation, you are enjoying the feel of the breeze against your sweaty shirt, listening to the bird calls, admiring the Fall foliage, and being in the moment, then you are engaging in positive, mindful cognition that is likely to be relaxing and rewarding. A third distinct possibility is that you will dissociate. That although occasionally attentive to external and internal cues, most of your internal dialogue or mental imagery is focused on something else entirely.

Any repetitive, overly rehearsed, habitual, or easily performed activity such as walking requires some cognitive control, but very little—they are known as automatic processes. When deep in thought you can be quite isolated from your environment and attend to it only when necessary; on your hike when you come to a stream and have to figure out how you will get across your predicament requires what is called controlled processing. But for much of the time you can be quite focused on your task-unrelated thoughts. If these are all variants of the same theme we call it ruminating; if the thoughts include anticipation of threatening or negative outcomes, we might call it worrying; and if the thoughts are of an ideal future we might call it daydreaming. You can also ruminate about the past and feel the pleasure of reminiscence (recalling good times) or the pain of regret. Because cognition is not bound to current stimuli, people can and do think back over past events and analyze them—what we call introspection.

If past experiences are unpleasant, or if they are unsatisfactory for whatever reason, all this reflection can be self-critical and self-deprecating. This produces further negative affect, or prevents those past event memories from gradually becoming more neutral. Clark and Wells (1995) suggested that this is one mechanism that maintains social anxiety. Earlier in this book we were all for maintenance, but when the behavior pattern is aversive, we want the exact opposite. It is a bit like what in simple conditioning we call incubation (Chapter 5)—but here dwelling on the unhappy features of past experience prevents the negative feelings related to that experience from slowly fading away. Although we can learn to put negative thoughts out of our minds, there are usually too many cues for that to work for long. Associated thoughts, similar negative moods arising from a different current experience, reminders in the form of people or phone conversations, Facebook photos or news items—these are all the sorts of triggers that can reactivate negative memories. So what we need to do is neutralize them in some way or reevaluate them. This is what cognitive therapy is all about.

Cognitive Processes

A very different way of approaching cognition in psychological science is to think of it as the meat in the sandwich—the bit that always has to come between afferent (sensory) input and efferent (motoric) output in any higher-order activity. This refers to *processes* such as the interpretation we place on events, our rapid assessment of the meaning of a social exchange, our calculations regarding an appropriate response, and our appraisal of our capability of making one. Certainly, some responses, at a basic reflexive level, are automatic, rapid, and unmediated. Both elicitation and conditioning of these reflexes can take place without awareness. Other slower responses, even emotional patterns, follow a hypothetical appraisal sequence whereby an individual judges an event, perhaps compares it to previous events in memory, and makes a decision as to how to respond—although none of these operations is necessarily at a conscious level (Lang, 1994).

A popular clinical model of cognitive processing, this time in social contexts, was proposed by Dodge (2011). If a child is aggressive, to paraphrase Dodge's work considerably, it is because he or she regularly misattributes the intentions of a peer as hostile. If a child regularly judges a smiling face as ridicule rather than friendship, then it makes sense clinically to try to alter those erroneous judgments. Of course we could equally try to teach the child restraint behavior, even if the peer *was* making fun of him or her. That would be adding a new mediator to behavior between the possible provocation and the response. That would be handy because just sometimes your attributions are correct, and so it would be generally sensible to test them rather than either totally responding to them or totally negating them. It is very natural for these mediational processes (self-control or restraint) to become the target for therapy.

There is a further proviso to these cognitive process analyses: we typically represent them as conscious judgment or appraisal processes and we may even suppose there are internal verbalizations, something like the child saying "That kid is making fun of me." But of course the emotional flash of anger [or joy, or fear, or any other feeling in the Behavioral Inhibition System/Behavioral Activation System/Flight–Fright–Freeze System (BIS/BAS/FFFS)] occurs so fast that whatever these mediating processes might be they are certainly not inner speech. Guthrie (1935) rather unfairly poked fun at Tolman (1932), the originator of cognitive explanations of simple learning, suggesting that when his rats came to a choice point in a maze they would sit down, buried in thought. His rats, however, were not scared or angry, just hungry. With emotion it may be that this assumed interpretation of events also occurs very rapidly; Beck (1976) believed so, describing them as "automatic thoughts." That may be well and good, but the experimental evidence contradicts the causal intermediary of anything resembling thought. Zajonc (1980) made it very clear that affective reactions to stimuli can occur without cognitive or even perceptual encoding. Such operations are independent of, and come later than, emotional responding. It seems likely that there is a continuum from unmediated reflexive responding, through unconscious, implicit appraisal processes, to slower, careful, reflective judgments before responding: from reflexive to calculated; from hot to cool.

There is also not much conscious cognition happening with well-rehearsed overt activities and daily routines. The rich stream of our everyday consciousness seems to be capable of occurring regardless of the concurrent overt activity. This means further thoughts and the feelings they evoke (such as worries, attitudes) are not constrained by physical conditions and realities. You cannot think about your finances and your grandchildren at the same time, but if you broaden your thoughts to worries about future employment, your finances and your grandchildren can both be included as relevant features of the internal dialogue. Separately the two themes may be neutral (finances) and joyful (grandchildren), but the more complex compound thoughts might make you worry about how to provide for your dependents. Clients often report they have difficulty containing their thoughts and preventing them from running into each other and causing distress. Ironically, a high level of emotional arousal contributes to unfocused thought, so many clients are trapped in a vicious circle.

People often do not like their thoughts, especially if they are doubts or repetitive thoughts such as "maybe I'll harm my baby"—the sorts of obsessional, unacceptable, alien thoughts that are described by Lee and Kwon (2003) as ego-dystonic. In this case it is quite common practice in therapy to encourage clients to stop such thoughts or exchange negative, distressing thoughts for more positive ones. But as thoughts are not constrained, this is quite difficult to do. "Thought stopping" as the therapeutic techniques is called, or deliberately not thinking about something, often has the opposite effect. Daniel Wegner (1989) is credited with exploring empirically the well-recognized notion that if you are asked *not* to think about something—such as a white bear—you end up thinking about it even more. This is usually conceptualized as a rebound effect. With overt behavior, as explained in the previous chapter, reduction of one response can be aided by encouraging an alternative behavior, since, as explained in the previous chapter, it is not literally possible to do nothing. We might imagine, therefore, that to suppress a thought, focusing on other distracting thoughts, would be a sensible tactic, and this is exactly what Wegner and colleagues have shown (Najmi, Riemann, & Wegner, 2009). This is still hard to achieve with thoughts, as multiple competing and contradictory thoughts can be held more or less together or in rapid succession.

In clinical work, there has long been an intense focus on thoughts judged by therapists to be irrational. However, clients do not seek treatment for irrational thoughts or erroneous beliefs. We can be thankful for this, as most of us engage in irrational thinking much of the time. A large part of modern experimental cognitive psychology, especially the bit related to reasoning and judgment, is concerned with telling us how bad we all are at being rational in uncertain situations (Tversky & Kahneman, 1974). Lots of people have magical thoughts, read horoscopes, believe in conspiracies, think Barack Obama is a Muslim, and deny the Holocaust or climate change. If we look at the biases and cognitive distortions that psychologists have identified the list is considerable. A Wikipedia (not, I hasten to reassure the reader, my usual authority on any topic) article entitled "list of cognitive biases" (http://en.wikipedia.org/wiki/List_of_cognitive_biases) identified 103 named biases in decision making, probability estimation, beliefs, social distortions, and memory errors.

Cognitive therapists are quick to notice six of these: arbitrary inference (what Dodge found aggressive children do); overgeneralization; its opposite, selective abstraction; catastrophizing; personalization (incorrectly relating external events to oneself); and black or white thinking. It is when irrational self-relevant thoughts and blatantly erroneous social beliefs cause unnecessary distress that people become clients. If we can convince them that the belief is incorrect (it is not true they are unworthy, or unlovable, or responsible for some accidental disaster), then their distress should be reduced. As long as the erroneous belief is the cause of the negative feelings and not the other way around, correcting the belief should be therapeutic.

Certain stimuli and events are objectively unpleasant, but the individual's response to them is out of proportion to their level of threat due to cognitive deficits, misinformation, or lack of information. Children with needle distress, who react emotionally to having injections, illustrate this quite well. They often have erroneous beliefs, revealed in drawings as well as statements, that the needle will go right through them or that they will bleed to death (McIvor, 2011). These beliefs can easily be corrected by explanations designed for their level of comprehension and understanding of biology. However, if the child has had an extremely painful experience with an injection, lumbar puncture, blood sample, or indwelling catheter, information alone will not alter the conditioned fear (Chapter 5).

Introducing Cognitive Therapy

Epistemologically cognitive interpretations of human functioning tend to share certain broad philosophical assumptions. One is basically an existentialist view that humans are driven by a need to make sense of their experiences, often referred to as meaning making. We use prior knowledge to give meaning to new information. A second assumption is that of human agency, best articulated by Bandura (2006). A core human property of agency, he argued, is the ability to reflect judgmentally on our own thoughts and actions.

With the emergence of cognitive therapy within such a paradigm, interest in changing client's thoughts became very widespread. Originally the kinds of thoughts that needed changing were those that seemed intrinsically harmful to the client because they were erroneous or irrational and thus led to negative feelings. No one would consider sadness, even for quite a long time, after severe loss such as the death of a loved one, to be pathological or something that should be changed. Losing your job is punishing and would make anyone angry, worried, depressed, or all three, but if later you are unwilling to apply for new positions because of a core belief that you are worthless, that is dysfunctional. Feeling down only because you think you are of no value, or scared only because you believe the world is threatening, reveals errors in thinking. Thinking errors, such as drawing the wrong conclusions from limited evidence, or being able to recall only negative memories, can be corrected and altered. So the new trend called cognitive therapy was really about word constructions—about internal dialogue, beliefs, labels for things and people, expectations, and inferences, all decoded in words, and amenable to change by other words. From this slightly folksy introduction as to why cognitions might have a central role in effecting therapeutic change, we can see that there are three clearly different meanings of the term cognition.

(1) One meaning that is widely encountered in clinical work, refers to the *content* of your thoughts, especially self-referent beliefs. Clinical interest arises from the assumption that the content of a thought precedes, influences, or causes emotional states and overt behavior. The thought "I don't know how to respond in a social situation" or "Other people might reject me" or "I might be evaluated critically" seems to cause feelings of social anxiety—although only if being perceived as competent or being socially accepted is very important to you. It is a causal process in exactly the same way that the thought "I'd like a piece of toast" serves as an internal cue causing you to stop what you are doing and go and make some toast, especially if you are actually hungry. That thought, however, will not make you upset, unless you are out of bread.

Conscious, maladaptive thought content as the target for therapeutic change came to prominence largely through the work of Albert Ellis and Aaron "Tim" Beck. Ellis (1962) suggested that clients tended to have thoughts that were irrational or illogical: you might have failed in one particular task but to conclude that you *are* a failure is crooked thinking and leads to an unwarranted emotional reaction. The thought that if you are not perfect all the time you must be a total failure is irrational. Ellis called his therapeutic remedy rational-emotive therapy (RET), and he was very opposed to people's "oughts," "shoulds," and "musts." The philosophical basis for his approach also included ideas such as humans are natural scientists, who create their own meaning, and attempt to use rational thought to judge the likelihood of future events. He contended that the goal of therapy was not simply to change the content of clients' self-defeating beliefs and absolutist demands, but to alter their philosophical suppositions. Clients have to realize that they create their own emotional distress by believing their own irrational thoughts. They can choose to make these less disturbing, be more accepting of uncertainty, reduce their "discomfort anxiety" (the feeling that they *must* not feel uncomfortable, or that they *can't bear* being disliked, or that they *can't deal* with criticism), and actively work at modifying their thoughts, feelings, and behaviors (Ellis, 1971).

This emphasis on thoughts not having the status of edicts is similar to the tenets of Acceptance and Commitment Therapy (ACT), although ACT's justification is different, basically proposing that thoughts do not in fact determine (cause) behavior (Hayes et al., 2006). Beck's (1976) original position focused more specifically on those particular thought errors that lead to feelings of depression—overgeneralizations about the world and our ability to control our destiny. These were the beginnings of cognitive therapy, although the basic ideas were in keeping with many features of conditioning-based behavior therapy. Staats (1968), for example, had explained in detail how words and images influence actions and emotions.

(2) Beck's metatheory was far more intrapsychical, however; inner dynamics generate depressed and anxious moods. He proposed the construct of schemas—not just a shorthand collection of information around a construct, but as integrated patterns of ideas, beliefs, and their related emotions. Although speculative, the schema notion is basically a response-interrelationship model. There is plenty of evidence that cognition and emotion are interactive and intermingled in the brain (Izard, 2009). Maladaptive, long-standing schemas, often acquired during childhood, do appear to become an ingrained component of our personality (Young, 1999). The tight bundling of semantics, verbal constructs, and intense feelings resembles what Mischel called "hot cognitions" (Metcalf & Mischel, 1999).

(3) A third and rather more complex meaning of cognition is the psychological analysis of information processing ("cool" cognitions)—how we attend to, select, interpret, store, and retrieve information. This is sometimes called the rational system, as opposed to the emotionally driven experiential system (Epstein, 1994). Attentional and memory processes are not usually available to consciousness, thus they are very different from the *content* of cognition in the sense of Ellis's and Beck's positions. It was not long before psychologists studying these processes saw information processing as especially relevant to human problems. Distortions occur not just in the incorrect content of a conscious thought, but in the unconscious processes of appraisal, judgment, inference, and perceptual sets. If your attention is attuned to external threats from the environment (you are hypervigilant to danger), your visit to the shopping mall is likely to be more anxiety provoking than if you are focused, like most other people, on getting a good-fitting pair of shoes. Recognizing that there are dangers in the world, even in shopping malls, is not irrational, but always looking out for them is maladaptive. If people allocate too much of their attention to themselves in a social situation then too much of the very complex visual and auditory information inherent in such situations will seem self-relevant in a negative way, and thus create anxiety (Clark & Wells, 1995).

Today it is often these processes that are the focus of therapeutic change, rather than the content, because the processes control the content. For example, if during the past week you had two failures and five successes, but infer "I am a failure" because the two failure experiences are more salient, more easily recalled (retrieved), more firmly stored, and the successes are misinterpreted in a more dismissive way (attributable to chance—revealing an external locus of control), then the depressed feelings are really due to those process distortions, via the misrepresented content. The cause is the erroneous processing, even if the resultant content (the thought of "failure") directly elicits the melancholic feelings. In other words you do not reflexively feel depressed because you have experienced a failure, nor do you choose to feel depressed because you are not controlling your irrational thoughts; no, it is faulty processing of information due to memory and judgment errors that has distorted your appraisal of events and the meaning you ascribe to them.

(4) Self-reflection is a highly adaptive meta-cognitive skill. This points to a fourth and fairly important meaning to cognitive change, one sometimes referred to as meta-cognition—thoughts about your thoughts. Meta-cognitive strategies as a means of change have arisen from a number of sources. The most obvious is that just as words control behavior through a process of learning, so inner speech (words said to yourself) can control behavior as well (Staats, 1972). Pavlov (1927) referred to this feature of conditioning as the "second signal system." It was Meichenbaum who really popularized this principle when he showed that impulsive, overactive children could approach academic tasks more successfully using self-instruction, in which they had to tell themselves to go slow, be more careful, take your time, and try to figure out what the task is (Meichenbaum, 1977; Meichenbaum & Goodman, 1971).

About the same time, educational psychologists became interested in what it was about children with mental retardation that made them poor learners. Typically developing children, when asked to memorize information at school, spontaneously use strategies such as cognitive rehearsal. Children with Down syndrome do not. But they can be taught to. It was soon demonstrated that children with intellectual disabilities could acquire internal strategies and mnemonic devices to help them learn academic tasks (Brown & Campione, 1986).

If together these four phenomena represent cognitive causal mechanisms, planned change might incorporate a raft of different elements. One is modifying basic processes (if cognitive process no longer distorts judgment, you could not conclude you were a failure). Another is altering content to render your dominant internal dialogue and word usage more accurate or less distressing ("it is not true I'm a failure; I'm a success"). A third is making the negative content less potent as a trigger to emotion (you still say to yourself you are a failure, but you do not let it bother you). A fourth is reorganizing complex thematic schema comprising memories of past incidents and all the related feelings (failure of a college course, of a marriage, and making a bad investment with the associated feelings of frustration, pain, and self-recrimination are all interconnected to our identity as a failure). A final change method is teaching self-talk as a regulatory and problem-solving strategy ("what do I have to do to succeed in the future?"). Although clearly cognitive in focus, we will not examine the self-talk, meta-cognitive approaches in detail until the next chapter, when we look at the whole issue of self-regulation. So the present discussion will revolve around the other four. Because all these approaches currently coexist in what is accepted as cognitive therapy in the literature, making a simple analysis of clinical change methods is just a little complicated.

Changing Words and Thoughts

Various early behavior therapists did not see the cognitive revolution in psychotherapy as particularly new. Systematic desensitization, the earliest of the well-established behavior therapy techniques for altering the emotional valence of object, situations, and events, typically exposed the client to a hierarchy of fear-arousing stimuli by means of vivid imaginal thoughts (Wolpe, 1958). Almost all conventional psychotherapy involves words and the power of words to change overt behavior, thinking patterns, and emotional responses (Staats, 1972). It is the case that early behaviorists tended to think of words as stimuli, whereas the cognitive approach tends to think of words as information, but the distinction can be quite subtle. Inner speech, reflection, internal dialogue, rumination, call it what you will, can easily bring about short-term behavior change. If you are sitting alone and you start thinking about pizza and how good one would taste, that may well be the antecedent event for going to the phone and ordering a pizza delivery. It does not explain where the thought came from, but the process of influence is not that different from a member of the family coming in and actually saying "let's have pizza tonight, would you call up and order a delivery?"

Beck's (1976) cognitive therapy, did, however, address many novel sources of influence. The basic theory is simple, although the details are complex. Certain forms of psychological distress, especially depression but anxiety disorders as well, are caused by negative cognitions, arising from errors of thought (e.g., overgeneralization: "Nobody likes me") and errors of information (e.g., incorrect inference: "She said she was too busy to join me for lunch, so she must not like me"). These conscious cognitions are emotive in content (like beliefs or attitudes) and tend to be personal or interpersonal. That is to say we might consider that someone who believes in the literal biblical account of creation has irrational cognitions, but these would not typically be the target for psychotherapy.

Because negative thoughts lead to emotional distress by rendering everyday situations as threatening (causing anxiety) or hopeless (causing depression) or blameworthy (causing guilt), aspects of cognitive therapy focus on changing the things clients say to themselves. This is done by Socratic questioning, persuasive communications, and exercises in which new words are practiced. It is important to understand that cognitive techniques are not arguments, in which the client's verbal habits and peripheral beliefs are challenged directly. Ironically, one of the major methods for countering unduly pessimistic or generally erroneous expectations is, in conjunction with the client, to work out convincing ways of testing the client's hypotheses and assumptions by performing behavioral experiments.

This is what Beck called collaborative empiricism. Agreed upon tasks, requiring behavior change in meaningful situations with careful observation of the outcome (reactions from others or our own subsequent feelings), are carried out by clients as "homework assignments" in the natural environment (Tee & Kazantzis, 2011). Unfortunately, people with seriously distorted thoughts, such as people with obsessive–compulsive tendencies, can and often do equally distort the implications of any observed outcomes: "OK, it is true I didn't get a coronary this time, but I was lucky; I might next time." That is a direct quote from a 25-year-old client of mine who had an unreasonable dread of having a heart attack if he engaged in any strenuous exercise. He had been declared totally healthy by a cardiologist and the agreed homework assignment was to take a short leisurely walk. This young man regularly brought me newspaper stories of top athletes dropping dead on the gridiron. I soon abandoned rational homework assignment as an intervention plan.

Furthermore, depressed clients do not explicitly trot out the three fundamental beliefs that Beck called the cognitive triad. You discover that these seem to underlie some of their thinking based on the types of content that dominate the client's discourse. This is equally true when identifying irrational beliefs the way that Ellis would have had us do. Clients, at least in my experience, do not start off by sitting down and saying things such as "I must be successful in order to feel as if I am a worthwhile person." Instead, what happens is that when you find they are spending long hours in the office that this is interfering with family life, and you suggest they take the weekend off or steer them to make the same suggestion, you get resistance in the form of an argument or a negation: "But I couldn't possibly do that." The therapists finds out why by asking what would happen if he just did take the weekend off, and what would happen if he didn't get some work finished, and what would happen if the client lost a sale, and so on. After systematic probing with "what if?" questions, the client will eventually say something such as "If I don't work hard all the time I won't be successful" and eventually "If I'm not successful I'd feel like a loser" and from there to "I must be successful in order to feel that I am a worthwhile person."

Correcting Erroneous Responsibility

In Western culture the dominant religions such as Catholicism and Judaism place a great deal of emphasis on taking responsibility for our actions and the induction of guilt for morally proscribed transgressions. I have already argued that guilt arising from punishment plays a large role in inhibiting socially sanctioned behavior. It is therefore not at all surprising that guilt is a dominant but irrational feature of those traumatic experiences that can cause symptoms of posttraumatic stress disorder (PTSD) and depression. I recently saw on U.S. national television a graphic interview with an injured veteran of the Iraq war who was returned to Iraq as part of a rehabilitation program. Five years earlier he had been wounded in the shoulder; his lieutenant had rushed toward him to help him and had been shot dead. This soldier stated that he had constant nightmares and saw his officer's face every time he relived the incident. He stated that he felt overwhelming guilt that this man had been killed on his behalf. Sometimes guilt is experienced from being the only person to survive a terrible disaster. Similar phenomena are regularly encountered in women victims of sexual assault; they wonder if they had somehow contributed to the rape in some way. Society adds to such burdens by often blaming the victim. And sometimes people who are responsible for terrible accidents that were entirely fortuitous are consumed with ongoing guilt and self-recriminations.

The strategies used to reduce guilt are essentially persuasive discourse, known as cognitive-processing therapy. But they are not just arguments—the persuasive communication is targeted at the common distortions seen in survivor guilt, such as ascertaining whether the person actually did something that went against their values. Kubany identified the most important distortion, which he called "hindsight bias" (Kubany & Ralston, 2008). This occurs when knowledge of an outcome distorts our memory of what we knew before the outcome was revealed. Typical statements revealing this bias are "I should have known better," "I should have seen it coming." Clients are shown through repeated examples and analogies that their judgment of the traumatic situation is based on what they know now rather than what they could reasonably have been expected to know at the time.

Changing Schemata

There are cognitive errors that seem to involve deficits in information processing rather than in just active reasoning processes. Information processing is not conscious and does not depend on words. It includes errors such as distorted memory processes (selective recall, for instance) and imperfect information processing (such as too much or too little selective attention). If current situations are judged according to our memory of similar situations in the past, it indicates that the meaning we make of events, particularly social and emotional events, is partly a function of how past experiences, particularly negative ones, are stored in autobiographical memory. If as a result you are wary of intimacy, of sexual advances, of aggression, or of commitment, reconstituting those memories should be one way of changing current behavior. A host of possible change mechanisms arise from this simple observation. Past experiences are rarely wholly negative, so they can often be reinterpreted as valuable learning opportunities, such as making you a more sensitive person, or, as in childbirth, the memory can be the joy of the baby rather than the pain endured. Revisionist history is not only good for politicians and dictators, it is a significant coping strategy, and makes it possible to develop a coherent self-identity.

Yet there are contexts in which the new inferences are much more subtle than this and involve our subjective experiences of reality and our awareness of the perspectives of others (theory of mind). Fonagy (see Bateman & Fonagy, 2011), coming from a psychoanalytic rather that a cognitive therapy perspective, argues that some clients, notably those diagnosed with borderline personality disorder (BPD), confuse their feelings in a situation with the probable thoughts and feelings of others in the situation. Calling this a deficit in mentalization, clients are taught to make more accurate mental representation (cognitions) of their own and other people's emotional states.

The clinical deficit can be nicely understood by an example I once heard Fonagy present at a symposium. He described observations of mothers with BPD playing with their children. One mother was playing nicely with her young daughter, but after a little while, as toddlers are wont to do, the little girl wandered away attracted by another toy in the playroom. At this point the mother said, "So, you don't want to play with mommy anymore?" By personalizing an incorrect inference the mother was also failing to teach the daughter authentic understanding of feelings as we would hope to happen in "emotion talk" described in Chapter 1.

Changing How We Experience Thoughts

A widely used cognitive strategy called decentering is based on an attempt to help clients recognize that individual schemata developed historically and their own thoughts are not reflections of absolute truth or reality. Some of us are happy to say to our friends, "what an idiot I was," but we recognize it as an exaggeration, a figure of speech. But with clients who are depressed, criticizing themselves in this way influences their mood and actual self-perception. The goal of decentering is to demonstrate to the person that thoughts are just thoughts. This can be achieved by mindfulness training in which the fact that a person is having a thought is acknowledged, but the indicative meaning of the thought is minimized. This, in turn, can be achieved by many different mental rehearsal strategies including classic Zen meditation (focusing intensely on one object), verbalizing the thought and accepting that you are having it, and refocusing attention on what you are actually doing—in therapy this might be slow breathing or muscle relaxation, and in life it might be the things you have to be doing concurrently, such as teaching, kicking a field goal, or nursing the baby.

Unwanted Thoughts and Images

Most people will have experienced being deep in thought when driving a car and realizing that for the past 10 minutes or so you were completely unaware of the traffic, the signs, and the roadway—you were just driving on autopilot. Probably everyone has had the experience of dissociation during a conversation with someone on a topic in which you are not terribly interested. You are nodding and agreeing at all the right places but you are not attending to their words—your thoughts are entirely elsewhere, maybe focused on some aspect of the person's appearance, but more usually focused on some totally irrelevant theme of interest or concern to you that is quite different from the topic of the conversation.

People with social anxieties, especially those seeming to stem from fear of negative evaluation, often attend excessively to how the person might be judging them. Occasional dissociation when in social contexts, or when driving a car, is not in any way harmful, although it can be annoying to the other person if detected, or dangerous if your reaction times are slowed. But extreme degrees of dissociation are emotionally disruptive, especially if your thoughts are unpleasant, angry, or negative. The great thing about engaging in rich everyday activities such as social conversations, long walks, playing tennis, watching TV, chairing a business meeting, or whatever you do, is that these activities can and should engage your attention and prevent unpleasant rumination. But because thoughts can run on their own parallel stream, many clients do experience this separation between their internal dialogue and their daily activities.

Thoughts and fantasies represent, therefore, a special type of psychological event in that they are not fully regulated by external environmental events. Social influences are more limited because thoughts are inherently private. In fact, thoughts are never known to anyone else unless they are expressed in words, either spoken or written. It is easy to change what someone says; it is much harder to change what they think or what they think about. So too with fantasies that involve inner sensations that are based on memory, or generated de novo by imagination, but that can be entirely separate from the stimulus array of the environment at the time the images are being generated. Images became used in change strategies early in the history of behavior therapy because people can produce them and they have stimulus properties and elicit emotional arousal almost as readily as the real event itself. Someone who is snake phobic can experience considerable amounts of anxiety simply by imagining a snake, or thinking of a snake (in words), or changing the valence of a harmless situation, such as a walk in a field, by generating a belief that snakes might be present. One of the best developed techniques for making the stimulus of a feared object or event less anxiety producing is to encourage the client to imagine the feared object while in a safe situation such as the therapist's office. The convenience and controllability of these imaginal hierarchies of ever increasing anxiety triggering capability is exactly what made systematic desensitization such a popular and effective therapeutic strategy.

What if trying to suppress your unwanted thoughts has the rebound effect that Wegner (1989) described? Could your worrying thoughts and ruminations that cause distress actually be made worse by deliberately trying to not think about them? You might be able to distract yourself for a while, but when that no longer works you are even more distressed than before. Some people seem to worry about their worrying, not unlike the fear of fear concept we have encountered already. It is not that they have more negative thoughts than before. Rebound effects mean the distress (anxiety, depression) caused by these returning thoughts is greater than before (Roemer & Borkovec, 1994).

This rather simple idea—for a few people the struggle against their problem *is* their problem—has given rise to a cluster of recent psychotherapeutic strategies, all converging on the concept of acceptance. At first blush the idea of acceptance as a therapeutic goal seems odd. You're having panic attacks? Don't fight them, just accept them. But of course the raison d'être of all acceptance models is that the acceptance results in the problems being ameliorated. Viktor Frankl's (1967) "paradoxical intention" has been well used in psychotherapy: encouraging clients to bring on their anxiety and to stop trying to evade or cope with their distress. This is a technique that seems to work particularly well for people who for social or experiential reasons find their manifestations of distress distressing.

Savoring, Mindfulness, and Meditation

Much of cognitive therapy has implicitly been focused on thoughts that are judged by others—particularly your therapist—to be irrational, erroneous, overly emotive, or inappropriate in some way. Clients are more likely to complain of difficulties tolerating certain thoughts and feelings. But the stream of consciousness, or the stream of experience, need not be dominated by negative thoughts, worrying thoughts, or rumination on what is wrong with your life. If your attention can be focused on positive external experiences, as well as internal feelings such as the pleasure of sexual satisfaction or feeling replete after a wonderful meal, then the psychological emphasis is more on enjoying pleasurable sensations than on tolerating negative ones.

This phenomenon of conscious attention to the experience of pleasure has recently been described in the literature as savoring (Bryant & Veroff, 2007). It is the perfect word for what we mean, psychologically. It is about concentrating on the enjoyment of the rich mouthful of a full-bodied Australian shiraz rather than gulping down a beer, or, since I have nothing against beer drinkers, actively feeling the pleasure of a cool beer on a hot summer day and admiring the condensation on a cold glass. Savoring involves a temporal sequence: you can anticipate an imminent pleasurable event ("we've got a 2003 Barossa Valley shiraz in the cellar that will go perfectly with the steak"), be in the moment while it is happening, and recapture some of the enjoyment by positive reminiscing ("wow, wasn't that a fantastic shiraz we had last night? I can still taste those blackberry and cherry flavors"). Not surprisingly, savoring has become a major concept in positive psychology. People who habitually savor life experiences are more contented, more optimistic, and less depressed than those who do not.

One of the very useful things about positive psychology as a movement is that when applied to the change we are trying to accomplish in psychotherapy it makes it possible to focus on beneficial outcomes far beyond simply surviving the negative (Seligman, 2002). We can return to a much earlier chapter in which I was examining the sorts of outcomes we expect with therapy: surely it is something more than symptom reduction, coping with negative feelings, or managing emotions? Positive change that results from truly effective therapy should mean something more than minimizing the negatives in life.

Savoring can, of course, be taught. It would be a very useful strategy to add to whatever other therapy you are doing. It is hard to know if people who are depressed, unhappy, and anxious are that way because they do not savor life's marvelous experiences, or whether having these predominant emotions makes it hard to savor anything. Part of what we mean by these conditions as clinical entities is that the person emphasizes the parched thirst and not the cool beer. After a sufficient period of time, however, it seems likely that many clients have stopped even trying to savor, or do not enjoy access to the social interactions that can facilitate it. Sharing the shiraz with your lover is going to bring greater pleasure than drinking it alone—as long as it is not your last bottle. In my past practice, I always noticed that as clients showed improvement they began to describe positive experiences, using sensory language and rich descriptions of positive sensations. Now, because the topic of savoring has become much better understood and studied, I personally would not wait until it begins to happen, but would try to start clients with exercises designed to get them to attend to and focus their concentration on pleasurable life events. This is slightly different from mindfulness and is carried out for a different purpose.

Although the cognitive processes relating to both meditation and mindfulness might be quite similar, the use of these two in planful therapeutic change is quite different. They have both recently become extremely popular ideas in therapy, especially cognitive–behavioral therapy, despite being very ancient practices of Buddhism and other Eastern psychologies. As therapeutic methods they really belong in the following chapter on self-influence, as the therapist can teach the principles and encourage clients to practice these cognitive skills, but for them to be effective they have to be utilized in situ by the client. As far as we know, they are not like the types of cognitive revelations—insights, for example—that happen in the course of therapy as an intense interpersonal interaction.

I said earlier that it is not literally possible to do nothing and so too it is literally impossible, when awake, not to engage in thought, and if those thoughts are upsetting, distress continues. However, it is very possible to focus attention on abstractions so completely that the troubled internal dialogue and vigilance toward negative events can be suspended. Meditation can achieve this. It brings attention to objects, internal sensations, and ideation so as to observe them without analyzing them. Buttle (2011) invokes the importance of working memory, which is hypothesized to have a central attentional system assisted by two slave systems, one verbal and one visual/spatial. Meditation can involve concentrated attention on a visual stimulus (object), but more often involves the repetition of a word or sound that allows for the prevention of intruding thoughts.

The recent resurgence of interest in mindfulness has a slightly different purpose (Segal, Williams, & Teasdale, 2002). Within ACT, the purpose of mindfulness training for clients is to disrupt the connection between a thought and an action or a thought and a feeling (Baer, 2010). Whereas in conventional cognitive therapy the goal is to change thoughts, the goal in ACT is to allow thoughts of any kind, but to make them irrelevant to how we feel and behave. There is an equal purpose in focusing attention on a feeling state, such as anxiety, and in a sense savoring it as a feeling rather than resisting it and trying to suppress it or get rid of it. The rationale for this is based on the importance that ACT theory places on the presence of experiential avoidance (intolerance of distressing feelings: anxiety sensitivity, for example). We might argue that experiential avoidance is characteristic of only some clients' personalities. But for those for whom it is a major component of what is maintaining distress, the strategy is logical.

Mental Imagery and Metaphor

Some versions of mindfulness training are very similar to other older methods in psychotherapy and behavior therapy that have made use of encouraging clients to conjure up mental images of tropical beaches and warm log fires that elicit feelings of peacefulness and calm. The behavioral interpretation is of the mental image as a stimulus, a direct substitute for the real object or event. In systematic desensitization, essentially an extinction procedure, the feared stimulus patterns are presented in imagination rather than in vivo, although a few clients, not used to this kind of experience, find it difficult to generate vivid imagery and report that they know they are thinking about a situation but cannot visualize it in their "mind's eye." When they can, the internal generation of an image, often with other sensory properties in addition to visual representation, is capable of eliciting the same distress in clients with phobias as external events can (Lohr & Hamberger, 1990).

It was not long before behavior therapists used the stimulus properties of mental imagery in other ways. In particular, the generation of highly negative images was used as though they were the aversive unconditioned stimulus (evoking, fear, disgust, shame, and so on) to be associated with positive but undesirable stimuli (the conditioned stimulus) in order to degrade them and lower their appetitive valence. A common presentation in this form of covert sensitization, as it is called, for someone with a drinking problem might be the following: "imagine yourself having a drink at a bar; now imagine that the booze has made you throw up, right on one of the other customers; it's revolting, puke is all over the bar and barman. Everyone is looking at you in disgust, cursing you and calling you names." In addition to the association between drinking alcohol and vomit, it was argued that that kind of scene also represented something like covert punishment—imagining the behavior being followed by imaginary negative consequences (Cautela, 1977).

Aversive images can also be used as a self-control device. One of my clients was a teenage boy who had been arrested for making obscene phone calls and for exhibitionism. The Honolulu police had caught him exposing himself in a suburban backyard and had brought him back to his parents' house still undressed in order to deliberately humiliate him. As just one component of a complex plan for change, we used the powerful imagery of him being arrested, handcuffed, and put naked in the back of the squad car and being marched up to the front door of his house as a negative stimulus complex to counteract some of the urges he was still having to go out and expose himself. If he felt the urge to roam the neighborhood he was asked to imagine this highly painful and embarrassing scene. If he resisted the urge, he was instructed to switch to relief—focusing on a new positive and optimistic image of himself being congratulated by his parents for overcoming temptation and of going to the high school ball where he meets a girl of his own age who seems to enjoy his company (covert reinforcement).

Positive imagery is more pleasant to use therapeutically. Mentally simulating positive interactions with others increases more tolerant attitudes (Crisp, Husnu, Meleady, Stathi, & Turner, 2010). For clients who can generate vivid imagery the potential of emotive imagery to evoke counteractive feelings is considerable, especially as the imagery can be tailored to their cultural and religious icons and symbols. When the Teenage Mutant Ninja Turtles were popular, Friedman, Campbell, and Evans (1993) encouraged a child who had to endure unpleasant medical procedures to fantasize himself as Leonardo, with magical powers. Imagining himself as a superhero allows the fearful child to enact the feelings and deeds of someone brave. Aspects of Buddhist meditation encourage adults to imagine that they are in the form of a deity, promoting compassion and kindness. With adults, vivid symbols serve as emotive primes, activating positive emotional schema (Evans, 2010).

Imagery and role playing are helpful ways of encouraging children and less verbal people to acquire self-management skills. A standard practice when teaching young children a relaxation procedure is to ask them to pretend they are a rag doll, all loose and floppy. To teach young active children to inhibit impulsive behavior you teach them to stand absolutely still like a stone statue (on the playground this is the game of Statues), or to play Red Light/Green Light (called Grandmother's Footsteps in Britain). To help children self-sooth you have them imagine they are a kettle and the water is getting hotter and hotter and is about to boil in a cloud of steam. Turn down the gas, switch off the power, unplug the kettle, and feel the bubbling water cool down. In Hawaii we always asked children to think of the volcano Kilauea Iki they all knew about, and to feel the tension inside them like the hot lava about to erupt and then use imagery: "Now let the lava cool and subside, the volcano is not going to explode today; it is perfectly natural for lava to get hot, but it can drain back into the earth through little crevices where it is cooled by the rain water that trickles out to help all the lush vegetation grow on the sides of the mighty mountain of Kilauea. *Kahili ikaika*, stand strong like that mountain; let the lava cool."

Metaphors

Metaphorical language has always been used in psychotherapy (Lakoff & Johnson, 1980). Idiomatic language represents complete communication since it conveys the pattern of cognitive (words and images) and emotive associations of dominant schemata. From an assessment perspective, listening carefully to clients' discourse provides information on their idioms of distress: "not being in balance," "out of sync with the rest of the world," "my thinking is coming unglued." After an hour of initial assessment of a 6-year-old girl with hard to pin down severe tantrums and outbursts of violent aggression, her father remarked as they were leaving my office, "Maybe it's time to splash the holy water around." I asked him to come back in and explain why he thought his daughter was possessed. He laughed nervously, but then for the first time specified that it was the vacant look in her eyes when her rages began and the fact that they did not seem to be triggered by frustration, but were preceded by repetitive jiggling of her foot. Immediately I had a new hypothesis, later confirmed by a pediatric neurologist: this little girl was having complex partial temporal lobe seizures, innervating her limbic system according to the electroencephalogram (EEG).

Recently metaphor has become a popular topic in cognitive–behavioral therapy (Stott et al., 2010). If the therapist tries to alter or replace self-perceptions through the use of metaphor, the strategy becomes a potential change process. The essential idea is that autobiographical memories will be altered and new patterns of association built up, generating revised automatic thoughts and assumptions. Even processes of change and prospects for future outcomes, as I stated in Chapter 1 and as we shall encounter again in Chapter 11, are often metaphors that shape beliefs and expectations, sometimes in unpredictable ways. Envisioning the therapist as a life raft will not encourage a client to swim to safety. The client who has been sexually abused and now perceives herself as permanently scarred may have a concept of possible change different from the client who now perceives herself as Zena, warrior princess.

Therapists use metaphors to clarify arguments and information that they hope clients will better accept and understand. Metaphorical language aids communication in the same way that figures of speech in poetry and prose are able to evoke mood and feeling more fully than propositional language can. Suggesting to a parent that she is like a mother hen conveys a sense of overprotectiveness that might be more evocative than if you stated that she is exercising too much control over her children's striving for autonomy. However, clients' understanding of a therapist's metaphors may be very different than intended: "mother hen" just as easily conveys futile lack of protection from attacks by predators. When professors agree to take a doctoral student under their wing, are they implying gentle mentoring or are they shielding the student from the heartlessness of academia? Metaphors are highly culturally specific, and thus not always suited to the client's unique history of images and associations.

Perhaps most concerning of all is the fact that metaphors depend on analogy, and analogies, by definition, are never perfect matches of the phenomenon so described. ACT therapists like to have clients think about being trapped in a hole in sandy ground that they are trying to dig their way out of with a shovel. The more they dig the more the earth caves in around them. The intent is to convey to clients the idea that their own struggles to manage distressing feelings are actually making it less likely that they will overcome their distress. Combined with that explanation, the metaphor is expressive; by itself it is a bit misleading, especially if the client tends toward literality. It is difficult to see metaphorical discourse in therapy as a principle of change rather than yet another technique for conveying therapeutic influence, the purpose of which must still be specified. On the other hand, because metaphors typically evoke emotional imagery, rescripting clients' metaphors (proposing alternative, more benign ones) should reduce one source of ongoing negative internal stimuli. The client with chronic pain who describes the pain metaphorically as "being branded with a red hot poker" can actually visualize the poker and the seared flesh. Reducing the words and images and replacing them with images of cooling, of healthy tissue, and of the gate closing on the pain nerves should assist in pain management (Frazer et al., 2002).

Implications

An emphasis throughout this book on constructing the alternatives to the things we want to change applies equally well to changing cognitions. Distressing thoughts need to be replaced with alternatives. It cannot be assumed that after cognitive change people will just change from being depressed or anxious caterpillars and suddenly emerge as happy, jolly butterflies without a care in the world. We need to think much more carefully about the likely and appropriate alternatives, just as we must when reducing excess, challenging behavior in people with intellectual disabilities, or helping offenders change from criminal activities to socially appropriate ones.

What are these alternative cognitions? For thoughts whose content is irrational and self-deprecating or driven by hindsight bias we want people to be more optimistic and reasonably capable of evaluating their own successes and contributions. [Not too capable, as most of us would be depressed if our self-evaluations were too accurate—depressed people are called sadder but wiser (Alloy & Abramson, 1979)!] For ruminations we want to be able to switch off task-irrelevant thoughts and be able to focus more mindfully on the present or future activities and the things we really want to do and the goals we want to achieve (Kabat-Zinn, 2003). And that might include savoring the present so that the full richness of any current experience can be appreciated and enjoyed. If the current situation is a sad one, we want to be able to have enough empathy that we are mobilized to help others. For worries, we need to be able to replace them with constructive plans and to take action to try to solve the specific things we worry about. For memories that contain strong association with fear or guilt or regrets we want to be able to reevaluate them, facilitating recall of the more positive elements of the experience. For the imagery and metaphorical language we use in everyday conversation and definition of our self-identity we want new scripts, more accurate metaphors, and words and images that are more closely analogous with reality. The movement known as Positive Psychology comes much closer to the ideal of helping clients develop the affirming alternatives to negative ideation. Seligman's original theory focused on what he called "authentic happiness."

Throughout this book I have been attempting not to describe any particular method of therapy. In presenting the major principles of changing cognitions, however, it is difficult not to do so. This is because cognitive therapies have to a large extent created their own principles of change rather than drawing on the more fundamental theories of how cognitions interface with general psychological functioning. Some leading theorists, such as Teasdale (e.g., Barnard & Teasdale, 1991; Teasdale, 1999), have managed, after the fact, to place a more rigorous psychological interpretation on the methods of treatment that were developed on the fly by clinicians such as Beck. Others have reversed this process. For example, Hayes (2004) has a sophisticated radical behavioral perspective constructed around principles such as stimulus equivalence and relational frame theory. His now very popular therapeutic techniques were supposedly derived from theory; however, many observers have been hard-pressed to see the logical derivation of techniques such as mindfulness from the theory (Arch & Craske, 2008; Leahy, 2008). Indeed, mindfulness was first introduced into cognitive–behavioral therapy by Linehan, following a totally different set of theoretical assumptions. However, Hayes's theory and clinical techniques, touted as a "third wave" in cognitive–behavioral therapy, would not actually be considered by him to be part of cognitive therapy at all, nor of belonging in this chapter. In some ways I would agree with this: the most obvious rationale for mindfulness the way it is used in ACT is to decouple any connection between a thought and its associated feeling. The most obvious rationale for acceptance training is that for some clients (but by no means all) the aversiveness of negative emotion exacerbates their distress ("experiential avoidance").

One of the intriguing features of cognitive therapies is how they all encourage overt behavior change. In treating depression, Jacobson's approach was to promote the performance of once enjoyed activities: "behavioral activation" (Jacobson et al., 1996). Beck's approach encourages clients to test their hypotheses by seeing if negative consequences followed approach behaviors. And Hayes's techniques are called "ACT" rather than A.C.T. in order to emphasize that clients need to commit to engage in new actions. None of this negates the importance of changing schemata, only that direct evidence from new experiences is possibly as important as verbal persuasion by a therapist. Furthermore, in the next chapter on self-influence, we find that all the things therapists do can potentially be done by the individual alone. There are, as Mark Twain said, many ways to skin a cat.

9

Self-Influence

> The Camel's hump is an ugly lump
> Which well you may see at the Zoo;
> But uglier yet is the hump we get
> From having too little to do.
>   (Rudyard Kipling, 1919)

Rudyard Kipling had a solution for dealing with negative moods he claimed all children and adults will experience on occasion: not to mope around but to get out into the garden in the sun and the wind and dig *"till you gently perspire"* (Kipling, 1919/2008). Apart from being a bit rude about camels, his advice recognizes two important principles of change: first, engaging in busy behaviors is helpful because inaction and idleness are aversive (Hsee, Yang, & Wang, 2010), and second, we should be personally responsible for changing our own moods when, as Kipling described it, "We climb out of bed with a frowzily head, And a snarly-yarly voice." The previous chapter was all about a special form of social and experiential influence in which our conscious thought processes, as well as nonconscious processing of information, might be altered therapeutically in order to change our feelings and actions—our moods and overt behavior. But people are also fully capable of changing their own behavior and do so all the time, often by allowing themselves to realign their cognitions and understanding as a result of deliberately creating new experiences. People work all on their own toward goals, learn new skills, cope with adversity, self-calm through meditation, resist social pressure, deliberately expose themselves to anxiety-provoking situations, use distraction to manage pain, listen to music to chill out, pray to gain courage, read to find new ideas, and fight depression with mindfulness, to name but a few.

These are the very things for which many seek therapeutic treatment, so there may well be a subgroup of the population that does not have effective skills for managing its distress or maximizing its quality of life. They are the ones who become clients. Even "wicked problems" such as alcohol dependency can show substantial rates of amelioration without any professional treatment, and half of these involve low-risk drinking rather than abstinence (Dawson, Grant, Stinson, Chou, Huang, & Ruan, 2005). By watching Supernanny on TV, or reading her book, parents can correct their previous practices and self-initiate her "cycle of change" by increasing praise and positive attention to their children (Frost, 2006). There is a certain irony in realizing that our clients in professional practice are the people who are the least able to change on their own, and yet encouraging self-change and promoting autonomy are quintessential values in clinical psychotherapy.

There is an unusual feature of this topic and that is the dualism that is inherent in the concept of people "changing their own behavior," which implies that their personhood, their self, is different from their behavior. It seems to suggest that there is a self-mechanism—the real you—that can direct what you do and how you act. Logically there cannot really be two separate entities—yourself and your behavior—but we try to make this distinction all the time. We frequently hide our true feelings, or say something and think the opposite. It is an inevitable consequence of human consciousness: to be aware of yourself and aware of others' awareness. When someone accuses you of a negative action, you might reply, "I'm sorry; I didn't mean to do it." When a with-it mother corrects her young son, she might say "That is a very naughty thing to do. I'm not criticizing you, I'm criticizing your behavior." When a manager is complaining about a worker's error, she might say "I'm surprised at you not following the safety regulations—you should know better than to act that way."

To avoid dualism it is necessary to have a more careful model of what it is we mean by people regulating or managing their own reactions and behaviors. Knowing that repertoires are interrelated, behavioral psychologists attempted to address this need by thinking of self-control as engaging in one action, called an enabling behavior, which makes a new action more or less probable. To remember something in the future, tie a knot in your handkerchief while you remember it now, or if you are not quite so old-fashioned, enter a reminder in your smart phone; knowing you will not be able to resist the allure of the Sirens' song, do as Ulysses did and tie yourself to the mast before you hear it. Anticipating that going to a party alone will elicit considerable anxiety, individuals with social phobia will contact a friend with whom they feel really comfortable and ask the friend to come to the party with them. Conscious that she will have a difficult time resisting buying cute clothes for her granddaughter, the grandmother who is trying to save money will window shop the children's stores in town without taking her credit card with her. When clients can be made aware of their susceptibility to certain environmental influences they can be taught the value of self-directed anticipation and hence avoidance of situations that might lead them astray. (When we do so clinically it is called relapse prevention.) I do not want to be too precious about the dualism issue, however—it is simpler to call all these actions self-influence rather than the cumbersome phrase "enabling behaviors."

As so much of our behavior is already self-directed and planful, a clinically important form of self-influence is self-control. This is when you actively resist performing desired actions or acting on urges because you are aware that doing so could be harmful (having a second helping of ice cream; giving the finger to a driver who has cut you off), socially unacceptable (yelling at a subordinate at work), illegal (speeding when in a terrible hurry), or contrary to your values (making a pass at an attractive person who is not your partner). Self-control such as this typically involves deliberate strategies to resist temptation and suppress reflexive responses. Self-regulation of emotions learned during socialization, however, is different and does not always involve deliberate, overt strategies but acquired unconscious competencies in shifting attention (distraction), self-soothing, and regaining equilibrium. Adaptive regulation of emotion does not involve simply suppressing emotions. It also involves increasing emotional arousal and exaggerated expression when the situation requires it, such as when playing an imaginative game, encouraging others in the team, or delivering a lecture on a dry topic. These emotion-regulation competencies are learned in early childhood.

The behaviors we call active coping strategies are classic examples of self-change at least in the short term: performing one accessible action in order to manage others that are less under voluntary control. The fundamental idea that behaviors are the independent variables for other behaviors emerges again. Not long ago I heard Larry King interview Chelsea Handler, a late-night talk-show host. During the interview, while she was explaining that much as she loved her work she found it very stressful, she remarked, "Pilates keeps me sane." Everyone would know what she meant: it was a figure of speech in which she was extolling the virtue of a specific physical and mental exercise routine (emphasizing control of posture and breathing) to cope with stress. Most of us know how to engage in one set of actions to manage another.

A Paradox: Influential Therapists Promote Self-Change

All therapists should encourage clients to pursue effective self-change strategies. To explain why this is so it is necessary to go back to the therapeutic framework—the context within which therapy occurs, and where generalization and maintenance are vital, as is some sort of cumulative trajectory of clinical improvement. Most therapists I have encountered give clients encouragement for the future by emphasizing that it is they, and not the therapist, who is bringing about the desired change. I certainly have taught and practiced this kind of interpretation. We may tell clients that they are embarking on a journey (metaphors rule!) for which you the therapist are merely providing the roadmap and the compass: "As the journey may be difficult, other supports might be needed—for example, medication could be useful at first, just like a good walking stick might help you over the difficult initial stage of the journey. As you become more confident, fitter, or the path becomes easier, you can stop using the walking stick and stop using the pills. And you will not need me as a therapist forever either: once I have shown you the road and you are strolling confidently along it, I will wave you goodbye; all I want is a postcard when you reach your desired destination."

Such figurative discourse is neither a trick nor deceptive. The implications are accurate in many ways. Clients cannot rely on the therapist being at their side and offering advice and encouragement and support for any length of time. At some point therapy has to be terminated and that will usually occur well before the client is totally free of all the concerns that brought him or her into treatment. Even more importantly than that, this kind of discourse underscores the need for clients to gain independence, right from the start of treatment—they will have to do many things on their own. They must begin to practice self-change in order to become more autonomous, relying only on natural supports such as friends and family. These are well-accepted values of professional intervention and change.

A client with depression can be given a homework assignment within one or two early treatment sessions. Clients are asked to generate alternative, "glass is half full" kinds of statement to replace pessimistic, hopeless forms of cognitive content, and to practice saying these things at home. That is clearly a self-change strategy by definition, even though the strategy has been suggested to them, perhaps even required of them, by the therapist. Another interesting kind of "do-it-yourself" suggestion in therapy comes from a further metaphor encouraging independence. This analogy was originally proposed by Michael Mahoney (1976). His contention was that good therapy involves exploration, careful self-observation, and the testing of hypotheses. Essentially this is the same as the scientific method, and so clients could really think of themselves as scientists. This is a particularly useful metaphor when the therapeutic goal is to challenge erroneous and illogical beliefs. If someone with a social phobia has a strong belief that he or she will be negatively judged by others and rejected in social situations, then it is a very obvious strategy to encourage him or her to test this out. Seeing what will happen when you try something—in this case a social overture to someone—is just like the scientific method of testing a hypothesis.

Self-change often involves attempting something different and noticing and being interested in what happens. Whether done by clients on their own, or encouraged by a therapist, the two principles of this sort of discovery by trial and error are exactly the same. First, it must be seen as a trial, so even a negative outcome provides you with information (just like any good science experiment)—success is judged from trying, not from the outcome. Second, it has to be a fair test of the hypotheses. If you are a socially phobic teenager you cannot properly check your hypothesis that you are likely to be rejected if you test it by approaching the most popular, high-status student in the school and ask the student to be your prom date. Rejection, if you are a bit anxious and not very socially skilled, is highly probable. Instead, you have to select a more promising person (but not another shy one) who you like and ask that person to join you at Starbucks for a caramel mochachino after school. You might still be rejected (fine, that's information), but the chances are less likely. As a therapist you can explain all of these variables to your client and help design a fair experiment. In self-change the client has to figure them out for himself or herself. Either way it is up to the client to initiate the easier, higher probability behavior in order to make other behaviors in the chain more probable. It is easier to approach a peer socially when it is just an experiment, or it is just for coffee, yet it facilitates a more difficult, less probable set of behaviors, such as a more formal invitation for a date.

Basic Principles of Self-Modification

It should not come as a surprise that when explaining and arranging change there is nothing fundamentally different between planning it yourself and putting yourself in the hands of a therapist to plan it for you. In other words, self-modification is not a principle of change at all but a tactic, one that by definition means a therapist or other change agent is less directly involved. In therapy, the therapist implants an idea or proposes an activity that he or she thinks the client is capable of and that will have the effect desired. Clients either cannot generate new ideas or do not know these means–ends rules and cannot apply them in problematic situations (individual skill differences described in Chapter 4). So when clients are taught self-change as a general set of principles, they are really being taught the rules that make easy, accessible Behavior A more likely to result in a change in difficult Behavior B.

Behavior A is a usually a matter of rearranging your social or physical environment to better meet your needs. But thinking back to the discussion of different structural relationships among behaviors, the "change A to change B" is rather simplistic. Sometimes Behavior A will set the occasion for Behavior B, sometimes it will be a prerequisite, and sometimes it will be incompatible with Behavior B. Emotions illustrate this last principle quite well. The physiological expressions of emotion are often not under voluntary control, however emotionally well-regulated you may be. If you faint at the sight of blood, gag when presented with a food associated with chemotherapy, or experience anxiety in a social situation, you cannot simply tell yourself not to feel this way. You cannot tell children to stop crying the same way you can ask them to stop hitting their sister. But fortunately the autonomic nervous system seems to have its own checks and balances in the form of homeostatic control. Deep muscle relaxation is incompatible with—reciprocally inhibits—anxiety; sexual arousal dampens down fear (unfortunately, the reverse is also true); anger subsides over time through exhaustion; REM sleep overcomes stress.

Self-Help Manuals

To obtain a sense of how psychologists systematically promote all of those rules, we only need to examine the foremost textbooks designed to teach individuals (not just clients) how to change their own behavior. As in clinical practice, these works often start off with the assumption that the individuals have an excess behavior that they consider undesirable and that they would like to engage in less, or that they have a deficit behavior that they would like to increase in frequency. In one the most successful of these books—Watson and Tharp (1977)—the examples given are wanting to exercise more, do more homework, eat less, watch less TV, quit smoking, have fewer marital arguments, and reduce the frequency of temper outbursts. These are hardly the most significant emotional and social problems that bring clients into therapy, but if we cannot understand and change the simpler behaviors it is unlikely we will be able to understand and change the most complex ones.

So let us summarize the main suggestions for self-change. Basically, you first have to decide what is changeworthy and set a goal. Then you have to do one of two things to modify your own behavior: arrange for new or different stimuli for the identified behaviors (stimulus control) or arrange for new or different consequences for these behaviors (self-reward). (Behavior is controlled by antecedents and consequences.) At the same time, you have to fight off that evil force, procrastination. Finally, you have to have some way of obtaining feedback (monitoring your progress), which can also be reactive.

Setting Your Own Goals

When someone is consciously attempting a self-directed change program, their goal is usually fairly specific—they want to exercise more for health reasons, they want to lose weight for their niece's wedding, they want to save money for a trip overseas, or they want to spend longer hours studying to improve their grades and gain admission to medical school. Mischel (1973) saw self-regulation and planning as one component of a social–cognitive dimension of personality. The importance of goals for motivating change has already been explained in Chapter 3, and from this analysis effective goal-related conditions can be suggested, for which there is a reasonable amount of evidence (e.g., Lutz, Karoly, & Okun, 2008). The individual has to value the goal, think about it positively, and feel it is attainable by his or her own effort (self-efficacy belief). The individual has to decide whether the desired level of the goal is strictly personal ("I'll feel better if I shed five pounds") or is based on social comparison ("I'll look better than my brother, the father of the bride, if I lose weight before the wedding") or social norms ("A healthy man of my height and build should weigh 180 pounds, so I need to shed 10 pounds"). A measurable outcome for our self-change program allows consistent self-monitoring of outcome (weight) and of strategy (number of hours at the gym this week). Specifying the goal in terms of a positive approach enables the individual to feel satisfied when progress is being made and not be self-critical when progress is slow.

Personal goal setting is confounded with motivation to change. In addition to determination to achieve a particular outcome, other influences are intriguing. Contracts, or any verbal agreement to do something, are considered obligatory in our legal system. A public statement that you intend to change seems to operate in the same way. Not surprisingly, within therapist-directed change programs, written contracts became a popular behavioral intervention. These can be between a teenager and his or her parents, or between distressed couples, and they usually contain specification of the rewarding consequences of the desired action. But they can just be between the therapist and the client without any stated contingency. You can also write your own contract with yourself, specifying precisely what you plan to do.

Why is it that a public commitment to change seems to make it easier to adhere to a personal change plan? Maybe more social support and encouragement are elicited that way. Maybe it comes from the fact that in many cultures we are taught as children the importance of finishing something we set out to do. In New Zealand society, as is probably the case in many others, it is especially important not to be seen as a "quitter." Agreements to do something are considered very important—if you do not follow through on a commitment you are "letting the side down." In New Zealand, when prominent public figures are caught doing something wrong they almost always say "I let myself down."

Self-Management of Antecedents, Consequences, and Priorities
Stimulus Control

It is difficult for me to see how someone could be a successful agent of change (either for yourself or, as a therapist, for others) without a reasonably good understanding of how environmental cues, including those from your own internal proprioception, elicit, evoke, or trigger reactions. We have seen earlier that the vast experimental literature on classical conditioning tells us much about how, through association, the significance (meaning) and the valence (affective properties or attitude) of stimuli can be changed. Although in terms of underlying mechanisms in the central nervous system the basis for this change is most probably networks of stimulus–stimulus connections, the reality for any of us as individuals is that certain stimuli come, through learning, to elicit responses just as readily as in simple, unlearned, reflexive circuits. Similarly, in instrumental conditioning, a discriminative stimulus—one consistently signaling the availability of reinforcement—comes to control behavior with high degrees of reliability, such that the operant will be performed only in its presence [Staats' Attitude–Reinforcement–Discrimination (A-R-D) concept]. Less obvious in either paradigm is that other external and seemingly irrelevant cues arising from the environmental context also come to control behavior.

Because most simple habits that we would like to eliminate happen automatically, there are essentially two strategies for extinguishing them. One is to change the context in some way so that the triggering stimulus is no longer quite the same or quite so available. This is the rather unfortunate Victorian strategy of smearing bitter aloe on the child's thumb to eliminate thumb sucking. It has been claimed that in treating childhood enuresis, changing the cue complex of the bed, such as raising the end of the bed on a couple of bricks, reduces the likelihood of wetting (Turner, Young, & Rachman, 1970). The other, preferred method is to evoke an incompatible response to the triggering cue. It seems that this is approximately how the bell and pad method for treating enuresis works as the internal cue of the full bladder comes to elicit waking up, the response elicited by the loud bell ringing the moment the child starts to wet the bed (Doleys, 1977).

If feasible, the therapist encourages the client to deliberately practice an alternative, incompatible response in the presence of the cue. In a habit problem such as trichotillomania, for instance, there are good case studies in the early history of behavior therapy in which clients would be taught to deliberately get hold of a hair, feel it in their fingers (the stimulus usually triggering the response), and then instead of plucking it, deliberately opening their fingers, letting go, and putting their hand down (Taylor, 1963). Some have argued, quite reasonably, that actually these kinds of strategies also change the cue complex simply by focusing conscious attention on the task. There are lots of responses that have become automatic that are interfered with by consciously thinking about performing them—as illustrated by the old joke that the way to paralyze a centipede is to ask it which leg it starts off with.

Mindfulness exercises can be taught first in formal therapy contexts, but then the clients are asked to practice and to use the techniques on their own during critical moments. There are various strategies used in mindfulness training, such as body scan (the person lies prone, systematically goes over all body parts, and focuses on that part of the body), sitting meditation (classic lotus position), mindful movement, which is essentially Yoga, walking mindfulness, which involves focusing on and being aware of our changing environment, and focus on an image of a mountain with its aloof strength and isolated beauty. All of these areas of focus can be taught directly, or learned via a CD.

The goals of mindfulness training with people with substance abuse difficulties are to reduce the "automatic pilot" effect in which behaviors just occur without much prior thought or choice, being more aware of triggers, greater acceptance of discomfort, and developing an overall lifestyle in favor of recovery (Hsu, Grow, & Marlatt, 2008). As those with an addiction tend to focus on and be overly influenced by the urge to use the substance, a specific image is used in the mindfulness training—riding a large wave on a surfboard—you can "surf" the urge like a wave, stay on top of it, and know that it will eventually fade away like all waves—part of the ebb and flow—so stay with the wave, ride it out. Drug abusers are given a specific mnemonic called SOBER, which stands for stop, observe, take a mindful breath, expand (focus awareness on external stimuli, not internal feelings), and respond (choose an appropriate, adaptive response). Cravings are reduced by both formal and informal practice.

The reason I introduce these very effective habit control procedures in the discussion of self-change is partly that anyone can come up with these procedures on their own but also that if taught the general principle by a therapist it is then very much up to clients to practice and make the necessary changes in their own natural environment. A very good example of this is the essence of Bootzin's well-established stimulus-control method for changing patterns of insomnia (e.g., Bootzin, Epstein, & Wood, 1991). It is not the only component—after all anxiety about not being able to fall asleep the night before an important event is a classic example of that "fear of fear" phenomenon (worrying interfering directly with what you are worrying about not achieving—sleep). But the stimulus-control argument is that going to bed (snuggling under a warm blanket and turning out the light) or just lying in bed must be a cue simply for falling asleep, not for reading a book, having a brief rest, watching TV, thinking about plans for tomorrow, or any other activity incompatible with sleep. Thus, the client is prescribed a simple practice routine that prohibits any activity in bed other than sleep; a client who cannot fall asleep quickly must get up, get out of bed, and do those other tasks such as watching TV or reading a book somewhere else in the house until feeling sleepy again. Bootzin has commented that any time this approach has failed it is almost always because the client did not follow the instructions to the letter. The actual procedure is not complicated—anyone can learn it from a book. But the principles need to drive the method.

Self-Reward

One of the interesting things about self-reward is that because of the process known as "reducing cognitive dissonance" we can seek and obtain satisfaction from actions even if they do not actually result in the intended positive consequences. The wry comment "experience is what you get when you don't get what you want" vividly conveys one way we can justify to ourselves a certain level of nonreward. The phenomenon of sour grapes, often seen as the classic illustration of cognitive dissonance reduction, reveals a possible mechanism of such reduction, namely adaptive preference formation. This is a little like an acquired taste—by repeated experience, preferably in a socially engaging context, we come to enjoy things (Mexican peppers, single malt Scotch, jazz, abstract art) that we originally found unpleasant or strange. Edmund Burke (1759/1909) told us long ago: "A man frequently comes to prefer the taste of tobacco to that of sugar... but this makes no confusion in tastes, whilst he knows that habit alone has reconciled his palate to these alien pleasures" (p. 2).

We do know that people who are depressed do not engage in much self-reinforcement (Fuchs & Rehm, 1977) and happy children are more likely to self-reward. Clients, whether seeking new rewards on their own or being encouraged by a therapist to find new sources of satisfaction, need to focus on the enjoyment that comes from a good book, meeting friends, a great wine, a magnificent symphony, a deep conversation, or a brilliant touchdown in football. As shown in Chapter 6, rewards for humans are not so much the objects themselves as the pleasure we draw from them. An item from a well-known self-reinforcement questionnaire (Heiby, 1982) is "When I do something right, I take time to enjoy the feeling."

So that is one meaning of self-reward: allowing yourself to enjoy your own success, even when you were not that successful. But for a long time there has been another more literal meaning. This is when after doing something you set out to do, you overtly reward yourself with a treat of some kind. The odd thing about such a strategy is that if you are rewarding yourself you presumably have free access to the treat, so why would this function as reinforcement? There is no imposed contingency rule. You can just help yourself any time you want. But our socialization seems to play a defining role in not rewarding yourself for poor performance. Children acquire internal standards and are not satisfied until they are met. Mischel found that American children will not help themselves to a freely offered reward if they themselves do not believe that they deserve it. And if you guarantee them a reward for any easy task, such as hitting a large bulls-eye with a dart, they will deliberately make the task harder, for example, they will step much further back from the target (for a summary, see Mischel, 2004). Exactly where these internal standards come from is less clear, but doubtless skilled peers, parents, teachers, sports heroes, and religious faiths are all among the social agencies that define high standards to which children should aspire.

I do not believe that self-administered reward operates psychologically the same way as external reinforcement, but it does seem to help change behavior by reducing procrastination (see below). The lesson from all self-modification books is to encourage readers to set up a reward program for meeting their behavioral goals. As a therapist it is quite entertaining to encourage clients to do the same. They look at you quizzically. But if they actually do it, they are learning the principle of positive consequences, allowing themselves to recognize success, and have something amusing to tell you about the next session: "I went to a movie on Friday to reward myself for not screaming at the kids all week, just like you told me to!" Note too, that just as people can reward themselves, so they can punish themselves. This can be emotional, such as self-blame for something not really that bad. Some therapists have tried the idea of asking the client who is trying to exercise restraint to hand over a sum of money; every time clients break their own rule and transgress, the therapist sends a percentage of that money to the client's most disliked charity. Clients can set up their own self-punitive rule exactly the same way. There are reports that this is an effective strategy, but I would not bet the farm on it. Most of these demonstrations of change principles are little more than generalized social conformity.

The Thief of Time

There is surely a stage of change that Prochaska and DiClemente missed, and that is the one in which the individual starts to take action but finds there are other priorities demanding more immediate attention. This stage is known to some of us as the principle "never put off 'til tomorrow what you can possibly do the day after." Procrastination is an interesting example of self-regulatory failure because it is so common, and known so well to most us (except the ultraconscientious), that its potency challenges all of the rational strategies usually included in discussing self-change. Steel (2007) conducted a fine meta-analysis of the large volume of research on procrastination. He concluded that neuroticism per se (anxiety) is not the issue. But dithering is something we do when in conflict in aversive situations. We procrastinate when tasks are aversive, so a possible strategy is to find ways of making boring tasks more challenging and difficult tasks a little easier. Conflict often arises when rewards are delayed, so setting shorter, intermediate, more easily achieved goals should benefit us and our clients. A number of people are less able to stay motivated when rewards are deferred, and they need to be able to generate more immediate ones.

In Chapter 3 I introduced the motivational construct of intentions. Disruptions to intended activities can seem like procrastinations when in fact they are often unavoidable. From a self-modification perspective our intentions—written, spoken to others, or just thought—affect our daily routines and activities, as opposed to our big life goals and dreams of possible selves that influence long-range plans and aspirations. Everyday intentions are easily disrupted by sudden circumstances—an e-mail demanding attention, a phone call request from a friend, a sudden moment of self-efficacy doubt, or a sick child at home. It has also been noted in the experimental literature that environmental cues unconsciously prime associated concepts, which can then interfere with the intended action (Gollwitzer, Sheeran, Trötschel, & Webb, 2011). If someone around you talks about sleep, tiredness, or being drowsy, for example, you would be unaware that this has primed you to take a nap later rather than work on finishing an assignment. Gollwitzer and colleagues suggest that an antidote to unwanted conflicting influence of primes is to form "implementation intentions." These simply encourage you to specify very precisely the when, where, and how of an intended course of action: "I'll finish my essay on positive affective priming this afternoon, in the library, using the materials I have stored on my laptop under 'psychology: self-regulation.'"

Procrastination can also be reduced by increasing our expectations of success. Self-efficacy is certainly relevant here, and these beliefs are open to social influence. Being surrounded by cues that are related to the task that must be completed is another stimulus-control strategy to reduce temptation. Making the less desirable behavior more automatic, part of a regular daily routine, also combats procrastination. It should also be possible to condition positive affect to effort itself by reinforcing effort with intermediate rewards—a glass of a good red wine for every five assignments conscientiously graded is one of my own strategies.

The Reactivity of Self-Recording

If you think back to Chapter 2 on understanding and defining change you will recall the argument that relying only on questionnaires and self-report instruments is not a particularly good way of measuring change. But they are convenient for therapists who should always be monitoring client progress in order to adjust and moderate treatment variables in a more effective manner, particularly if there are periods of apparently little change, as early change seems to lead to better outcomes. Behavior therapists in particular like to ask clients to estimate their own degree of change, using some sort of arbitrary scaling procedure. Examples are the Fear Thermometer in which clients estimate their level of fear from 0 (none) to 100 (the most intense it can be), and subjective units of distress (SUDS) in which you ask clients to report on a scale of 1 to 10 how distressed they are, or, as in solution-focused therapy, how close they are to their positive goals. Evaluating progress in this way is something clients can do for themselves and conveys useful ideas about self-reflection and being aware of improvements, which can be received in a mindful way regardless of how small they may be.

Changes can be small, but they should not be too slow. Advocates of "precision teaching" from the Skinnerian tradition (e.g., Lindsley, 1992) have identified the practical importance of continuous monitoring of behavior, since that provides a true and direct measure of change in the form of variations and fluctuations. If you plot the acquisition of a skill over time you will see improvement and a smoothed graphic line can then be fitted to show the trend and extended to make it possible to predict whether a desired instructional goal will ever be reached in a given amount of time (White, 2005). If it is good for therapists to monitor progress, then presumably it is equally good for clients who are engaged in self-change—being their own therapist—to monitor their change as well. But when this happens, we have a very curious outcome. Keeping track of your own change actually helps to promote the change. This reactive effect of self-monitoring is of interest, not only because it helps get results, but because of what it tells us about the change process. Formal self-recording is more than simply noticing your own behavior and thoughts.

There are a number of mechanisms at work underlying the reactivity of self-monitoring. We know about them because of a steady line of research interest on the topic over the past 30 years or so by Rosemery Nelson-Gray and her colleagues (e.g., Nelson & Hayes, 1981). First, we can see that a good measure of any phenomenon is the ability to detect change before it is more obviously noticeable to the human observer. If you are treating your child for a fever and taking his or her temperature with a clinical thermometer every few hours, you will be able to detect that the temperature is coming down a degree or so at a time long before the child starts to feel better, seem less feverish, or is sweating less. If you are on a weight loss plan it may be a few weeks before you really notice that you can tighten your belt one more notch or wear a pair of jeans that have not fit you for a while. But if you have a reasonably accurate and consistent bathroom scale, you can easily detect a weight loss of a pound or two a few days into your diet (Wilson & Vitousek, 1999). In this example, however, we have the inevitable down-side of any procedure that fails to consider the larger picture: if clients are made overly conscious of their weight and are overly concerned about losing it, then monitoring could obviously be counterproductive—unreasonable expectations may not be met and a sense of failure could be generated. So the first basic advantage of self-monitoring is detecting small positive changes that are greater than expected to avoid disappointment. To see those small changes when taking a measurement you have to remember what the values were the time before. The easiest way to do that is to record them somewhere, as in a diary, or better still on a graph. In this way you obtain feedback.

Second, formally recording change helps the individual confirm that he or she is on a change program. It is far harder to ignore the fact that you are trying to quit smoking if you have to write down every time you have a cigarette. This is an additional reason why self-monitoring is reactive—it cues the need to stick with your change strategy. There is a third, related but probably much more influential source of influence and that is the way in which the self-record helps define the desired goal of the change program. This influence comes under the general class of having incentives—clearly specified positive goals that you are striving to accomplish.

A fourth, and certainly the most powerful influence, is that the demonstration of progress, however small, is highly intrinsically rewarding. If the goal is being able to run successfully in the New York marathon, the problem is that this reward will come only long after initiating the exercise behaviors designed to achieve it. But seeing that your completion time for running 5 kilometers is decreasing and your heart rate at the end of it is becoming slower and slower constitute immediate rewards for the effort of getting up that day for your early morning run.

If that is so, then we might worry that excessively frequent monitoring of your heart rate will have the opposite effect, because fitness level does not usually change that much in a single day. Monitoring your weight on the bathroom scales neglects the fact that because of natural fluctuations in body weight you may actually find that you have gained a pound, not lost one. This negative feedback and potentially punishing consequence will be less likely to occur if the individual has set a realistic level of fitness or degree of weight loss over a realistic period of time. Then a straight line between the present and this desired endpoint will reflect a reasonable slope and it is perfectly acceptable for your physical accomplishments or weight to fluctuate around that line as long as the general direction is being maintained. Good clinicians warn their clients that change is never perfectly linear and thus try to mitigate the negative effects of slow or erratic progress. Self-change clients need to be informed of this, either from a manual or from using their own common good sense and knowledge of change.

I have used the examples of fitness and weight measurements during a diet not because I am advocating dieting but to illustrate these points, since it is something with which many people are familiar. They may not be drawing graphs but they will be carefully noting small degrees of improvement. If they are going to a gym, the weight that they can bench press keeps going up; getting feedback on this has the same cueing, incentive, and reward function as described, just as long as the expectations regarding degree and rate of change were realistic to begin with. Self-help programs are prone to failure when individuals set goals for themselves that are difficult to actually attain. The thing about reward is that nothing is rewarding unless it satisfies a desire. In the laboratory we create that desire by starving the animal—remember that in all operant research the animals is usually at about 80% of its normal body weight and 24 hours away from its last free feed. No wonder it is easy to shape lever pressing in a rat or key pecking in a pigeon. But human desires are not that objectively or biologically determined, and are almost always based on a socially designated standard. Ten cents an hour is not a meaningful reimbursement for someone who is well off, and seeing a two pound weight loss is not a meaningful reward for someone who expected to drop 15 pounds in a week.

This proviso is even more salient when the clinical disorder itself is one of distorted expectations of what is normal, typical, or socially desirable. The classic clinical syndrome in which this occurs is anorexia. Anorexia can be usefully thought of as a variant of all body dysmorphic disorders, which are characterized by an inaccurate or highly distorted image of what you *should* look like or what a particular body part should be like. Perversely, the anorexic client who needs to be gaining weight is often contented only with an unreasonably low weight. Gaining a few pounds during an intervention program is hardly reinforcing for someone with those standards. This may explain why some types of problem are not easily amenable to self-change, as there is no external agent, except maybe a nagging parent, who is setting the bar at a realistic, attainable, and healthy level.

To end this brief excursion into the rather fascinating realm of self-observation and monitoring, it can be affirmed that it is often a simple and effective tool in promoting change. But only if we think about and understand the mechanisms of the effect can it really be used to its full advantage. Self-monitoring as an exercise does not have some intrinsically magical properties that will make it effective; it is not a treatment. In Jarrett and Nelson's (1987) study of cognitive–behavioral therapy (CBT) for depression, the self-monitoring component did not produce change directly, but what the clients were monitoring (dysfunctional thoughts) was a necessary precursor to them learning to distinguish "thoughts" from "facts," generate more logical alternatives, and test their beliefs and hypotheses—common components of CBT for depression. Self-monitoring is not always directly reactive but may be a rather important attentional variable that is an essential precursor to other change strategies. Asking clients to keep charts and diaries and put graphs on their fridges has to be done with a clear understanding of what we are hoping to achieve. Thinking about mechanisms of change will assist in that purposeful planning. Self-monitoring is just part of a much broader effort to gain a deeper understanding of what really controls your behavior.

Exercising Restraint

Having stated that the principles of self-change are not very different from therapist-directed change, I now have to qualify that claim. The qualification derives from an important distinction in psychological process, one we have already encountered. Some actions, such as simple habits, are quite *automatic*. They just get performed in the right context without much thought. Other actions are *controlled* and require the utilization of cognitive resources such as focused attention, contemplation, and planning. These are called executive functions. Strack and Deutsch (2004) theorized that we have an impulsive system, in which stimuli are judged according to emotional and motivational valence, and a reflective system, which is much slower acting and represents our personal standards and aspirations. It is pretty obvious that across many client groups and types of clinical problems people get into trouble when the impulsive system overrides the reflective system, especially for toddlers, teens, addicts, and criminals.

I mentioned the topic of inhibition when considering the neuropsychological substrate of certain profound personality differences related to emotional behavior. The inhibitory system discussed allows emotional behavior to be regulated, to be dampened down, just like lowering the amount of oxygen will cause a fire to burn less brightly. I have also touched on inhibitory conditioning, in which we learn a tendency not to respond. There is, however, yet another important meaning of inhibition in psychology, one essential to all purposeful and coordinated action, and that is a mechanism allowing for the suppression of a prepotent response, whether a reflex, an impulse, or an inappropriate thought. Without this mechanism you would not be able to coordinate motor activity, cross a street safely, turn down a second helping of your favorite dessert, or hold your tongue—stop yourself from telling your boss what you really think of him or her.

It may be that inhibiting such actions requires the same neural circuits as the Behavioral Inhibition System; however, many clients seek treatment to change highly specific impulse-control disorders ("road rage," gambling, addiction, violence—these sorts of problems) rather than for some overall modification of their dominant personality style. We need to be able to stop behaviors selectively before or as they start rather than to inhibit all action, what some have called a "global brake" (Aron & Verbruggen, 2008). And the inhibitory mechanism may be different from simply changing or extinguishing a habit at a behavioral level. It is an active neuropsychological process of stopping an incipient action before an unwelcome, unsafe, or socially inappropriate overt behavior occurs. If it is, and we need to employ it selectively, this mechanism has to come under voluntary control. It is the *expression* of unwanted behaviors we wish to purposely inhibit, despite a strong action tendency. Furthermore, needing to inhibit impulsive motor actions—looking before leaping—is not always essential. Motivation plays an important role, with some individuals tending to emphasize speed over accuracy in performance of any kind. Seizing the moment is often beneficial.

Exercising restraint requires stopping yourself from performing an action directly, not through avoiding temptation in the first place, eliminating cues, or any of the other behavior control strategies that have already been explained. Instead of showing self-control by not buying the box of chocolates, or reducing temptation by means of portion control (taking a smaller helping of food than you might normally do), you should be able to stare at the array of delicious chocolates and not take one, or leave half of a scrumptious pasta in the plate and put down your fork (e.g., Tsukayama, Toomey, Faith, & Duckworth, 2010).

Obviously all children learn to exercise varying degrees of self-restraint from a very young age, as they are taught not to grab hold of what they want, to wait for a promised treat, and to cease a fun activity when it is time to do something else. Parental strategies to achieve this are varied, from punishment to promises to simple self-regulatory strategies such as taking a breath. If explicit strategies are acquired, children will be able to use them when needed. One of the best understood and researched strategies is the encouragement of verbal mediators, such as Meichenbaum and Goodman's (1971) self-talk for inhibiting impulsive behavior. Before responding immediately when presented with a task or a problem, it is possible for children to learn verbal strategies such as saying to themselves "take your time," "don't jump in right away," or "let's see now, what do I have to do?" These verbal mediators, if they are used, can be very useful self-regulatory skills. An outpouring of research on self-instruction further confirmed its usefulness therapeutically (O'Leary & Dubey, 1979).

Talking to yourself is a key self-regulatory mechanism for emotion constraint as well. Teaching anxious children to talk their way through a crisis is a mainstay of Kendall's Coping Cat program (or Coping Koala if you are an Australian kid) (Kendall & Hedtke, 2006). The mechanism is not obvious, however. If you are an American driving in Britain, repeating to yourself "keep to the left" provides a cue for conscious actions that override automatic habits. Does "Keep calm and carry on" work the same way? From sports psychology we do know that self-talk is more likely to enhance novel, fine-motor task performance, compared to well-learned, gross-motor tasks. Motivational self-talk ("let's go," "I can do it") improves competitive performance, whereas instructional self-talk ("keep your eye on the ball," "follow through from the shoulder") is useful when learning new skills (Hatzigeorgiadis, Zourbanos, Galanis, & Theodorakis, 2011). Self-talk is clearly not just one thing. Words you say to yourself are stimuli that trigger responses, focus attention, increase self-confidence, and combat disruptive thoughts.

In a series of inventive studies of self-control, Mischel demonstrated that if a child is trying to resist eating a forbidden treat, imagining how good it will taste makes it harder to resist. Distraction, thinking of something else entirely, is a more effective method (Mischel, Shoda, & Rodriguez, 1989). Mischel's studies were conceived around a closely related topic—delay of gratification. The ability to resist an immediate impulse is just a subcomponent of self-control in which there is an implicit choice between immediate gratification (often through a small reward, in Mischel's studies just one marshmallow) and later gratification (often through a larger reward). The option is thought to resemble many experiences of life in which delaying gratification has considerable longer-term benefits, and so the phenomenon in the everyday lives of clients involves variables such as accurate knowledge of the possibilities and judgment regarding the likelihood of actually receiving the deferred reward. If we look simply at the moment when the response to the immediate reward is being resisted, then we are back to talking about inhibiting a prepotent behavior. In addition to showing that imagining consuming the reward was deleterious to such restraint in 4-year-old children, Mischel demonstrated that active distraction, such as playing with a toy, was beneficial.

Certain games and activities encountered at home and at preschool are better than others in helping to develop executive function skills, which are made up of inhibitory controls, cognitive flexibility, and mentally holding and using information. The latter skill is necessary for children to follow a story being read to them, and doing so without pictures might aid working memory (keeping a subset of necessary information in mind while engaged in a cognitive activity). Family games requiring taking turns rather than always letting the younger child go first are the sorts of learning opportunities that prepare children for preschool. Parents who encourage imaginative play, as a further example, have children with better emotion regulation skills, possibly because imaginative play allows emotional reactions to occur in a safe context and regulating their intensity is necessary to preserve the fun activity (Galyer & Evans, 2001). One preschool curriculum, Tools of the Mind, has been developed based on a variety of activities thought to promote executive functions, such as talking out loud and telling yourself what to do (Meichenbaum and Goodman's suggestion), dramatic play, and games such as "Simon Says" that emphasize the need to attend and to inhibit impulsive responding. There is evidence that programs using Tools of the Mind do increase competence on similar tasks found in the standard educational curriculum (Diamond, Barnett, Thomas, & Munro, 2007).

Therapy targeted at increasing executive control over impulsive behavior has not yet gained much clinical traction. One reason for this is that for many syndromes the dynamics of the response interrelationships (Chapter 7) overwhelms the reflective system. After drinking alcohol, or being sexually aroused, or excited by a big win when gambling, executive functions may be directly impaired (when drunk) or just too weak (when highly aroused). In these situations people may need a lot of practice with working memory. Following this sort of reasoning, Houben, Wiers, and Jansen (2011) showed that problem drinkers could reduce their alcohol intake following intensive training with tasks that enhance working memory.

Acquiring good emotional self-control and inhibitory skills is clearly essential. What is especially interesting from a self-change perspective is whether children and adults can learn conscious, applicable strategies that can be used deliberately in situations of temptation, emotional arousal, or provocation. We have much less information in this regard, although self-talk has certainly been widely applied therapeutically. Anger management programs represent perhaps one of the best examples of attempts to teach restraint, although how effective these programs are is still uncertain. Anger management typically involves a whole raft of procedures, but the essential component of feeling the anger but not expressing it—particularly through violent behavior—is the key requirement. This is quite a different set of principles from finding ways of reducing anger in the first place, by avoiding confrontational situations, for example. Anger can be diminished through generalized stress reduction, such as relaxation training. Surely everyone notices that when they are stressed at home or at work they are more likely to fly off the handle with minor provocations.

Coping Strategies as Self-Change

The words *problem solving*, *coping*, and *strategies* appear with great frequency in the treatment literature, and often together. Regardless of the exact wording, the implication is clear: we are referring to deliberate, purposeful efforts to regulate our behavior. These are typically cognitive (thoughts, ideas, plans), but to be effective they must be enacted in behavior. In addition to Pilates, your strategy for coping with stress at work might be to tell yourself that not everything depends on you, to share the workload by delegating better, to always take a full hour for lunch outside in the park, and sit in the hot-tub with a glass of sauvignon blanc when you get home. You could, probably more effectively, solve your problems by quitting that job and finding a less stressful one with a kinder boss, but that might be quite impractical. And what if you discover your coping skills are generally deficient and the next job is equally stressful? Much of psychotherapy involves finding out what strategies clients have and are missing, why they do not use the ones they have, if they are using them why they are not working, and weighing the advantages of one strategy against another. There are very few clinical concerns in which treatment should not have coping strategies built into the intervention plan.

What we generally refer to as coping strategies logically represent only a special case of self-change skills. Coping, by definition, implies dealing with adversity. Adverse circumstances might be environmental, such as a natural disaster, social, such as a divorce or the loss of a loved one, or physical, such as having cancer. In every case the adverse circumstance causes emotional distress and it is with this distress that we attempt to cope. We might, in some circumstances, be able to deal with the cause of the distress. If it is caused by losing our job, finding another one is the best of all possible coping strategies. Many adverse situations have already happened, however, such as a flood, being in a war zone, or having a fatal illness. In these situations prior prevention might have been a useful thing, but moralizing about prevention is less useful than focusing on those skills needed to cope with negative consequences despite adverse events having occurred. Similarly, it will not benefit your future adjustment if you focus too much on wondering why these bad things have happened so undeservedly to you and feeling hard-done by. One of the acceptance parables used by ACT therapists is to point out that you cannot control the hand you have been dealt, but how you play your cards is up to you.

The discussion once again runs the risk of being repetitive. This is because almost anything a therapist can do for a client, a client can do for himself or herself. One way to keep potentially overlapping topics somewhat compartmentalized is to think that at times we are talking about a psychological mechanism and at other times we are talking about its mobilization as a therapeutic tool. Emotive mental imagery is a perfect example. Mental imagery has the potential to regulate emotion, in both directions, as was discussed in the previous chapter. If the therapist teaches the client to use emotive imagery as a self-soothing strategy ("Imagine yourself lying under a palm tree on a tropical beach listening to the distance sound of the surf"), and the client does so, then it becomes a self-initiated intervention. Lee (2005) proposed that clients can be taught to generate a particular kind of image, that of a "perfect nurturer." The image can be anything the client wants: an angel, a fairy-godmother, Mother Nature, or some deity. The image evokes feelings of warmth, self-acceptance, and compassion (Gilbert, 2009). Another powerful strategy is to encourage clients to write about the higher values that define them (religious beliefs or personal relationships).

This self-affirmation focuses their sense of personal worth and integrity and buffers them against the kinds of daily stresses that interfere with coping and self-regulation (Sherman & Cohen, 2006).

Self-Help Therapies

One of the driving forces behind the emergence of community psychology was the importance of giving psychological knowledge away. There will never be enough professional therapists to act as agents of change for the number and variety of everyday and more serious problems that befall most human beings during their lifetime (Sarason, 1974). George Albee (1990) was the most effective and penetrating critic of psychotherapy as a limited resource, advocating a move away from this model toward an emphasis on prevention, community support, environmental modification, and using many of the other principles of change being presented. These principles can be communicated in many ways, the most common of which is still the self-help book (including videos and other media).

To the extent that self-help books describe therapeutic processes based on sound psychology, it would seem that they should really be the first line of defense. In terms of public policies and effective resource management, people who want to change should start by reading and following a good self-help book written by a reputable professional. Only if that fails to have an impact should the next stage be entering individual or group psychotherapy. Many would agree with this position. Yet it raises questions for a theory of change: is following a self-help book actually self-influence, or is it really no more than psychotherapy delivered by a therapist but through the written word? And to complicate the question still further, does not conventional psychotherapy involve a great degree of self-initiated modification? It seems that it is becoming obvious that the clear differentiation between self-treatment and other-treatment delivery is a very murky one, at the level of understanding change.

The mosaic of extant self-help therapies has been ably presented by Watkins and Clum (2008). Many interesting conclusions are drawn. Therapists can recommend books that promote sound scientific knowledge and discourage those that do not—diet books, detoxification, and chelation for autistic children are all especially misleading. Several self-help books stand out when they teach useful skills, such as how to read food labels or how to teach children with autism to make choices. When self-help books are used without the active guidance of a therapist outcomes tend to be less successful, so readers could be disappointed. However, whatever successes are documented have at least been achieved in a very economical fashion. Good self-help therapies draw from principles of self-regulation—the very things we have encountered in this chapter, such as setting goals, dividing them into more immediate versus more distant ones, and monitoring and rewarding progress. Conversely, there continues to be a need to ensure much greater cultural sensitivity if self-help books are intended to reach diverse groups.

Implications

Many tenets of self-regulation have been described and you wouldd be excused for wondering whether people do not already know these basic principles? I have suggested that clients tend not to or they would not be clients, but that is quite an oversimplification. A better way of conceptualizing individual differences in self-regulation is Rosenbaum's notion of "learned resourcefulness," defined as a "repertoire of behaviors and skills by which a person self-regulates internal responses that interfere with the smooth execution of an ongoing behavior" (Rosenbaum, 1990, p. 144). When our automatic reactions fail to meet our outcome expectancies (goals) resourcefulness is needed. Rosenbaum argues that in addition to techniques we need to have a general belief in our ability to self-regulate: I suppose we could call that self-self-efficacy. It is enhanced by self-affirmation strategies that remind us of what is truly important.

With respect to techniques, the topic of self-monitoring—which of course we do much of the time in an informal way—brings to our attention some of the fundamental mechanisms of change, especially cueing and feedback. Cueing is a bit like getting reminders for initiating behavior or inhibiting it (if it is an activity we would like to reduce). What has become clear in this chapter is that these reminder cues can be external, but in the absence of external cues they can be generated by people themselves. The two are often connected. Therapists provide external cues and can do so very explicitly by strategies such as calling clients, e-mailing them, or sending them a text message to remind them about a given exercise or activity. When the client knows this is going to happen, and when the client desires not to disappoint the therapist, the expectation of the external cue become the internal prompt to self-cue. So self-cueing of behaviors is rarely completely independent of the external environment. Any strategy that helps link these two thus turns out to be useful, such as following a checklist (Gawande, 2010), having the daily schedule for the family prominently posted on the kitchen wall (one of Supernanny's favorite interventions), or having the therapist's suggested goals for the week written into your schedule on Outlook.

Feedback is an equally fascinating causal element for behavior change. Feedback is hard to discriminate from rewards or reinforcement. The usual difference is that feedback provides information that the organism (otherwise known as the client) has done the right thing—performed correctly, performed to a certain standard (or not)—whereas reward (which provides feedback) dispenses pleasure for doing the right thing or meeting a standard. In self-regulation we recognize that the individual decides what is right and sets his or her own standard.

It is hardly surprising that cueing and feedback can have very deleterious consequences for those individuals who are overly vigilant, which pretty much defines a great deal of psychopathology. Socially anxious people are always monitoring possible feedback from others regarding their acceptability. People with obsessive thoughts are generating far too many cues (worrying thoughts) for checking and repetitive behaviors that have to be performed. Conversely, there are problem areas in which individuals do not cue their own behavior (in schizophrenia, often) and are insensitive to social feedback (in Asperger's disorder). Damned if you do and damned if you don't, so having some appropriate level of cueing desirable behaviors and getting (via self-monitoring) just the right amount of feedback to guide future actions seems to be the happy medium. As will be touched upon in the next chapter, therapists need to think carefully about how to support clients to achieve this balance.

For clients, Nezu converted the teaching of skills to solve your own problems into a formal treatment protocol. Which only goes to show that the self-delivered versus therapy-delivered distinction in helping people change is a bit of a false dichotomy. If the therapist teaches a client to problem solve, or teaches coping skills, or teaches a strategy for self-management, the point at which intervention is internal versus external is very blurred. If the client is taught self-help or self-control skills or reads about them in a book, where is the source of influence? The complexities of direct social influence will be the focus of the next chapter.

10

Social Mediators and the Therapeutic Relationship

The nature of many therapies can be quite vague, especially in the eyes of the public and especially when the goals are nebulous. Consider, for example, comments about therapy made by Alexa Joel, the adolescent daughter of superstars Christie Brinkley and Billy Joel. She told the reporter that she sees her therapist regularly and now "I'm in a Zen good place" (Hamm, 2010, p. 80). "Therapy allowed her to step away from the pressures of her life and dig deep: 'there was always somebody there I could talk to'" (p. 80).

In an earlier chapter on response interrelationships, as well as in my excursion into self-directed modification, I suggested that much therapeutic change consists in developing an understanding of means–ends relationships at the behavioral level. To change one aspect of behavior, change another: usually a more basic response pattern. And to effect change in that, promote change in a yet more fundamental response, one which forms part of the hierarchical structure of response repertoires and personality structures. A similar model can be applied to patterns of social influence. Because our emotional experiences as well as our daily patterns of living are so bound up in social relationships, we may need to construct the processes of change as first changing individual relationships (especially between therapist and client), then changing the social interactions with significant others, such as parents, spouses, and teachers, then changing relationships with peers and primary social groups, and finally extending this to broad social contexts such as communities, networks, and cultures. Thus, we can imagine that there is a continuum of restorative influence from the therapeutic relationship, through "mediators"—to be discussed in this chapter—and thence to groups and communities, to be discussed in the following chapter.

Social psychology is predicated on the influence of social conditions on all behavior—a kind of social ecology in which general environmental circumstances can be more precisely specified as each person's social landscape. The same physical environment, such as our neighborhood, will differ in social influence for the different people within it. A collective, sociological term for positive social resources within an individual's landscape is "social capital." Although there are many different possible elements to social capital, the essential currency is trust between people and bonding within social networks. Various possible measures of social capital exist (Spellerberg, 2001), but commonly used ones for youth include community cohesion (e.g., shared community values), informal social control (e.g., willingness of adults to intervene), and positive relationships with adults (e.g., having people at your school that you can approach). These are the three components of social capital that Evans and Kutcher (2011) found to militate against the negative health and social influences of poverty in low-income neighborhoods. What is so interesting for planning change is that to some extent these areas can be the target for intervention efforts.

At the other end of the social influence spectrum is the individualistic, one-on-one relationship with a mentor, therapist, or counselor. The nature and the role of the therapeutic relationship are probably the oldest and most venerable of all the topics that surround the analysis of psychotherapy and how it works and what about it makes people change. Because all approaches to therapy include some sort of relationship, it is frequently claimed that all forms of therapy have more in common with each other than they have differences. Most books about therapy start with this topic, rather than waiting until Chapter 10. However, there are good reasons for representing the therapist/client relationships as a highly specialized element of all social influence.

There are many synonyms for the relationship, such as the "therapeutic alliance," "rapport," or "moments of intersubjective meeting" (Stern, 2004). It is absolutely certain from both client reports of their experiences and therapist descriptions of their own and their clients' reactions within sessions that there is something very distinctive and emotionally meaningful about this relationship. It differs from other social relationships, such as friendships or romantic relationships, and from other professional relationships, such as with a lawyer or medical doctor. So intriguing is this special alliance that it has acquired a certain mystical quality—thought to be difficult to define or objectify. In addition, there is a long-standing assumption that it is the relationship itself that brings about change, just like a pill. So ingrained is this view that studies showing that the greater the number of therapy sessions the better the outcome have been referred to as revealing a "dose–effect relationship" (Howard, Kopte, Krause, & Orlinsky, 1986; Kadera, Lambert, & Andrews, 1996). But that analogy makes little sense if we think carefully about the actual communicative transactions that take place during therapy sessions.

Therapeutic Processes

Interacting with a therapist is a new experience for most people and like any other social experience considerable new learning inevitably takes place. When we examined the nature of clinical change in Chapter 2 the focus was on the outcome of intervention—how a process is put into effect that leads to the desired differences in individual functioning. Yet interacting with a therapist is a process that also changes clients, especially when the interactions are emotive, meaningful, and intense, such as self-disclosure. If that degree of influence is sufficient to start changing the client positively, we can see why the therapeutic relationship is considered so relevant to good outcomes. Could the social learning that takes place as we interact with the therapist be part of that whole chain of *if...then* relationships representing the causal sequence from initiating something different in our life to achieving the long-term benefits we desire? Clients begin to think that change is possible, that someone understands them, that there is hope that goals can be attained, that they have taken the first step to a new life, and that important values are affirmed—these can be the thoughts and feelings following the first session.

In educational research, especially higher education, there is a concentration on student engagement, which predicts academic success. Engagement is a motivational variable, encompassing interest, passion, and commitment. Clients differ in the extent to which they engage in psychotherapy, and the extent to which the therapist, like the inspirational teacher, can foster that engagement is a motivational variable tied to the rapport between therapists and clients.

But there are other processes to consider when trying to understand the complex role of the relationship as a *cause* of change, one of which goes back to some very early ideas in behavior modification. The question behaviorists posed was basically this: Is it possible that in the therapeutic interaction, therapists—quite apart from introducing "treatments"—are unwittingly (both to themselves and to the client) shaping certain behaviors by means of a social influence process such as selective attention, social reinforcement, and differential communication? Take any description of experienced therapists in action and the social influence could not be clearer: "The expert counselor was attentive and interested in the [client]. He looked at the [client]; he leaned toward him and was responsive to the [client] by his facial expressions, head nods, posture, and so on. He used hand gestures to emphasize his points" (Strong & Matross, 1973, p. 28). The question is whether the therapist's verbal and emotional approval is contingent on approved client responding, and the answer is that it is and thus shapes the client's discourse in quite noticeable ways (e.g., Salzinger & Pisoni, 1958). Working in Spain, Froján, Montaño, and Calero (2010) showed that cognitive–behavioral therapists' verbalizations that were judged to be reinforcing usually followed a series of "discriminative stimuli" that were questions requiring client answers during assessment phases. Then quite long periods of information were offered: "I'll try to explain to you why you react in the way that you do..." (p. 926). In treatment phases, reinforcement followed instructions only after the clients had agreed to try a suggested strategy.

Independent of the attempt to introduce a formal and planful treatment, the social context of therapy moulds and alters the client's behavior. It might be added that the client's social interactions shape and alter the therapists as well, and over long periods of therapeutic practice therapists will undoubtedly have their interactional styles subtly modified by the kinds of approvals and successes they obtain from clients. Psychotherapy, apart from everything else, is a mutual social influence process, what developmental psychologists call transactional regulation (Sameroff, 1991).

Behaviorist interest in how therapists shape clients, however, has mostly just faded away (Salzinger, 2008), probably due to the field shifting from concern with process and principles of change toward a focus on technique. Today, novice psychologists learning cognitive–behavioral therapy are likely to have a very good grasp of a validated treatment protocol, but not know much about the literature on social contingencies in therapy nor fully recognize how clients are influencing them. They may use social reinforcement principles in interacting with clients, either deliberately or fortuitously ("that's really great; I'm proud of you; what an effort you must have made; let me make a note of that; that must make you feel good about yourself"), but they would rarely see it as part of treatment, unless perhaps the client was a child with a disability. If asked to describe their treatment plan they might say they are going to do cognitive restructuring, but they are unlikely to say that they intend to differentially shape rational utterances by the client—a process needed for cognitive restructuring to occur.

Without broad principles of change it is also possible for therapists to be unaware of the complex interactions between therapist's feedback and client's self-identity. Encouragement and social approval seem straightforward until you remember that some clients crave the assurance and predictability arising from knowing oneself (Pinel & Constantino, 2003). They need feedback that is not too discrepant from what they recognize and understand about themselves. Other clients, with a strong desire to feel good about themselves, will need feedback that is affirming (of the "that's really great" variety). Personality, self-identity, reinforcement (feedback), and the therapeutic relationship are not separable elements of change—they all interact.

Incidental (Implicit) versus Planned (Explicit) Influence

It is undoubtedly true that the quality of the therapeutic relationship affects the outcome. However, the magnitude of this effect may be proportionate to the degree of planful influence that can be exerted, either in contexts in which very explicit treatment goals must be met or in which there is a clearly effective intervention design in place. Two simple corollaries follow: (1) when the client's goals are largely interpersonal and self-exploratory, the magnitude of the therapeutic relationship's influence will be relatively greater; and (2) when the planful part of the treatment is relatively weak or ineffectual for the type of problem being addressed, then the therapist–client relationship will be relatively more important. It is not possible to answer the question "how important is the therapeutic relationship?" in the abstract—it depends entirely on the nature of the treatment goals and the potency of the planned components of the treatment.

An analogy can be made with classroom learning and teaching. Teachers who are skilled at relating well to children and creating a warm and exciting classroom atmosphere are able to greatly increase children's academic learning (Evans, Harvey, Buckley, & Yan, 2009). But if the teacher has no curriculum and no focused program of instruction, even the warmest most interactively gifted teacher will not achieve much in terms of student's academic progress. On the other hand, with an excellent curriculum that is faithfully adhered to, even teachers who are not very skilled at engaging the children emotionally will be able to produce reasonable academic learning outcomes. However, with an excellent curriculum and well-structured lesson plans the teacher who is harsh and abrasive and who treats students unfairly will not obtain good learning outcomes. In addition to academic outcomes, there are many other possible gains from a year of classroom instruction, such as acquiring social and emotional competencies. Because these are not usually in the curriculum, the best likelihood of children acquiring such skills is from a socially and emotionally competent teacher. Hopefully the lesson for psychotherapy is clear: if the goal of therapy is incidental change, learning about yourself and others from the intensive interaction with a caring human being (the therapist), then of course the gifted, warm, empathetic, and genuine therapist is likely to produce good results.

The variables here are (1) the proportion of incidental learning to planned learning, (2) the degree of effectiveness of the structured or planned learning, (3) the nature of the therapeutic goals (whether targeted behavior change or interpersonal exploration), and (4) the social and emotional skills of the therapist. These skills, by the way, are unlikely to be universal—what works well for one type of client will not work equally well for someone with a completely different personality. Interpersonal exploration is not a bad thing in which to engage and in every therapeutic encounter there will be opportunities for clients to discover things about themselves and why they are the way they are.

The Relationship Debate

When behavior therapy first began it was thought that the therapeutic relationship was immaterial. This position was asserted mostly to distance the approach from the more traditional psychoanalytic and humanistic schools of thought, which argued that everything meaningful in therapy was due to the relationship. But once behavior therapy overcame this initial rigid stance, it was obvious to everyone that the relationship was very important, if for no other reason than it determined the degree to which the therapists could get the clients to do the sorts of things that would bring about the changes in behavior they were seeking.

Terence Wilson and I wrote a number of articles proposing that the relationship was critical because the therapist represented not only a "reinforcement machine" as the operant behaviorists liked to call it, but also a cue complex that allowed behaviors to be elicited under the controlled conditions that would bring about change (e.g., Wilson & Evans, 1977; Wilson, Hannon, & Evans, 1968). For instance, we pointed out that exposure-based interventions, relying on extinction processes, required clients to experience difficult feelings at manageable levels. The positive therapeutic relationship offers a generalized "safety signal" that counteracts experiential avoidance. I have not heard anyone challenge this perspective, but it did not get fully integrated into the discourse around behavior therapy and even less so around cognitive therapy. Where we do find echoes of this idea is in models of the therapeutic relationship as being an attachment relationship, recapturing the secure relationship between a young child and a caregiver; from this safe base potentially dangerous and threatening experiences can be explored.

It has become popular to argue that the relationship accounts for most of the effect of therapy and the specific technique being used is proportionately less important. Wampold (2001) has made this argument in an influential book. But is it logical? If we follow the Wilson and Evans argument that the relationship is the vehicle or the context in which a formally planned treatment is delivered then it would not be possible to compare the effectiveness of the treatment in the absence of its delivery mechanism, or to study the delivery mechanism in the absence of something worth delivering. Going back to my previous suggestion that verbal psychotherapy includes emotion talk, allowing the learning opportunities of clients to increase their emotional competence, then the therapeutic interaction constitutes an active learning condition. If we add the radical behavioral perspective that the relationship allows for the implicit shaping of social and emotional change, then that shaping is the therapy and the relationship serves only to make it more potent. Relationships that do not serve to implicitly influence behavior are of little value, except that like any other friendly social interaction they are pleasant and desirable and bring satisfaction to the client.

An added complexity in the relationship debate is that a greatly enhanced relationship between therapist and client can emerge as a *consequence* of effective treatment, not just the other way around. One of the advantages of approaches such as behavior therapy is that they can be quite morally and judgmentally neutral. A careful case conceptualization of clients' circumstances offers an explanation for their behavior that makes sense, but does not imply that they are evil or stupid or "going crazy." Explanations do not exonerate clients from responsibility, but clients can see how patterns have developed without making self-deprecating, negative judgments about their character. This often provides a sense of relief and with it a deep appreciation of the therapist (Orbach, 2005).

Two other therapeutic areas in which the importance of the relationship seems to be still neglected today is treatment for people with significant intellectual disabilities and the rehabilitation of clients who are offenders. I have already criticized the fortunately brief professional enthusiasm for aversive control of challenging behavior. It seems inconceivable that any therapist genuinely interested in treating a child with both a disability and very difficult behavior could set up a highly aversive and technically distancing automatic shock device (Linscheid, Iwata, Ricketts, Williams, & Griffin, 1990). Although aversives have essentially been banned from practice due to to agency and professional guidelines grounded in civil liberties legislation, we still have very regimented procedures for shaping simple behaviors in children with autism and other developmental disabilities, in which the focus is strictly on the method, and the relationship between the client and the applied behavior analyst is rarely mentioned. This occurs despite the clear demonstration when viewing tapes of trainers engaged in the process that a definite relationship develops between clinician and child, which could be greatly enhanced if it were specifically a component of the method, such as we might see in many varieties of play therapy. In play therapy the clinician is highly responsive to the direction of the child, which is then reciprocated. This is an excellent example of transactional relationships, but one in which the therapist deliberately allows the child to take the lead in the emotional tango that is purposeful play.

With respect to criminal behavior, think back to Ward's Good Lives Model (Ward & Marshall, 2004). What is the underlying set of values implicit in a model that perceives offenders as seeking a universal array of human "goods"—happiness, agency, inner satisfaction, family, and romantic and community relationships? Plainly this encourages clients to make their own decisions, decreases some of the stigma associated with criminal behavior, and shifts the therapeutic alliance in a positive direction: "The fact that the offender is viewed as someone attempting to live a meaningful worthwhile life in the best way he can in the specific circumstances confronting him, reminds therapists that they are not moral strangers" (Ward et al., 2007, p. 93). Clinical language, one of the defining features of the therapeutic alliance, needs to change: "relapses prevention" becomes "change for life" and "personal deficits" become "intimacy building."

My assertion is that psychotherapy—including CBT and applied behavior analysis—is a social influence process. This is an old perspective. It is hardly novel. But if it is a social influence process the therapist must have the power to influence the client. Where does that power come from? One answer is from the emotional relationship itself; another important origin is the expectancies of the client. A third related idea is a reinterpretation of the placebo effect: that both therapist and client play out *roles*—the role for the client is to come in sick and to go out well (Krasner & Ullmann, 1969). Clients usually know what they are supposed to do: you come into therapy with a set of problems, talk about them, maybe talk about your past and your family, try out certain things that the therapists recommends, gradually come to feel much better, and finally walk away from therapy free of the original problems. The role for the therapist is to offer culturally recognizable forms of analysis, encouragement, discussion, and advice. If both parties stick to their roles, all will be well.

Relationship-Based Strategies That Promote Change

In this complex analysis of social influence in therapy, I have made the argument that only in narrow circumstances does the forging of a relationship with a therapist promote meaningful change directly. At the same time, without such a relationship, the strategies that constitute psychotherapy are going to be much less effective. For one thing, you may never as a therapist get to understand your client's needs and true feelings unless there has been sufficient trust developed. If safety is assured the client can disclose, without fear of judgment or criticism, what are often socially unacceptable, secret feelings or disturbing, even repulsive behaviors.

When it comes to treatment, trust is again essential. Some intervention strategies involve directive efforts to promote very difficult change outside the therapeutic environment. An additional feature of the therapeutic relationship is that there are things transpiring in therapy that promote change in unexpected ways. Let us consider a few of them, simply to try to make the point more tangibly.

Expectations

Most adult clients and many children already have a distorted perception about psychotherapy that has been shaped by the popular media. The expectations are for a nondirective, counseling type of experience with perhaps elements of psychoanalysis thrown in for good measure. However, contemporary, evidence-based interventions, as likely to be carried out by clinical psychologists, are nothing if not directive.

Clients rarely expect that therapy will require them to make significant efforts to change, and this clash between client expectations and the likely modality of therapy makes it harder to implement effective behavior change (Seligman, Wuyek, Geers, Hovey, & Motley, 2009). When CBT therapists talk about "psychoeducation" they usually mean providing a client with information about the designated syndrome. They may go somewhat beyond this and try to explain in technical language the origins and the controlling variables, which in turn will provide a rationale for the treatment plan they are about to recommend. It creates a story that allows therapeutic actions to be justified and seem logical. It provides a common focus for discussion and future communication. When client and therapist share the myth, I would suggest, progress occurs. However, it would also be sensible to prepare the client in a yet more fundamental way: be prepared to change; therapy is designed to make you different.

Making Social Commitments to Change

It is assumed that change will be more likely if the client makes a public commitment to change, despite the fact that saying and doing are totally different things. Some therapists will ask the client to sign a written contract, agreeing to perform certain actions or to desist from others. Where there is a strong therapeutic alliance, the client will be less likely to want to disappoint the therapist and to be more ashamed if some agreed upon change is not implemented. Promises to do something are established very early in child development as important covenants and expectations in our culture. "But you promised..." is a significant, guilt-inducing reminder for a child, maybe even more so for a parent or spouse, when an agreed upon action has not been performed. A common context for still more public agreements is group work, in which the client is encouraged to make the commitment to the whole group. This kind of technique is common in treatment groups designed to change powerful habits, such as drinking alcohol, sexual excesses, and eating less (weight loss groups).

The Consequences of Early Influences

Past experiences shape and control present behavior. To some extent this was touched on when discussing personality, as personality is undoubtedly shaped by meaningful experiences. But there is something special about the influence of parenting relationships on children that carries on to adult life.

Right about now you may be thinking that I am implying that all therapists worth their salt should always ask adult clients about their mothers. Due to Freud and the psychoanalytic tradition this has become a sort of standing joke among the general public about what therapists hope to uncover. Nevertheless there is a great deal of modern evidence relating to certain very specific influences of parenting around how adults cope with emotion, form meaningful romantic relationships, sustain images of their self-worth, and possibly even how as parents themselves they manage the emotional relationships with their children. Much of this understanding comes from contemporary research in attachment: your early emotional experiences create what Bowlby (1969) called an "internal working model" of meaningful close relationships, both in the present and in the future.

Freud (1920) believed that in the relationship evolving between client and therapist there was a process in which the clients would tend to respond to the therapist in a manner similar to the way they would respond to their own father. (Note the explicit gender bias here; most of Freud's clients were young females and most early analysts were older males.) Freud called this process "transference" as the client transferred unconscious feelings and desires from the parent onto the therapist. There are many reasons why today we tend not to hold such theorizing in high regard; nevertheless it is difficult to discuss the nature of the therapeutic relationship as a vehicle for change without thinking about how it is possible that parental experiences from the past do color the way we relate to a therapist. This may be particularly true when the therapist emphasizes, as some do, their wisdom, their nurturing care, and their dominance.

There is another interpretation of the therapeutic relationship that appears to have as its primary scholarly function an attempt to keep alive traditional theories of unconscious influences. Cognitive therapy (the Beck tradition) has had the profound but not always recognized effect of relegating unconscious feelings to a back seat. Cognitive therapy stresses conscious processes—what you think (say) to yourself, what you believe, what you judge, and what you comprehend. It relies on the client's declarative memory processes, such as autobiographical memory, as seen when we ask clients to tell us about their past and we take more or less at face value the veridicality of their narratives. It could be argued that in cognitive therapy the critical relationship is the alliance between the client's rational self and the therapist's working, conceptual procedures (Bordin, 1994). But to some modern analytic thinkers (Fonagy, 1998) the therapeutic relationship involves implicit or procedural memory, similar to the way the motor system operates—we do not have knowledge of how we perform motor skills. In object relations theory "the therapist is a new object whose involvement permits a departure from past expectancies with other people" (Fonagy, 1998, p. 348). In this way the therapeutic relationship is similar to infant–parent attachment, with the potential to "alter implicit relational knowing... that may be imperceptible to either patient or analyst except, perhaps, for a sense of increased well-being when in each other's company" (p. 350).

Is it possible to think that early experiences that have now become dysfunctional for the client have a special place as targets of change? Might, for example, insight into how a reaction—even a transference reaction such as getting angry at the therapist—reflect a much earlier parental conditioning experience allowing the client to shed those emotional habits? Some of the parentally derived automatic cues we carry around can be very ordinary. My own mother, who was well-educated but nevertheless quite superstitious, was always concerned if someone spilled the salt and if so she would toss a pinch of it over her left shoulder. More than 60 years later I cannot look at spilled salt without experiencing a strong urge to throw it over my shoulder. We cannot pursue too many personal anecdotes instead of objective evidence, but I think that the point is clear. We do carry around unconscious emotional memories just as we have internalized all the positive, constructive lessons we learned in the past about how to manage emotion and cope with adversity within intimate relationships.

Problematic Behavior Occurs within Sessions

Most descriptions of how to do psychotherapy, from all theoretical persuasions, often presume that clients are involved in *reporting* the kinds of concerns and problems they experience outside the clinic in their everyday lives. What is neglected is how clients' difficulties are often enacted within the therapeutic setting. And if that is the case, it clearly means the therapy session itself is a learning opportunity, not just planning for the outside world. A client's social anxiety, interpersonal skills, attitudes and biases, poor anger management, child discipline practices, response to criticism, even mundane things such as time-management skills (punctuality), attentiveness, and dress sense are all transparently revealed. This, of course, is one reason many clinicians assert that it is challenging to work with clients with the diagnosis of borderline personality disorder because they may well enact their conflicts over acceptance and rejection in a confrontational manner during a session.

Cognitive–behavioral therapists use these in-session behaviors to change clients' dominant styles of interpersonal responding. This can be done fairly gently by giving feedback to a client, along the lines of "if what you have just said to me is typical of what you say to other people with whom you are interacting, I can understand why some of your relationships fall apart. Let me explain how what you said made *me* feel." It can also be done, as already stated, by differential reinforcement—attending to and praising the types of responses that are going to mediate therapeutic progress. In the case of people with a borderline diagnosis, treatment approaches such as Linehan's dialectical behavior therapy use the therapist's consistently accepting a client's erratic emotional mood swings as a direct learning experience. Therapists respond to clients so as to unequivocally demonstrate that not every meaningful relationship ends in rejection, and that criticism, if leveled, does not equate with emotional abandonment.

This general approach to in-session interactions being an opportunity for the therapist to both assess and teach the client directly has been called "functional analytic psychotherapy" by Kohlenberg and Tsai (1991). As part of assessment, the concept highlights the general principle of functional analysis. With a child having a serious developmental delay and challenging behavior we can begin to understand the function of that behavior by changing environmental conditions and seeing how that affects the behavior of concern. We might, for example, create a condition that totally accedes to the child's apparent wishes. If challenging behavior is greatly reduced under such conditions, the inference would be that the challenging behavior is serving the function of allowing the child to control his or her world. The exact same principle can be used in verbal psychotherapy. If the hypothesis is that the client is exceptionally resistant to control, or too sensitive to signs of anger, or does not handle feedback well, then directives, enacted irritation, and plain feedback can all be introduced purposefully to observe the client's response. And in case this sounds mildly devious and contrary to ethical principles of informed consent, this is exactly what every therapist will do anyway and has always done—probe the client's emotional and interpersonal life by slightly varying their own interactional style and observing the effects.

Emotions expressed within the therapy setting are highly revealing. In my culture, if clients cry and you hand them a box of tissues, they often apologize. And we reassure them that it is perfectly acceptable to show their feelings and to vent them. What we do not always explain to clients is that the therapy session is a wonderful opportunity to observe—to see how the client responds emotionally to different themes, to watch changes in facial expression and flushing and body language such as clenching fists, wringing hands, jiggling their legs, fidgeting with clothes, and to listen to how they express themselves. Hot, overarousing reactions and cognitions are being physiologically enacted right there during relevant social interaction, not coldly reported verbally on some paper and pencil instrument or questionnaire days later. Clients may not realize how closely they are under surveillance by good therapists

Relationships with Nonprofessionals

Much of behavioral psychotherapy involves other people being trained to be an agent of change for the target client. The relationship between that nonprofessional intervention agent and the targeted individual presumably replicates the same issues that are relevant for the relationship between therapist and client. The original formal emphasis on teaching other people how to change behavior came from a book by Tharp and Wetzel (1969) called *Behavior Modification in the Natural Environment*. In this book they explicated the argument and provided rich clinical examples of how when attempting to alter a target client's behavior it is essential to work through the medium of those individuals who actually have meaning in that client's life—friends, parents, other family members, and teachers. In certain circumstances it may be desirable to change the behavior of an intimate partner or spouse in order to facilitate change in the client—déjà vu, those means–ends relationships again. Such individuals will have established relationships and past histories with the target client that the professional therapist cannot hope to replicate. In behavior theory language such behavior change "agents" have access to the most salient cues and the most significant reinforcers for the client. The missing insight was that as a result of a meaningful relationship history, there would also be shared emotional experiences—caring feelings, love, and attachment needs. These components constitute the meaning of a positive personal relationship.

After the Tharp and Wetzel book, the recognition was soon entrenched that much of behavioral psychotherapy was going to be managed through training or educating mediators. In fact the basic idea does go back to some of the earliest demonstrations of behavior modification with people who were in long-term institutional care. If the nurses and orderlies and direct care staff in a psychiatric residential facility could be taught to shape positive behaviors and help extinguish negative ones, then the milieu of the psychiatric hospital could be modified in ways that made the environment itself therapeutic; that is, the general interactions with staff would change client behaviors for the better.

Again, however, in this large and rich literature on training staff (or any other mediator, be they teachers, parents, siblings, etc.) in order to effect positive behavior change in clients, there was little attention paid to the emotional elements of the existing relationship between mediator and client (Evans & Berryman, 1998). If the relationship between therapist and client in psychotherapy is so important, then surely the relationship between mediator and client must be equally so? And another insight seems to have been recognized only in passing. If the naturally occurring relationships in a client's life will have a potency that a therapist newly engaging with the client cannot hope to emulate, then surely all responsible individual direct psychotherapy should be looking at ways these natural influences can be mobilized to support the changes being targeted in therapy?

Support Staff

People with persistent and serious psychiatric disorders, such as schizophrenia, now spend much of their time in various types of community placements. This supported accommodation can be fairly independent, such as an apartment with a roommate or two, or might be a group home staffed by paraprofessional caregivers. If we think of the concept of implicit social influence, it seems logical that direct care mental health support staff play a potentially commanding role in providing ongoing informal rehabilitation opportunities for the residents of these many facilities. However, these caregivers are typically neither well qualified nor very well paid. In some countries such support staff receive various levels of training, often around safety, managing dangerous behavior, and facilitating the role of professional staff, who might be visiting psychiatrists or psychiatric nurses. In work I have conducted with colleagues Averil Herbert and Natasha Moltzen, we noted that the everyday social, emotional, and interpersonal skills of dedicated and caring staff were strangely considered less important than this pseudomedical role in which they were cast.

After spending many hours observing the typical, everyday interactions between support staff and clients in these residential facilities, Evans and Moltzen (2000) suggested that there were a few general principles of social interaction, which, if followed by caregivers, would provide excellent natural rehabilitative opportunities for the residents. Our six principles will be rather familiar if you have read this far, as they can easily be deduced from the most basic principles of change.

The first is acceptance, which refers not to unconditional liking or disliking of the clients, but to experiencing them as they are, as people. Often when a patient is overly distressed or angry, staff efforts are immediately directed at alleviating the display of these emotions, rather than "experiencing the moment" and not needing to control or direct the client's experience—with suggestions to the agency professionals regarding medication changes. A significant inverse relationship has been shown between level of warmth, as assessed by spontaneity, tone of voice, empathy, and interest in the client as a person, and relapse rate in schizophrenia (Ivanović, Vuletić, & Bebbington, 1994).

The second, related principle is the planned creation of a positive atmosphere in the residential facility. Atmosphere has already been discussed in the context of classrooms and schools—the principle is the same. Positive residences encourage patient autonomy and are warm and friendly; the staff members are fair and flexible and tolerate eccentric behavior. At the same time there needs to be expectations by the staff for the possibility of change. This is principle three. The staff will be seen to encourage clients to engage in novel experiences, discussing realistic but optimistic future goals, telling clients about opportunities in the community, and showing interest in client activities. Principle four is responsiveness: the staff members need to avoid attributing all of the client's behavior to illness.

The fifth principle is that of normalization. Although the community care model promotes integration for individuals with severe, persistent mental health needs, the stigma attached to mental illness often means that even when living in community homes, these clients are quite isolated from the typical activities of community life. Staff members need to encourage clients (to the extent that they desire it) to develop typical social relationships with people completely outside the formal mental health system. Finally, principle six, proposes that one of the roles of direct care staff is to teach new skills, but not in any formal sense, which is much better left to programs often available at community colleges. Clients can be encouraged to acquire alternative skills—to express feelings rather than being physically aggressive and to exercise choice. Clients, like the rest of us, benefit from honest feedback as well as praise.

In my experience, practicing therapists are quick to acknowledge the great importance of all those meaningful people surrounding the client with whom he or she has a relationship. Most therapists will make an attempt to analyze the influential social networks and try to assess whether the contingencies they present are likely to prove a barrier to client change. The caring husband who reinforces his wife's panic behavior by doing more and more things for her will quickly be recognized as someone whose actions require modification, if possible, because he is creating contingencies that run counter to the therapeutic efforts to encourage the woman client to expose herself gradually in vivo to fear-provoking situations. Therapists will also look for ways that new partner or parent behaviors can be added that will promote therapeutically targeted change. The supportive wife can make sure that she facilitates her depressed husband's initial efforts at doing more activities, even if her natural inclination would have been not to join him in these events. Thus, therapists will often try to mobilize the support of relevant others and try to access and restructure social networks to further the direct efforts taking place in therapy. But these elements are rarely seen as central to the treatment plan; they are seen more as adjuncts—good things if you can get them to happen. Yet it is possible, indeed likely, that these influences on behavior are much more powerful than anything the therapist can do in one-on-one therapy for 50 minutes a week. Nowhere is this more obvious than in parent training.

Behavioral Parent Training and Relationship Issues

Parent training is most often represented in clinical textbooks as though it were a distinct entity—a validated "treatment" that can be implemented when children's behavior is inappropriate: parents as therapists, not just as clients (Wahler, Winkel, Peterson, & Morrison, 1965). In Chapter 2 I suggested that behavioral parent training represents a precise example of influencing mediators to effect change in a perceived problem area. I also used this type of intervention to raise awkward questions about what it is we expect to change in parents. Clinicians typically focus on disciplinary tactics and parents' attempts to establish compliant behavior (McMahon & Forehand, 2003). It is therefore concerning that when direct, observable, independent measures of child change are made, behavioral parent training programs that purport to have a strong evidence base have not typically revealed substantial improvements in the conduct of the children (Thomas & Zimmer-Gembeck, 2007). Does that matter? If the children became clients because their parents were complaining, parental satisfaction is what we seek. Ironically, however, it is possible, indeed likely, that by making parents satisfied (giving them hope, making them more positive, increasing approach behaviors) family relationships improve and children do change—transactional regulation again.

If the behavior of children is altered by changing the characteristic behavior of their caregivers, it means that we need to consider all facets of the social–emotional interaction between parent and child, not simply the more obvious contingencies between the child's behavior and the parentally controlled consequences. Every major contributor to the parent training literature would agree with this statement, but only some have made it a key element of their intervention programs for parents and families. When programs do include strategies to enhance the parent (mediator)–child (target) relationship they have better outcomes (Thomas & Zimmer-Gembeck, 2007).

The basic components of discipline-focused behavioral parent training come directly from everything we have already examined under the rubric of instrumental conditioning. All effective parents shape positive behaviors (the ones they want to see) by modeling and reinforcing them. They discourage negative behaviors by a combination of extinction (planned ignoring, time-out), negative consequences (verbal reprimand, mild punishments such as loss of privileges), and, most useful of all, redirection (differential reinforcement of some other, preferred behavior). These contingencies have to be clear, explicit, and consistent in order to work, and that becomes one of the central tenets that a few parents need to understand and learn. Parent training also involves decreasing ineffective strategies, especially harsh discipline (spanking), threats ("if you don't come now, I'm going to leave you behind"), delayed and deferred punishments ("when your dad comes home I'll tell him what you've done and he'll deal with you"), unclear instructions, and double binds (sometimes laughing at bad behavior and sometimes expressing anger at it). Good parenting programs encourage mindful parenting with an array of different techniques to increase acceptance, even promoting recognition of the reality that it is possible to have mixed feelings about children's negative behaviors so that corrective discipline means no loss of love and understanding (Couch & Evans, 2011).

The change principles can be further refined. Assume for the moment that the focus of all parenting training programs is to encourage parents to use consistent positive discipline strategies and to discourage harsh (angry), punitive, and inconsistent ones. Inconsistency means different rules at different times, as well as not following through with a stated consequence. Family rules need to be based on moral principles, and directives should be clear, unambiguous, and fair, and reflect the things that the child likes to do. These positive approach behaviors are in turn reinforced by child compliance. Both parent and child become highly valenced, positive discriminative stimuli, the opposite of coercive traps.

That is the convoluted behavioral language encompassing the key dimension of parenting: the unconditional love and acceptance that the parent feels toward the child and expresses through word and deed. Children, in turn, feel secure and safe in their parents' presence, and are confident that when not physically around them (such as when the child is at preschool) their parents are nevertheless there for them. Securely "attached" children recognize that reprimands and punishments do not mean a loss of affection, but are meted out for their own protection, safety, and education. Children with a positive, loving relationship with parents will be motivated to please them, so that simple praise and attention are as reinforcing, if not more so, than material treats. Does all this not sound analogous to the benefit of a close, warm, working alliance between therapist and client in psychotherapy?

An additional parallel is the distinction that can be drawn between the relationship and what is done with that relationship—the more active techniques and behavior change strategies promoted by the therapist. In child rearing, is the relationship sufficient to ensure problem-free child behavior? Conversely, if the relationship between parent and child is not good, will teaching positive discipline skills work to improve behavior? Or, equally interesting, will such teaching lead to a more positive relationship? The answers are, respectively, "no," "sometimes," and "hopefully."

I cannot prove that my proposed answers are totally correct, partly because the research literature does not take all these concerns into account at the same time. The outcome variables for conventional parent training research are invariably negatively valenced: adults' rating of decreased negative behaviors (those being complained about). So we typically do not know if the training helped parents manage their anger and enhance their relationship with their children, or, if it did, whether the improvement was directly responsible for good children. What we do have evidence for, and which is fascinating in its implications, is that parent training programs, irrespective of type, reduce, at least in the short term, parental depression, anxiety, and marital conflict (Barlow & Coren, 2004). We do not know if this is because parenting programs render the child's behavior less stressful as it improves, or because they give the parents feelings of affirmation and hope.

Despite major gaps in the evidence, there are families in which children do differ in child temperament/adult style fit, in activity levels, in impulsivity, and in personality dimensions (see Chapter 7); such differences make discipline so much harder to establish. To this we need to add the further dimension of parents of very young children as teachers of emotion competence and self-control, confirming yet again the value of transactional models. Effective parents are able to adapt, since their ability to act as mediators of change shifts radically once their children become teenagers with much greater autonomy and less parental control. Adolescent/parent harmony requires negotiating agreement on family expectations based on moral, conventional, safety, and personal principles and decisions (Smetana, 2011).

Pointing the Finger Hampers Change

Regardless of the child's developmental stage, parents are sometimes seriously delinquent—those who commit acts of physical or sexual abuse or neglect their children's basic care. Thus, many parents interpret a recommendation for parent training as blaming them for the child's behavior, whether the clinician suspects they are complicit or not. Parents may want the therapist to fix their child and solve their difficulties. The profession is therefore faced with the classic problem that the parents are either the best possible or the most necessary mediators of change, and so they need to be encouraged to change without any implication that they are culpable.

By now you should be able to recite fluently the barriers and facilitators of such change: motivation to start, motivation to continue, program (especially trainer) appeal, practical and material barriers, social (especially spousal and family) support, and cultural (i.e., values) fit. Parents have to accept the need to modify their family interactions and the rationale for the benefit of parent training has to be convincing, so they are committed to making changes. Change is harder for parents with onerous child-care responsibilities, such as young solo mothers, or those who are financially strapped. The values implicit in the training model have to be culturally acceptable as well, and likely to be encouraged by family members, friends, and the local community, especially church congregations. In many societies, religious groups have distinctive ideas about child-rearing practices, so that, for example, some fundamentalist Christian sects are strongly in favor of corporal punishment, based on literal interpretations of the bible. Finally the initial skills or task requirements should not be too complicated and beyond the parents' capabilities to implement consistently. Their early efforts at changing their behavior should result in noticeable improvements (as defined by the parents) in the behavior of the targeted child. This is because happier children represent the most meaningful reinforcement to sustain the new family rules and protocols.

Parents need to be recruited as mediators even when the problems identified have no direct connection with discipline at home or school. It will be equally unhelpful, therefore, to hold parents to account for concerns such as habit disorders, shyness and social anxiety, phobias, apathy, and depressed mood. Family therapists, who tend to see the complex dynamics within the family system, try not to be drawn into labeling the child's behavior as either externalizing or internalizing, or into identifying either the child or the parent as the problem. No such judgment should be made when understanding that what needs to change is the relationships between family members. Family dynamics already complicate even the most simple parent training efforts. That is because mothers and fathers are different people who respond to different things the child does in different ways and have different attitudes regarding what the child should do and what the parental response should be. Anyone who has ever worked clinically with a family knows this is true. It is not always a barrier to the design of a change procedure, as parents do communicate, compromise, adjust, and reevaluate—most of the time. If they do not, then at least the child has to learn that there is more than one set of rules in the world.

Because they do learn so much about adults, children can be catalyst for adult change. In our work with teachers on the emotional climate of the classroom (Evans & Harvey, 2012), one of the striking findings was that students quickly learn about their teacher's personality, emotional buttons, and idiosyncratic rules and standards. Younger children sometimes interpreted punishments as their teacher not liking them. Slightly older children could see that punishments and other disciplinary procedures they disliked were designed for their own good. They realized that teachers who seemed to be angry were not necessarily so; and it was much more negative to realize their teacher was disappointed with them than to be punished. The oldest of the elementary school children were able to judge various discipline strategies, such as being asked to leave the classroom, as designed to help children manage their own emotions and to cool off, rather than being a punishment per se (Andersen, Evans, & Harvey, 2012). Family therapy is predicated on children's understanding of adults and their feelings, and how far rules can be tested and stretched.

Blame-Relief Encourages Zeal

Not everyone, however, agrees that a focus on the dynamics of family interactions is neutral with respect to blame—judgments apportioning responsibility. This is starkly illustrated in rival family-based treatment protocols for young people with eating disorders, specifically anorexia nervosa. One of the dominant protocols is called the "Maudsley approach" and is described as "family-based treatment" (Lock et al., 2001). But its proponents are quick to point out that this is completely different from family therapy, in which, they claim, the theory that parents are "enmeshed" with the eating-disordered adolescent implies blame and maligns parents. Instead they argue that parents are the best agents for change—instead of being concerned with family dynamics, the approach advocates "rallying the family behind the healthy adolescent" (LeGrange, 2005).

The Maudsley protocol requires anorexia to be considered an "illness." Parents are blameless—their coercive efforts are directly aimed at simply fighting the disease and not their daughters. The first phase of the protocol requires that the parents take control, monitor every meal, and insist on the adolescent eating more and gaining weight to a more normal level—weight restoration (Eisler et al., 2000). Once this has been achieved, the second phase involves slowly returning control to the young person. The third and final phase focuses on normal adolescent development, based on the grounds that while ill, the young person has missed common adolescent experiences, such as having a normal body shape, dating, doing teenage kinds of things, and negotiating changed relationship with parents. These are some of the aspects of adolescent behavior with which other treatment approaches start.

The families that are successful in implementing this draconian procedure become ardent supporters of the Maudsley program, true believers, probably due to cognitive dissonance. They have conferences, a website called Maudsley Parents (www.maudsleyparents.org), a complimentary monthly newsletter, and so on. Such devotion to a treatment method facilitates change through motivational zeal, modeling, social influence by communication and rethinking values—all the things on which we rely to promote change. But it also creates adherence to a formula—a faith in a method rather than an increased understanding of sources of behavioral influence and change that can be adjusted and modified according to circumstances.

Social Support

It is a truism that when distressed clients engage in psychotherapy and find a therapist who is supportive, nonjudgmental, caring, and competent, their immediate emotional reaction is one of relief. They feel safe. They may feel hopeful. Their mood will change, if only for a brief period of time. Again we encounter the influence of acceptance—clients feel accepted for who they are and the therapist communicates respect for the dignity of the individual, whatever their status. But to resolve stressful problems on a more permanent basis, life changes need to occur. Will the same general maxim apply in the case of positive nonprofessional relationships—what we call social support?

As a causal mechanism for change, the key difference between social support and social connectedness (which will be discussed in the next chapter) is in terms of the emotional and relationship intimacy that characterizes the former. Clients may have a long list of Facebook friends and spend much time texting and Tweeting, but still not perceive that they have someone they can turn to in times of crisis and need, both emotionally and materially. However, cultural influences, arising from the desire to belong and to identify with a larger group, shape and direct behavior irrespective of the low level of intimacy involved. It is for this reason that on-line support groups can be so beneficial. When people with a common need can share often immensely intimate stories, get advice and new perspectives, and receive encouragement and the awareness they are not alone, good, if perhaps not particularly specific outcomes accrue: hopefulness, feelings of efficacy, and strategies worth trying (Elgar & McGrath, 2008).

Much research on the nature of social support has confirmed that it is difficult to objectify—perceived or experienced social support is what is important for sustaining behavior change. Emotional support from spouses, family, and friends is surely similar to that provided by a professional therapist—having people that you can go to for assurance and sympathy. Social supporters need to be good listeners and empathic, at least if you are a woman and your support person is female—"tend and befriend" is the current catchphrase. Males seem to experience support even when their area of concern is not raised in conversation (Tannen, 1990). How your support network talks to you, discusses issues, and engages in advice giving versus simply listening and accepting, are all variables that determine the emotional benefits.

When a therapist asks a client, perhaps in passing, "have you got someone at home or in your life who you can talk to about these issues?" it is important to listen carefully to the answer. Robert Wahler (1980) provided a convincing illustration of just how crucial this is. He ascertained that for the young single women to whom he was trying to teach principles of more effective behavior management of their children, whatever potential social supports they had were negative: highly critical family members and threatening and coercive professionals such as child-protection workers. He called these mothers "insular," but the real point was not that they were alone on an island but that they were surrounded by circling sharks—unsympathetic family members, bossy social welfare staff, and critical neighbors. Understandably, in this context, these young mothers tended not to use the principles that they had been taught in the intervention. If we want new skills to generalize we have to ensure that there is a reasonably caring, well-informed social environment within which they are acceptable and can be practiced and reinforced. Stress from the many challenges of life can seem quite overwhelming at times if you do not have some degree of instrumental support as well—someone you can count on to look after your toddler for a few hours, lend you money to tide you over until payday, or give you a lift to the supermarket.

People who are designated as mentally ill represent themselves in negative terms that evoke stigma, as psychiatric labels interact with other people's ideas and prejudices about the "illness." Public policy responses to this wicked problem tend to try to counteract stigma in the general public by positive media messages about how mentally ill people need hope and understanding. It is undoubtedly a good thing to reduce stigma, but the way clients interpret and represent their symptoms to others is equally important. People who have never been depressed underestimate the emotional impact of depression and minimize its seriousness. Friends and relatives who have never been depressed may correctly perceive that encouraging a depressed person to be more active has therapeutic benefits, but if the depressed person is seeking greater understanding and more opportunity to express his or her sad mood, the mismatch can surely lead to conflict and lowered support (Vollmann et al., 2010). A therapist needs to pay attention to potential supportive relationships, as low levels of social support impede improvement in depressed people (e.g., Zuroff & Blatt, 2002).

With children the same general arguments apply, however the social support of interest comes really from parents, other family members, and teachers, until the child is an adolescent (teenager) when friends do become central. If we are considering children with anxiety disorders there is considerable research to help us understand how a parent serves to foster anxiety reduction or interfere with it. When a shy child encounters a stranger, or a child with performance anxiety has to take a test, parents can be supportive by suggesting strategies, clarifying the absence of threat, using positive, less emotive words, acting confident themselves, and not being overly attentive to anxious expression or rewarding avoidance (Thompson, 2001). This presupposes, however, that there is a strong attachment relationship with the caregiver, who is also not overprotective. When one of my students studied mothers interacting with their children who had to undergo an invasive and painful medical procedure, she observed large individual differences in the mothers' ability to mask their own distress, sooth their children in a compassionate rather than impatient way, and direct their children's attention elsewhere (Keene et al., 2003). Most important of all is that the support offered in such relationships somehow matches not just the needs of the individual but their preferred style of coping as well—accurate medical information is not helpful to a child who copes by avoidance (Melamed, 1983).

Expressed Emotion: Support That Isn't

Back in the late 1960s it was noted that family attitudes and communication often predicted "relapse" or the readmission to the hospital by patients with severe psychiatric disorders who had been discharged back into the community. The type of family response that seemed most damaging to long-term prognosis was a very subtle one that communicated some degree of hostility, negativity, or lack of acceptance toward the patient. This pattern was called "expressed emotion" and it could be assessed by a complex structured interview in which family members expressed, not overtly, rejection (the opposite of acceptance) regarding the individual patient who was now coming home to live with them (e.g., Vaughn & Leff, 1976).

Because expressed emotion was such a significant predictor of patient outcome, the phenomenon has been extensively researched (Hooley, 1985; Hooley & Hillier, 2000). But for all that, it seems to have been rather glossed over in all other areas of client care, and has been investigated seriously only in the original context—hospitalized patients returning to their families (parents, spouses, or children) for their on-going care. In fact, however, the phenomenon is really a part of what we have already been describing in detail: the people that we depend on for support need to be accepting and to be able to provide a social environment that is therapeutic—that promotes ongoing improvement and change for the better. Social networks can be rated for their intensity, or the degree to which an individual is induced to honor obligations arising from network ties, especially close-knit family bonds, intimate friends, shared interests, and tribal loyalties. Immigrant groups, for example, may sustain cultural expectations of obligation and reciprocity. Asian families migrating to New Zealand often place considerable pressure on their children to achieve at school on the grounds that they made a sacrificial move to a new country to give them a better life (Aye, Guerin, Evans, & Ho, 2000). Such networks can exert potent social pressure on clients, including criticism, sanctions for violating social expectations, and a web of unrelenting feedback. If people are relying on others, as they always do, for social support, these others have to be supportive. That may be the most important variable relating to generalization and maintenance of therapeutic change (Chapter 2).

There is one further way in which we can mobilize social influence as a direct aid to planned therapeutic change and that is to form treatment groups in which a number of people with similar needs or concerns are combined to collaborate together: group therapy. As there are so many different models of how group therapy might be conducted, I want to highlight only one issue related to change, as all of the principles discussed thus far are as relevant to groups as they are to individuals. Cultural expectations form a natural link with some of the matters described in the next chapter. *"Talk story"* is Hawaiian pidgin for a form of casual, often quite prolonged, seemingly unfocused social interaction involving relaxing, low-pressure catching up among friends, gossiping, shooting the breeze. Versions probably exist across many cultures. In the black community in the United States, a common form of naturally occurring support group is the *sister circle*. These involve friendships, extended family networks, and a strong sense of community. There is evidence that when formal interventions, say for anxiety concerns, are planned within sister circles a whole range of potent change influences occur, from sharing experiences, to music (gospel singing), to expressions of faith (Neal-Barnett et al., 2011).

Implications

For social relationships to be supportive they have to provide the support that clients need and can benefit from. This is true for all caregivers—parents, teachers, and especially therapists. As needs vary, it is the match between what is needed and what is offered that determines the benefit. Therapists might remember this, not only when assessing the potential capital of a client's social networks, but when judging their own relationship with the client. There are quite a few "shoulds," "needs," and "musts" in this chapter. Ellis would not have liked it at all. But of course I emphasize these imperatives because they show that values and methods of change cannot usually be contrasted—they are inseparable.

The ways that good social supports work to enhance change are very varied. In the depression example the implications were that conflict with friends and family might be reduced if depressed individuals are able to discuss mutual perceptions and feelings within their social networks. With other types of problems, with different dynamics, other influences pertain. For instance, it is quite often reported that people with eating disorders such as bulimia are especially sensitive to negative evaluation by their peers. Really good friends, it is assumed, are less likely to be critical and make negative evaluations and thus reduce the client's drive to thinness and enhance more realistic body weight ideals. The authors who have demonstrated this possible relationship in a cross-sectional study went on to suggest that prevention of eating disorders in college freshmen could be facilitated by community building activities that encourage the formation of early social support networks (Wonderlich-Tierney & Vander Wal, 2010); a neat illustration of increasing social capital as an intervention strategy.

It may seem that we have wandered a very long way from the therapeutic alliance with which this chapter began to the more general issues of emotionally meaningful social support. Thus, it might be useful to recap the major connections and parallels. As a value statement rather than a method of influence, therapists, support staff, and parents all help by showing unconditional positive regard—acceptance—for the client/service user/child. Another is that the therapeutic relationship has the potential to be a powerful emotional experience, one affecting both parties. In that way it is not unlike the emotional relationship between parent and child, or a meaningful close relationship between friends. But beyond that the comparison is not a good one—therapists are not surrogate parents. Similarly, the therapist is not the same as the client's friend. As family and friendship relationships seem so important to life satisfaction, therapists are advised to ensure that they are not offering a substitute to these. The promotion of naturally occurring affirmative social relationships that are supportive and have only positive expressed emotion is often an implicit goal of all psychological intervention.

Where the similarity between parent and therapist is noteworthy is in the way in which their influence on the other person (child or client) is both direct (shaping positive behaviors) and indirect (being a source of warmth, comfort, and safety). In other words, the need for emotional closeness is high both because it permits emotional growth (new emotion competence) and because it enhances the ability to influence the child or the client in other ways. It is not the same emotional experience for the client as for the child—but there are parallels. Parents need to be accepting and uphold standards in a generally non-judgmental fashion; therapists need to be accepting and selectively judgmental. Parents need to have boundaries, to offer honest feedback, to foster growing independence, and to avoid using their children to serve their own emotional needs. Therapists need to do all these as well. The mere fact of a relationship can teach important lessons about feelings, about intimacy, and about who you are. But without an intervention plan, a strongly allied therapist might really resemble a loving parent who does not understand simple positive discipline. A parent who has excellent discipline strategies but who does not feel close and loving and accepting might be able to maintain behavioral control, for a while. A highly directive therapist without acceptance and concern for the client might equally be able to promote positive behavior change, but not for long.

11

Culture as Behavior Change

What makes children happy? We all know the answer, but just to be sure UNICEF commissioned a study of children in three rather different European countries, the United Kingdom, Spain, and Sweden (Ipsos MORI & Nairn, 2011). Across all three countries the findings from 8- to 13-year-old children was consistent: "the message from them all was simple, clear and unanimous: their well-being centers on time with a happy, stable family, having good friends and plenty of things to do, especially outdoors" (p. 1). Where the children in each country differed was in the culture of the family. In Spain and Sweden family life appeared to be woven into the fabric of everyday life, whereas in the United Kingdom "we found families struggling, pushed to find the time their children want, something exacerbated by the uncertainty about the rules and roles operating within the family household. And we found less participation in outdoor and creative activities amongst older and more deprived children" (p. 2). Although all the children enjoyed popular brands of material goods for their social and symbolic value, these were not viewed as essential for their happiness. The children recognized that it was better to wait for and work for consumer goods than to be "spoiled." Yet the cultures clearly differed, with the British parents feeling considerable pressure to buy things for their children as compensation for their relative unavailability.

Culture refers to a set of beliefs, values, expectations, customs, symbols, and rules of behavior that are shared by a distinctive group of people (Fiske, Kitayama, Markus, & Nisbett, 1998). Even more importantly, cultures specify the rules of behavior—the actions that will be rewarded and the actions that will be punished. The classic observation in our field is how a new enthusiastic and innovative teacher is quickly put in her place by the culture of the school: "'That's the way we do things around here.' And she learns that cruel and unusual punishments await those who violate the cultural taboos of the school" (Barth, 2002, p. 6). Culture is learned and learned anew by successive generations. We are all social creatures and as a general principle we behave in ways that are similar to the people around us who are important to us—our in-group. These social groups can be varied, such as a workplace group, a sporting club group, an extended family group, or a school group. As a result of intriguing sociological research on social networks (Christakis & Fowler, 2009) we now recognize that we are all strongly influenced by people with whom we are connected in some way, even if we do not know them. Because cultural patterns are embodied in practices and institutions, social groups that regulate our behavior can also be large and impersonal but can encompass a group with whom we identify, such as a social class, a religion, an ethnic group, or gender (Cohen, 2009).

In clinical work when helping people change we consider all of these groups to be cultures, from the narrow circle, say, of three or four girlfriends with whom a teenager hangs at school, to the broadest class of, say, young upwardly mobile professional women. When we move from one cultural grouping to another, our behavior changes to fit with the expectations, norms, and standards of that culture. The extent of that fit, or the degree of adherence to the cultural rules, will be related to identity and our role within the group. You might be a teen identifying strongly with a particular clique at school, but your role might be that of the cynical maverick, whose behavior then reflects less conformity to that particular group and more rebellion, which defines your role or place in the clique. As long as the role is not overdone and you remain accepted by the group, you will remain in that culture and be shaped by it, even though the direction of action cannot always be predicted. Guerin (2003) argued that identities are not fixed beliefs residing within the individual, but are ways of talking and behaving that are shaped by the audience controlling access to resources. This is a useful framework, as obviously people have multiple identities and any discernible culture has multiple resources.

Colloquially we talk about some behavioral cultures as well. For example, we recognize that the oil company BP had a management culture prioritizing making profits over ensuring safety, or that some older teens and college students have a "binge drinking" culture. This too means that within an organizational or social network certain explicit patterns of behavior are accepted, even encouraged. Boastful or exaggerated stories of your inebriated state and previous night's exploits, and pictures of drunken behavior posted on the Internet, all provide encouragement and modeling beyond mere acceptability of excessive drinking. What are known as *behavioral regularities* are the commonly occurring patterns of behavior that develop in a cultural setting but that have no intrinsic connection to the aim of the activity, which is to have fun with your friends. The binge drinking culture also consists of *enabling behaviors* that are part of the sequence of getting drunk, but are not themselves drinking activities. Because bar prices for alcohol are inflated, young people will start out drinking at home or in apartments with friends and housemates. To do so requires planning and purchasing the alcohol from a discount liquor store some time before. If there are legally imposed age restrictions on the purchase of alcohol, the drinking culture normalizes low-level illegal activity by young people such as acquiring a false ID or persuading an older adult to purchase alcohol on your behalf. Changing individual behavior is difficult within this cultural context, and changing the culture through social policies and judicial sanctions—such as fines for industrial accidents on oil rigs, or raising the legal drinking age—is equally challenging because tactics that can be used for getting around these restrictions are sanctioned by the group.

The good news is that all broader human societies seem to share certain basic potentially uplifting properties. These can be summarized as (1) the centrality of social relationships, (2) the presence of status hierarchies, and (3) the reality that all cultures have a religion of some kind. The latter usually identifies rules and proscribed behaviors (morals), especially regarding reproduction, sexual behavior, gender roles, food preparation, and so on. Although individuals within a given culture will vary as to the degree to which these properties emerge as motivational forces, the three patterns have been neatly translated into their essential abbreviations: "getting along," "getting ahead," and the uniquely human motivational pattern "finding meaning" (Hogan & Bond, 2009, p. 579). Even if as a therapist you are targeting very specific behavioral change, it would seem sensible to have a component of your treatment plan in which each of these three elements is addressed in some way.

Changing the Client's Cultural Group

From this brief introduction it can be seen that culture is a construct capturing those diverse forms of social influence that extend beyond the more intimate personal social relationships considered in the previous chapter, while at the same time links us back to the socioecological (contextual) influences examined in Chapter 4 as well as the importance of goals, motives, and rewards. How are we to relate culture more directly to behavior change? One way to encourage people to change might be to get them to change the cultural group with which they spend most of their time—a classic ecological strategy. If your entire social reinforcement network consists of interactions within a criminal gang, no amount of the best psychotherapeutic programming in prison is likely to change your behavior from being a criminal to being an upright citizen. Remember Wilson's study of very high-risk offenders who were managing to desist from violent crime. Larger scale studies confirm that in the long term the strongest protective factors for violence are having close personal relationships with family and friends that involve engagement in positive activities—but not if these interpersonal relationships are with people who are themselves violent, drug abusers, or criminals (Ullrich & Coid, 2011).

For anyone trying to change, be careful who your friends are. Of particular interest to psychotherapy is that if the people in your client's social network—like a college dorm, or a rugby club, or a factory—are depressed, your client is likely to be depressed as well (Howes, Hokanson, & Lowenstein, 1985). It is a well-established finding that the mothers of children with significant behavior problems (such as conduct disorder) often seem to be clinically depressed (Goodman & Gotlib, 1999). I do not know if the mothers' depressed mood causes behavior problems or if it is the other way round, but I do know that if you hope to change the child's behavior by teaching the mother more flexible and positive behavior management strategies that is going to be difficult to achieve if the mother is depressed. What is so relevant to the present analysis is that, to make matters worse, when a depressed mother identifies her best friend, it transpires that that friend is often depressed as well (Patterson, 1974). Here is a perfect example of the implications of social networks for change, in this instance a negative one—maybe there is social support, but for the wrong behaviors, such as attributions of blame, negative labeling of the child, harsh consequences, and angry affect, all verbally expressed in conversation between the two depressed women seeking mutual approval.

Not that many years ago the dominant culture for married women in Western European countries promoted acceptance of a subordinate role. When depressed, unhappy, unfulfilled young women began to consult behavior therapists, it was quite common to attempt to teach them more assertive skills. Popular books for therapists and clients alike had titles such as *"Your Perfect Right."* Cognitive beliefs about the place of women in marriage and society were challenged in these female clients. In addition to attitude change around autonomy and independence, women were taught to be more competitive, to learn skills of negotiating fair treatment, and to assert their rights to equality in sexual relationships. Undoubtedly many women were positively influenced by therapists following these general dictums. However, it became obvious to clinical practitioners that unless there was some loosening of their in-group cultural norms, by older female relatives, by female friends, and by male partners and husbands, these alternative behaviors and values would simply result in conflict, possibly physical abuse, and sometimes separation, divorce, and the need to find an entirely new cultural group. Women's liberation as promoted within behavioral psychotherapy often came at a price.

Whenever a therapist tries to change a client, or clients try to change themselves, the effect that will have on the immediate cultural group has to be seriously considered. Although it may be difficult to get an excessive social drinker to switch from rum and coke to orange juice, it is a great deal more difficult if the client's drinking takes place in a social setting of heavy drinkers who regularly get together in a bar after work or after a sporting event. If such a client cannot easily change companions, then the client has to be taught two sets of ancillary skills. One set comes under the heading *assertion*: how to say "no," how to resist social pressure, how to take criticism and teasing, and how to maintain acceptance with a group and sustain social approval while at the same time violating its fundamental norms. The other set involves *exercising restraint*, which has already been explained in the chapter on self-regulation.

Encouraging clients to change their cultural group may not always be realistic, and in addition it may not lead to enhanced subjective well-being. We know this because people often experience unexpected emotional needs when moving to a new country and thus have to adapt to a new culture. We have already encountered the importance of the person–situation interaction, but culture research also demonstrates culture × situation × person interactions (Hong & Mallorie, 2004). Different cultures value different personality styles, that is to say the behavioral tendencies (dispositions) of the majority are reinforced (Rozin, 2003). If your own personality style fails to match that of the majority it is likely to lower your self-esteem and feelings of well-being (Fulmer et al., 2010). It is plausible that when people's activities are congruent with those of the people around them, "they exist in a shared reality that validates their daily experiences and reactions to events" (Fulmer et al., 2010, p. 1564). The opposite is also true. Such negative experiences are sufficiently universal that there is a popular layperson's phrase to describe them: "culture shock."

Another way to achieve change, one that has benefits for prevention as well as maintenance of change, is to address the behavioral culture of a specific group, using higher cultural values to justify such change. Within an indigenous culture such as that of Māori, for example, there are public health concerns about the prevalence of smoking behavior and the failure to comply with health screening programs and other regular medical check-ups. To make these two behaviors (one approach, smoking; one avoidance, not having check-ups) less acceptable in the culture, current public health advertising appeals to much more fundamental cultural values, specifically the importance of staying healthy in order to be able to be a strong family support—to be there for the children, who are treasures, and not to impair their health (through secondary smoking) or risk being unable to help them in the future (through premature death). The principle is sound—it is going to be easier for an individual to get a cervical smear or breast examination or to quit smoking if everyone in their immediate social group is doing the same and accepts its importance (Sieverding, Decker, & Zimmerman, 2010). Christakis and Fowler (2009) have provided many rich examples of how social networks influence health behavior, and thus health: "your friends' friends can make you fat" (p. 105). More to the point, your friends' friends help you go for health checkups.

How do we relate these broad ideas to the many other principles of therapeutic change that we have been examining so closely? From the UNICEF study that introduced this chapter, what are the implications for parenting programs, for reward contingencies, and for routines and time management? One tactic is to consider *mechanisms* of change that seem to be particularly relevant to the regulation of behavior by cultural demands and expectations. I will first consider imitational learning, or the role of modeling, since, as Tomasello (1999) argued, the ability to use information provided by others is essential for the evolution of culture. I then consider social networks (including the role of language communities) and connections that go beyond social support. I will propose "activity settings" as a key construct for planful change. These are mere samples of the possibilities of change mechanisms at the cultural level, but they were selected because they represent insights that are well within the possibilities open to both clinicians and clients in the enablement of change. Finally I examine psychotherapy itself as a culturally laden phenomenon and the "fit" between the culture of the client and the culture of the therapist.

Modeling: The Process of Connectedness

It would have been more conventional to include the topic of modeling in the chapter on learning. This is because of the profound influence of Bandura on behavior theory, social learning, and psychology generally. Basically, Bandura (1971) argued that imitational learning was an additional learning principle, that is to say, learning by modeling the behavior of others he considered one of the basic mechanisms of human learning. The classic studies that kicked off (another pun!) this entire disciplinary trend were his studies of aggression in children. If children merely observed someone acting aggressively (in the studies this was punching and kicking a blow-up plastic Bobo doll), and in particular if that person was rewarded for doing so, then the children observing this modeled behavior would be more likely to engage in it when they too had the opportunity to interact with the Bobo doll.

Like any other experiment, it is a huge leap from playing with a plastic doll that is designed to bounce back so that hitting it is actually the fun thing to do, to aggressing against other real children, who cry, run away, or hit you back even harder. But like all classic experiments its impact was based less on the details and more on the implication: we do tend to model the behavior of others, especially meaningful people ("role models"), who are seen to benefit from the action being imitated. Bandura's studies also came at a time when it was thought that you could reduce someone's aggression by venting anger. That idea came from loose Freudian notions that pent up feelings needed to be released. In the 1999 movie *Analyze This*, Billy Crystal, playing psychotherapist Dr Ben Sobel, encourages Robert de Niro, playing gangster Paul Vitti, to get his anger out by hitting a pillow, whereupon de Niro whips out a pistol and pumps the pillow full of lead. It is a clever spoof because laypeople know, despite Bandura, that venting makes you feel better, in the short run. Certainly in the movie gangster Paul Vitti said he felt better, but due to Bandura we doubt that rehearsing aggressive behavior would make him less violent.

One reason modeling never really stood up as a principle of learning is that in both the classic studies with the Bobo doll and in subsequent clinical applications of the principle, the behaviors that emerged were not really new responses that had not previously existed in the repertoire. Children probably did not learn how to be aggressive in the Bobo experiment; they simply learned that it was acceptable to be so. In any environmental situation we have to select stimuli to attend to from the "blooming, buzzing, confusion." Observing others has a straightforward stimulus facilitation effect, which is a pretty simple, basic form of social influence. If your mother fears heights you begin to notice heights rather than the view; if you watch the movie *"Jaws"* before going for a swim, shadows in the ocean become more salient.

Regardless of these nuances, modeling can be a very useful principle—we always need to know how we should behave, what is acceptable, and what the rules in this setting are. Modeling can influence behavior patterns implicitly—such as in cultural learning—or explicitly where the individual is clearly directed to observe the desired behavior and to imitate it. Earlier we saw that *imitation* is itself a response class and that some children need to acquire it. But if they have the capacity, showing someone what they should do helps them do it and thus learn it, especially if the model is credible, has high status, or is liked. These are the two basic elements of directed observational learning and they have applications in countless psychotherapy contexts, maybe all of them. If you want to know how to behave in a socially acceptable way, observe the behavior of successful others in the relevant society or social group that you admire, and then try to emulate it.

When we as a society or culture approve of the models, imitation is deemed a good thing. But when we do not approve we give imitation negative labels such as "bowing to peer pressure," "conformity," or "crowd behavior." By and large we all like to fit in—at least somewhere, although not necessarily in the mainstream. We generally want to conform to a social group, even if the group is nonconformist relative to the greater society. Fashion in clothing is one of the most striking examples: suddenly round about 2002 every young woman was baring her midriff, and then equally suddenly, they were not. Backpacks have always been convenient and attractive, but once they became de rigueur for American school kids they became indispensable equipment for students and mobile adults in every walk of life across the entire world. When I was in elementary school, playing with marbles was a popular craze for small boys; we had the most beautiful cat's eye marbles and boys who were good shooters had pockets bulging with highly prized marbles. But here's the thing. The marble craze lasted less than 2 weeks. It would start one day, not just in my school but across every school in the city, and everyone would be playing; then equally suddenly it was over and marbles were not seen again until the following year—it would be the worst social faux pas to try to set up a game once the craze was over.

This is just one personal example similar to the many that Christakis and Fowler (2009) marshaled to illustrate their work on social networks. They have described these connections so well it is best for me simply to quote them:

> Most of us are already aware of the direct effect we have on our friends and family; our actions can make them happy or sad, healthy or sick. But we rarely consider that everything we think, feel, do, or say can spread far

> beyond the people we know. Conversely, our friends and family serve as conduits for us to be influenced by hundreds or even thousands of other people. In a kind of social chain reaction, we can be deeply affected by events we do not witness that happen to people we do not know. It is as if we can feel the pulse of the social world around us and respond to its persistent rhythms. As part of a social network, we transcend ourselves, for good or ill, and become part of something much larger. We are connected. (p. 30)

An important feature of social networks is that they often have "hubs" such as popular celebrities. Paris Hilton is notorious, has a large following, and can easily alter fashion in clothing and style. This is despite the fact that she has no special talents; she is simply rich and famous. Other social network hubs can be iconic companies. You only have to pass by an Apple store in any city and you will see that it is always crowded with people exploring new products: the iPad-2 is not only a tool for social networking, it is also a positive stimulus connecting like-minded individuals. Ethologists might call these flocking behaviors. It is social networks that play a central role in determining the popularity of any behavior (Olfati-Saber, 2007).

Modeling and Emotional Contagion

Long before the extraordinary fascination and appeal of social networking sites, psychologists understood that a person's cultural identity, or their perceived connection to a wider group of kindred souls, was a major part of his or her sense of personhood. Identification might be with an ethnic group, a social class, a religion, a nation or a geographic region, or smaller units such as a club, a team, or a gang. If you want to observe strong emotions, such as elation or despair, you only have to watch the fans of a soccer club or football team that has won or lost a game. We have come to accept in psychology that loyalty, connection, and identification with groups of this kind help to define us as individuals, who we are, and where we stand. Yet these connections, whether via the Internet or through shared icons such as a flag or an anthem, although undoubtedly social, are very different from the immediate connections we have with others in our daily lives and who provide us with direct and tangible social support (Chapter 10). Social facilitation means that the mere presence of another can increase motivation or reduce fear—a phenomenon we make good use of in all psychotherapy.

There are some happenings within social networks and connectedness that are so emotive that it may be necessary to think of a special kind of modeling or imitational learning to account for them. The phenomenon I am thinking of is sometimes called group hysteria, in which people who do not necessarily know each other but are connected in some way begin to show identical fears (often in the form of panic behavior) or psychosomatic phenomena, such as a rash, nausea, or fainting. Christakis and Fowler (2009) suggest that the widespread fear in American schools about children having an allergic reaction to nuts provides a socially accepted everyday example, since the dangers of nut allergies to children are actually much less of a risk than, say, car or bicycle accidents.

Phenomena such as these, which have been reported across many cultural settings, suggest that modeling others' emotions as opposed to their overt behavior is a particular kind of imitational learning. Although Bandura did not consider such modeling specifically, later researchers certainly have, and this specialized form is now known as emotional contagion (Hatfield, Cacioppo, & Rapson, 1994). I am not sure that the negative connotation of the word *contagion*, which its medical links to infection, was ever really intended, since the definition by Hatfield et al. is "the tendency to automatically mimic and synchronize facial expressions, vocalizations, postures, and movements with those of another person's and consequently, to converge emotionally" (p. 5).

In other words, we share feelings when we observe other people's emotions, even though we have not shared the same causal experiences. In different contexts this might be called empathy, but in this model an effect based on actual mimicry and feedback from the mimicked responses is the proposed mechanism. The discovery of specialized mirror neurons as the enabling physiological mechanism for the effect has fuelled excitement among neuroscientists. Blakemore and Frith (2005) summarized the evidence that observing or even imagining a response activates the same motor neural programs that are necessary to perform that action. However, a reductionist account of empathy does not tell us much about why empathy is so limited in a few people and so unlikely to change behavior when we want it to. Yes, we might "cry at sad movies," or get "tense when...around people who are stressed out"; however, the implications for more permanent behavior change in therapy (Rosner, Beutler, & Daldrup, 2000) or in life are not obvious. But as soon as we have a concept we have a self-report scale to measure it—the two previous quotations come from the Emotional Contagion Scale (Doherty, 1997).

Emotional contagion phenomena provide a good example of the interaction between emotional predispositions, such as anxiety, and collective behavior in which social influences such as modeling are salient when there is *no* agreed upon culturally appropriate response to a situation. A rather intriguing illustration of this comes from an event that occurred among schoolchildren in South Africa in the year 2000 (Rataemane, Rataemane, & Mohlahle, 2002). Over 1400 students in Grades 8–10 experienced itching. The itching and scratching (using stones, walls, brushes, rulers, and pens) occurred almost exclusively at school, not at home. The itching was treated with antihistamine creams and the schools were fumigated and washed with antiseptics; entomologists found no biohazards. Prayers and washing with water that had been blessed by a faith healer reportedly made the itching worse. Once it was realized that this was a psychological phenomenon, strong public health messages, setting limits by the school administration, and asking those still itching to stay at home until it stopped ended the epidemic as rapidly as it began. The two major contributing factors—which demonstrate my general point—were (1) affected children were highly anxious about being infected and experienced hyperventilation, pins and needles, dizziness, headache, and fainting; and (2) the influence was by line of sight, with symptoms developing only when they saw others scratching.

In social contexts it is likely that imitation (modeling) is greatest under two key conditions: the closeness of the social network and uncertainty regarding appropriate or safe courses of action. A good example of these two interacting source of influence is provided by the behavior of voluntary vaccination, and especially immunization of children (Fu, Rosenbloom, Wang, & Nowak, 2010). Social networks (other parents of young children, general medical practitioners' patient registers, local district health nurses, attendees at early childhood centers, and so on) support the behavior of getting our children inoculated. The few families that fail to imitate this practice—known in public health settings as "free riders"—are protected from adverse consequences by "herd immunity." Sufficiently large percentages of a population immunize their children so that the infectious diseases are largely eradicated for everyone.

If, however, the number of free riders becomes too large, herd immunity disappears. This can happen if young parents now imitate an alternative social network, one of nonimmunizers. This new network occurs when highly connected people—such as the parents of children with autism or other parents accessing the same Internet information—are both uncertain about the risks of not vaccinating (as diseases become less common) and uncertain about the risks of vaccinating. This is precisely what has happened in countries such as Great Britain, where the widespread dissemination of myths regarding the dangers of the measles–mumps–rubella vaccination as a cause of autism resulted in the modeling of not vaccinating, such that herd immunity no longer pertains. This new imitative behavior results in the public health problem of increasing incidences of diseases once well controlled.

Language as Cultural Behavior

When we analyzed cognitions in Chapter 7, the focus was predominantly on verbal processes, the denotative meaning of words. Chapter 5 considered the connotative meaning of words and the manner in which internal dialogue and personal narratives influence emotional states and overt behavior. In this section we are more concerned with the social, communicative function of language. By changing language we change social relationships and from there perhaps we can change the behaviors and the contexts that cause us distress. Language is not a means to a behavioral end, it is an end in itself because it is a symbolic representation of the things everyone desires—security, acceptance, sharing experiences, love, and understanding.

Language carries the influence of culture on behavior in ways that do not require direct experience of phenomena, just as stories, fables, and myths carry the culture's collective memory of past events. The impact of the latter can be seen clearly in strongly bicultural settings such as New Zealand. Here the recent history of an iwi (tribe) can be readily encapsulated in a verbal concept such as "colonization," which conveys the connotation of loss, discrimination, and injustice that motivates groups of people to take actions to change their situation in spite of the fact that they never personally experienced the historical events (wars, land confiscation, suppression of cultural practices) directly. The former, somewhat more general case can be seen in psychology in many forms. An example I have always found pertinent is the verbal concept of "the terrible twos." In my culture it is common knowledge that 2-year-old children are difficult to deal with, a belief held even by people who do not have or know any 2-year-old children. Young children's actual behavior, when observed, will be judged more rapidly and negatively and responded to accordingly, just as acceptance of negative behavior can be influenced by totally different pieces of cultural lore that "boys will be boys" or "teenagers have raging hormones."

When considering in an earlier section the manifestation of "mass hysteria" it was clear that generally the interesting phenomena that have been reported have occurred in tightly connected groups somewhat segregated from other people, such as girls' schools, convents, factory workers, and hospital nurses (e.g., McEvedy & Beard, 1970). Psychotherapists are less likely to encounter such incidents directly. The cultural power of language, however, generates beliefs, common anxieties, and expectations that will represent a special case of distorted or irrational thinking. Such beliefs are hard to change when they are widely affirmed through word of mouth and the especially the media. In everyday parlance we call these notions "urban legends."

Psychologists, being skeptical by training, find it fairly easy to redefine occurrences such as memories of alien abduction as ordinary psychological events illustrating social influence and the ways we try to explain to ourselves anomalous personal experiences (Banaji & Kihlstrom, 1996). However, other urban legends, less implausible, can be readily accepted and thus unlikely to be challenged: they become common knowledge in a given culture, behavior patterns change, and the original threat is perpetuated. A common urban legend that emerged in the 1970s in the United States is that there are many dangerous people who deliberately try to poison children's Halloween candy or insert razor blades, needles, or shards of glass. The legend was created by the media and today everyone in the United States knows that children should not accept homemade treats or anything other than commercially wrapped candy when trick-or-treating (Best & Horiuchi, 1985). Children are given verbal warning by their parents and no one would risk challenging these "safety-seeking" behaviors, as they do serve the function of reducing a perceived threat.

Language encodes beliefs. Another class of widely accepted cultural beliefs, slightly different from more specific urban legends, involves stereotypes. Christine Sleeter (interviewed in Orelus, 2011) has shown from historical family records that the common American belief that white immigrants advanced their wealth and social standing purely by hard work and self-sacrifice is a stereotypic myth. Her own "pioneer" ancestors were sold arable land for one dollar after it had been confiscated from the indigenous owners. Given that stereotypes are so widely held in a culture, people accept them as applying to themselves. This has been documented by Claude Steele (1997) in a long series of fascinating studies showing the harmful effects of stereotypic threat. A good example is that because women believe the stereotype that females are less capable than males in math-related fields, their performance can be impaired when challenged by difficult problems.

The relevance for clinical behavior change is considerable as clients come with this level of cultural knowledge and "understanding" that is just as influential as the verbal distortions that are attended to and addressed by cognitive therapists. Indeed, clinicians might even share the cultural belief unless well versed in the empirical evidence from psychology and other social sciences. We may challenge irrational ideas that we recognize as such, but are less able to do so when we share them ourselves. Clinically relevant "distortions" are considered irrational because they are judged by the therapist as not universally held by the client's wider cultural group, although they may well be held strongly, and thus reinforced, by the client's more immediate social network.

A teenage client's attributions regarding external locus of control, for example, might be judged by a therapist as irrational and thus changeworthy, but might nevertheless be repeatedly validated by his or her immediate friends. An unexpectedly good grade on a test will not be seen as the result of hard work, good study habits, or ability if our friends only reinforce the discourse that "I was lucky that the test was easy and that I happened to know the answers to those questions." Because many teenagers tend not to like to boast about their ability, and even less about the intensity of their study efforts, external attributions to chance, luck, and fate are much more socially acceptable. As Guerin (2003) argues, language's primary function is to sustain social relationships. Social relationships are especially important to teenagers (or is that just a culturally held belief?), so discourse that maintains a social interaction is strongly reinforced. The cognitive therapist who hopes to challenge irrational beliefs that are not considered irrational by an influential cultural group has a long row to hoe.

Another major function of language is to get people to do things. Through language-transmitted communication some people try to directly influence others—the process of persuasion to a particular attitude, belief, point of view, or value. Dynamic Social Impact Theory embraces a substantial body of research demonstrating that the degree to which one person is influenced by a social group is a function of the strength, immediacy, and number of communications from others (Latané, 1996). Therapy is about persuasion. As a therapist you may, if commanding sufficient professional stature, be able to draw on strength and usually immediacy, but if a cultural group is providing a large number of opposite communications, changing an individual's beliefs and attitudes is going to be difficult.

Everyday Activity Settings

The daily schedules of ordinary lives are made up of a series of routines that fill the available time (this was discussed in more detail in Chapter 7). A similar concept in cultural theory is that of an *activity*: goal-directed behavior that occurs within implicit cultural expectations and social assumptions (Cole, 1985). Tharp and Gallimore (1988) called routines "activities" and the contexts in which they occur "activity settings"—"as homely and familiar as old shoes and the front porch. They are the social furniture of our family, community, and work lives" (p. 72).

There are four defining features of activity settings as a unit of analysis. The people present and available are the "who." Note the emphasis on available, as we have already noted with social support. If, as an illustration, you are a child growing up on the Upper West Side of Manhattan, your visits to the Natural History Museum may well be with your nanny rather than your parents. She is the "who." The task being enacted is the "what." The goal of the activity is at the level of "why"—the motive that depends heavily on the cultural and personal interpretation of the task. The nature of the activity as it unfolds—the form of the routine—is the "how."

When you get taken to the Museum by your father or mother the goal might be to increase your knowledge and understanding of science and nature. You would have the same overt activity as when you went with your nanny (walking around the museum), but how you do it will differ, perhaps focusing on specific exhibits, spending more time in front of them, having your attention directed to certain features, or being asked pointed questions. When you go with your nanny, however, the goal is to entertain you, or more likely to pass the time of day or to meet up with other nannies. You might still have fun and learn something, but the form of the activity will be different. Although not negating the possibility that nannies want children to learn and daddies want them to have fun, the fact that the primary goal varies will determine whether the activity is judged a success. The museum visit will be repeated by either caregiver if the parent sees their child has benefited intellectually and the nanny has met her friends without spending most of her time trying to control behavior. This is the reinforcement that establishes the activity as a regular one.

Because daily life is made up of a sequence of routines or activities, it can be seen that changing behavior requires changing activity settings. Because routine activities are comfortable, predictable, and generally work for us in terms of fulfilling everyday goals, even when major ecological change, such as a natural disaster, totally disrupts activity settings, people try to reestablish their routines to be as close as possible to their activities prior to the disturbance. Gallimore (2005) suggests that activity settings are difficult to change (and hence behavior is difficult to change) because while the *what* and the *how* of the activity may not be optimal, for the *who* (individuals or cultural group) the activity settings have evolved because they work just well enough and are predictable, familiar (as the porch and the old shoe!), and allow for feelings of control.

Gallimore has offered initial suggestions as to how activity settings (and hence behavior) might be changed. We have already seen that changing *who* the activities are done with is a significant contextual variable in all sorts of ways. However, Gallimore suggests that clarifying goals and sharing common ones will change perceptions of the task and how individuals within it interact. The museum illustration (based, incidentally, on closely observing children's behavior during recent visits to the American Museum of Natural History in New York) is still a good one. If it could be clarified that the goal of the visit is to teach the child more about the wonders of nature, it would be easy enough for the nanny to spend less time on her cell phone and, if she herself does not have the language skills and technical knowledge to engage in meaningful questions, to solicit help and interaction from the numerous well-informed volunteers and museum guides who are typically available (additional *whos*). (Parents of course can do the same, as their own technical knowledge might be equally insufficient.) Conversely, if the parent could clarify that the goal is for the child to have a good time and to want to return, then adding elements such as choice, a focus on the more interactive exhibits, and an ice cream in the cafeteria, would all alter the *how* of the parental museum visit.

Inevitably there comes a time when going to the same museum over and over again is neither enjoyable nor informative. Sometimes the *what* itself needs to be changed. In a sense, Gallimore, argues, changing activities is the same as innovation, and we have information from management principles as to how to foster innovation. The five commonly recognized principles should be familiar to you by now: (1) The innovation has to offer some clear advantage over the status quo—it has to be more effective and more reinforcing. (2) It has to be compatible with existing values and perceptions of needs. (3) It cannot be too complex and (4) it must permit experimentation—that is to say it needs to be able to be trialed, tested out before being adopted. And finally (5) the benefits (or the costs) must be clearly transparent—visible to those expected to use and accept the innovation.

For the therapist (no, we have not lost sight of the main point) this discussion highlights yet again some important principles, but this time within a cultural perspective. You need to find out as much as possible about the activity settings that contain and constrain the behavior patterns that have been deemed change-worthy. This is equally true for behaviors that are culturally commonplace but are not occurring for the client. For example, even though an adult client with an intellectual disability may have moved from an institution to a community placement, his or her accommodation will most likely not support the daily routines most of us take for granted—going to a movie with a friend, taking a long bubble bath, and ordering a pizza delivery. This is a principle formulated by Meyer and Evans (1989) when first proposing an educative approach to managing challenging behavior in such clients by enhancing the quality of everyday life. You need to clarify that the individuals relevant to that activity setting actually have the same goals. You need to see if any efforts are currently being undertaken to change activity settings. Are these efforts consistent with cultural values, and if so, can they form the basis of the innovations you propose, especially if these are likely to be equally successful as the established activity? Introduce these innovations simply as a trial, make sure they are not overly complicated, and look for ways of making the beneficial outcomes crystal clear, relative to the current situation.

Routines and Rituals

Whether we call the repeated events of everyday life "activities" or "routines" is of little importance compared with the recognition that "naturally occurring family routines and meaningful rituals provide both a predictable structure that guides behavior and an emotional climate that supports…development" (Spagnola & Fiese, 2007, p. 284). In families, emotionally relevant conversations, discussions of values and priorities, planning for the future, reading and story-telling—all highly culturally determined events—do not take place in a vacuum. They occur within the context of family routines and rituals. There is no firm prescription for how these are conducted. In some cultural and community contexts, for example, among Native Hawaiians, more conversation and emotion-relevant talk take place among siblings, especially when busy parents with large families rely on older siblings to provide substantial amounts of child care (Weisner, Gallimore, & Jordan, 1988).

Spagnola and Fiese (2007) propose that the difference between routines and rituals is as follows: "family routines are characterized by communication that is instrumental, involve a momentary time commitment, and are repeated regularly, holding no special meaning. Family rituals involve communication with symbolic meaning, establishing and perpetuating the understanding of what it means to be a member of the group" (p. 285). With their focus on early childhood, these authors explain how family routines at dinnertime involving conversation and meta-language regarding past events and future plans shape language and social skills. Bedtime routines that involve reading and stories enhance academic skills. When people get married or have babies, new routines have to be negotiated. Rituals such as saying grace, family gatherings, and holidays will tend to have a more direct cultural determination, but are highly variable within cultures. Having photographs and framed certificates on the walls, having family albums or electronic displays, or visiting a deceased family member's grave site will be represented differently across cultures, but some semblance of the common rituals will be universal.

The creation of predictable routines and meaningful rituals probably has positive benefit by giving parents a sense of self-efficacy and competency in parenting. Children involved in routines at home are more easily monitored by their parents, well-known to be an important antidote to delinquent and risky childhood activities. In addition, family rituals have symbolic value, are often celebratory, and create traditions that help bind families together in responsible and dependable relationships. Disruption of meaningful rituals can harm family cohesion; disruption of routines can be stressful and a hassle, but alternatives can and do emerge.

How does understanding these behavioral structures help us plan behavior change? Interventions must fit within the routines of people's lives. They must be consistent with their rituals. When people—and families, if you are working at the systemic level—lack appropriate routines to support the kinds of lives they hope for, they may need to be educated regarding the establishment of predictable routines. However, the therapist then has to ask questions as to why routines were impoverished in the first place (Fiese, 2006). Transactional models of family function illustrate how characteristics of the child alter his or her family environment and the environment equally shapes the child. The ways parents interpret their children's behavior can be changed, and routines can be realigned. The latter is especially important when events such as divorce, stepparenting and blended families, or having a child with a disability require that routines be renegotiated.

Culture and Psychotherapy

It has long been assumed that therapists from the same cultural background as the clients will be better equipped to help them change and thus achieve better outcomes. It makes intuitive sense that people from the same general culture share implicit knowledge of routines and rituals. But life is not that simple. When I first started to supervise Māori clinical psychology students in New Zealand I rather naively thought that they would be especially comfortable working with Māori clients, with whom they would have shared knowledge, and would be able to establish an easy rapport and supportive working alliance. I was wrong. These supervisees told me in various different ways that their Māori clients often treated them with suspicion. Some clients thought that these new young clinicians had "sold out" by working professionally in a mental health facility that was clearly based on European New Zealanders' ideas and values. (In fact the mental health service models were even more alien, being essentially derived from Great Britain and the United States.) Other clients found the language and assumptions of cognitive–behavioral therapy (our standard trainee mode) to be disconcerting, regardless of who was delivering the treatment. A small number of Māori clients were embarrassed that their knowledge of Māori cultural rituals and practices was not as sophisticated as that of the Māori student trainees. And finally, the trainees, whom one would certainly consider bicultural (at home in both Māori and European New Zealander contexts) and able to think and feel according to broad Māori perspectives or world views, were not themselves intimately familiar with all of the specific expectations and practices of other iwi.

Just as an indigenous ethnic group needs to have behavioral skills that permit functioning in different cultural settings, so anyone moving into a new cultural context will find it alters the dynamic of previously familiar contexts. In describing what it was like for young African American woman returning to their families after having gone away to college, Gilford and Reynolds (2010) explained how they were "perceived as stuck up or out of touch, or were told that they were now 'acting White'" (p. 13). These same young women were identified on the basis that they had been "parentified" as children—growing up in single parent households in which the sole parent, for many different reasons, was dysfunctional and placed parenting responsibilities on the older child in the family. Such family responsibilities and expected duties are a common feature of many cultures as well as a result of exiguous circumstances within families. Going to college was a way of physically and behaviorally breaking out of that highly restricting environment. At the same time the desire to help their families and crack the mould more permanently enabled them to be very successful as college students despite the challenging social environment.

Culture means a set of implicitly held assumptions, beliefs, and expectations regarding what activities are normal, acceptable, desirable, and admirable, and shared and accepted by a particular group. If you belong to that group, those cultural norms and values will profoundly shape and determine your behavior—adaptations often known as social contagion. It can, of course, be hard to separate the influence of the group (contagion) from the tendency to connect with people similar to yourself (homophily) (Leenders, 2003). What makes the influence of culture so profound is that we are rarely aware of these contingencies until we attempt to function in a new culture with very different expectations. This reflects the old adage that the fish does know that it lives in water. A complete theory of change would need to explain how cultures influence behavior, but as this book is only about planful change, it is necessary to examine the relationship between culture and planned psychological treatment only briefly.

Cultural Competence, or Knowing What You Don't Know

A widely recognized difficulty for ensuring culturally competent change programs is that the forms of behavior considered abnormal vary across cultures and societies. Putting this in simpler and more meaningful terms: will someone who is depressed in Japan behave in the same way as someone who is depressed in Finland? Pluralist models tend to think that the pathology is the same even though it might be expressed in slightly different ways. A second important way that culture has been considered is in the way the *client* approaches therapy, especially when the therapists is from a different culture. Will it be possible to forge a meaningful relationship, and will the therapist's model of psychopathology and causes of distress be compatible with the worldview of the client?

Recognition within psychotherapy of the importance of culture has grown considerably in the past 20 years or so. Yet it would be fair to say that cultural diversity is still very much an afterthought, given that professional psychotherapy is still a phenomenon of Western industrialized societies and within them is dominated by the ethnic and cultural "European/Anglo-American" majority. There are basically just a few ways that culture has been addressed, even by those genuinely interested in cross-cultural psychology and counseling. The most prominent is something like cultural sensitivity or awareness on the part of the therapist. Often called cultural competence, it relates to how a therapist of one cultural group, typically the dominant one in any given society, can appreciate the values, expectations, goals, and needs of clients from another culture, usually a subordinate one. Cultural competence requires skills in understanding other cultures in a particularist manner, and yet not stereotyping clients by assuming they represent their cultural norm (Sue, 1998).

Avoiding expectations based on stereotypes is easier said than done. This is because in terms of words spoken therapists are not likely to be racist, yet in practice professional behaviors (judgments made, decisions reached, and strategies designed) might nevertheless reflect what are called "implicit attitudes" in the experimental literature. One of the classic studies in this regard comes from education. Wright (1992) observed teacher–pupil and pupil–pupil interactions in class and on the playground in multicultural English schools with teachers fully committed (verbal behavior) to principles of equality. The observed behavioral biases were not necessarily based on negative attitudes; for example, Asian children were expected to be compliant and motivated to learn, although less able to socialize with other children. Black children (African-Caribbean), especially boys, were the most frequently reprimanded. Teachers' differential responding was reflected in the way children interacted with each other, something I also found in observational studies of how children with disabilities were treated differentially in highly positive, inclusive classrooms (Evans, Salisbury, Palombaro, Berryman, & Hollowood, 1992). The children and their parents in the Wright study felt such injustices keenly, resulting in more negative classroom behavior and parental complaints to the school. Despite the conscious good intentions of the school staff, they interpreted these complaints as efforts to cover up and deny the bad behavior of the black boys.

To mitigate the potential harm of both negative and positive stereotypes might require some sort of recognition and celebration of individual differences within a well-defined cultural group. The alternative—deemphasizing intergroup distinctions—is known as color blindness. This color-blind approach to promoting tolerance and inclusion is the basis for many social policy attempts to advance equality and reduce prejudice. The message that race is irrelevant and we are more similar than different sounds like a constructive one for reducing bias. However, there is growing experimental evidence that the message distorts social judgments, minimizes meaningful ethnic differences, and actually increases racial bias (Richeson & Nussbaum, 2004). A *value-diversity* message may be more helpful for changing prejudicial thinking: the emphasis should be on recognizing differences, appreciating them, and seeing how racial differences "make each of us special" (Apfelbaum, Pauker, Sommers, & Ambady, 2010, p. 1588). Another possible antidote to therapists making erroneous assumptions about clients is to keep focused firmly on culture but to appreciate the multiple cultures to which any client will belong. It is very easy, for example, for a client's ethnicity to override considerations of other group affiliations, such as socioeconomic class, religious faith, and age (in particular, generational divides such as college student, new parent, grandparent, or retiree).

Culturally Responsive Therapy

I have borrowed this phrase from education, where the concept "culturally responsive pedagogy" has been a significant focus of school reform for 30 years (Villegas, 1991). The goal is to develop instructional practices that are tuned to the skills, talents, cognitive styles, language traditions, and motives of minority students so that they are given a fair chance to learn and succeed in school. There are numerous good examples documenting the benefits of this strategy for responding to the needs of the diverse student populations characterizing schools in many parts of the world. Culturally responsive pedagogy is designed to redress the power differentials emanating from social discrimination and disadvantage.

The provision of mental health services can be seen as exactly parallel. There seem to be very few places in the world in which minority rights have been robust enough to assert that minority cultures can address uneven power only by providing their own services for their own people. In New Zealand, however, there are such examples. This is because the right to manage—have "sovereignty" over—their own affairs was enshrined in a formal treaty, which, although somewhat shakily at times, has maintained its legal force. Thus, in New Zealand, there are some Māori services for Māori clients, just as there are Māori schools for Māori pupils. In these situations culturally responsive therapy (or pedagogy) is essentially moot.

In spite of this apparent solution to a complex need, the reality remains that most members of cultural minorities, even in New Zealand, will access services (and education) in settings designed by the majority culture and so the need for culturally responsive procedures remains paramount. In addition, members of minority cultures have a right to choose. If they choose a "mainstream" service or approach it is still essential that the service selected be responsive to their needs. Thus the argument returns full circle: how do we best achieve this responsiveness? The answer will explain why this long discussion is relevant to the issue of change. Do we have to do anything to our change plans (therapy) to make them more effective for diverse cultural groups? Are the principles of change I have been espousing culturally specific? Or are the principles sound enough, but they have to be translated into practical strategies in a way that accommodates cultural specificity? There are two main elements to culturally responsive therapy.

Setting: Inside the Comfort Zone

The first of these is that the setting, the context, the therapist, the therapy, and the whole idea of therapy have to be acceptable and meaningful to the client. Clients have to stay in treatment; they have to return for more sessions or further exposure to the altered conditions. They have to feel positive, safe, and understood. If you are a client, therapy has to feel right for you. That alone is a very major accomplishment. Are public mental health facilities designed so that people from a different culture feel immediately, "yes, this is for me"? And because we all come from some set of complex cultures and we all access variable services we all know that feeling when we encounter it: the doctor is a young women like you are; the receptionist knows how to pronounce your name and tells you about the buses without assuming you own a car; your therapist is an older man but he seems awfully relaxed around your two boisterous preschool children; even though you have trouble paying the bill you are treated with respect; your car mechanic can diagnose the problem without making you feel like a complete idiot. It does not have to be a perfect match or even a close one—just enough to stop you from running out of the room screaming. You feel assured enough to give it a chance.

So universal is this feeling we have a popular layperson's phrase for it: you are inside your comfort zone. There are lots of simple ways of ensuring that feeling. If your culture is one that tends to start formal proceedings of any kind with a prayer, then starting a therapy session with prayer will feel right. In Māori culture, for example, it is very common to begin an activity with a *karakia* (a prayer), even when the participants in the activity are not especially religious. It is a ritual and it has emotive properties. As such, a *karakia* can be considered a positive affective prime. Would we suggest this interpretation to a religious client? Probably not—which is no more deceptive than hanging your framed university and licensing board credentials on the office wall. These too are primes—for some people, evoking schemata of competence and credibility.

Process: Getting Out of Your Comfort Zone

The second main element is that the new experiences—the conditions or process of therapy—have to be able to change your unique patterns of responding according to your thinking and learning style. This is hugely more difficult to achieve than ensuring therapist and therapy acceptability, for all the reasons we have already examined around cognitive flexibility, resistance, or fear of change. Almost by definition planful change—therapy—takes people outside their comfort zone. No matter how seemingly detrimental their current behavior might be—to their goals, their happiness, and their relationships—the problematic behavior must be serving some sort of function for them or it would change on its own accord.

Once we express the circumstances of treatment like this, what has it got to do with culture? Surely the point just made is no different from saying that therapy needs to be particularized according to the unique goals, predilections, emotional resources, and so on, of the individual client. And have we not already seen that according to the available evidence, such individualization is not that crucial? The difference now is that that particular finding has not been replicated across cultural groups—the individuals within a given culture may have enough similarities that the conditions of therapy have a good chance of producing change. This may not be true across grouping of clients representing very different cultural styles, such as being an interdependent culture as opposed to one favoring independence. Furthermore, by looking at this issue through a cultural lens, the therapist's own assumptions about what's what in the world suddenly become especially relevant. We have not spent much time in psychotherapy research exploring the extent to which the therapeutic translation of a principle rests on an implicit cultural assumption. This is so difficult to examine because almost by definition we are strongly tied to our own culture—we just don't know what we don't know.

There are many illustrations of how difficult this is. One of the hardest things for scientific researchers engaged in, let us say, outcome research to recognize is that even scientific method itself is culturally shaped (Chamberlain, 2000). I am always disconcerted when the criteria for what constitutes truth and knowledge in modern psychology, which I accept unconditionally, are not universally regarded as defining sound evidence. Scholars from indigenous cultures frequently ask "Who decides what is evidence?" This skepticism regarding Western science is often driven by painful recognition that methods that are supposed to work do not always work for their people. The problem is that the causes of such failings are hopelessly confounded by the issues discussed—people being outside their comfort zone even before the intervention has begun. When a person has power over others, as therapists do, analytic perceptual style becomes even stronger, so that there is a greater focus on disposition than on environmental contexts (Guinote, 2007).

The focus in the psychotherapy literature is often on the supposed differences between cultures; however, I consider that the *principles* of behavior change are essentially the same across all cultures. Think about the absolutely critical influence on children that has been mentioned a number of times: how adults shape children's emotional development and emotion skills. The goal of having children who are emotionally competent is common across cultures. The processes whereby this is achieved, such as teaching, modeling, and having a distinct meta-emotion philosophy, are also universal. This is known as an etic position—pan-cultural. But the socialization practices are very different across cultures so that whether children are expressive or reserved, labile or stoic, empathic or ego-dystonic, and everything in-between, is entirely culturally determined (Kitzmann & Howard, 2011).

Where we have to be extra cautious in practice is with respect to the power differential when a therapist is a member of a dominant cultural group. Ensuring that our expectations of appropriate emotion expression are unbiased and that the behavior change is in the best interests of the client and his or her community takes more than cultural competence. It requires strategies that reduce the power imbalance. These include respect for the less dominant group's standards of evidence, practices that acknowledge the harm caused by institutional discrimination and historical injustices, and support for professional services delivered for and by minority ethnic groups, especially indigenous peoples (Evans, Herbert, Fitzgerald, & Harvey, 2010).

It may seem as if issues such as these go somewhat beyond the scope and reach of this book. But if you were to think of the prominence given say to motivational theories, or the importance of the therapeutic relationship for promoting client change, then the opportunities as well as barriers provided by cultural justice are surely substantially greater. Can we truly expect meaningful change against the powerful backdrop of the culture of poverty or the culture of alienation arising from the destruction of indigenous peoples' way of life and traditional economic opportunities? Duran, Firehammer, and Gonzalez (2008) evocatively describe the effects of oppression and loss on Native American communities as "soul wounds." We have long accepted that effective psychotherapy requires trust; liberating commitments go much further. Planful change requires understanding context, history, and barriers to social justice (Comstock, Hammer, Strentzsch, Cannon, Parsons, & Salazar, 2008). Fundamental inequities in the cultural context negate trust and understanding, and thus cannot create the opportunities for meaningful change.

Where there are power differentials across cultures (especially gender and ethnic groups), being in a subordinate, powerless role creates distress and contributes considerably to emotional disorders. But generally, even the most challenged cultures have strengths to be celebrated. Nowhere is this more beautifully illustrated than in recent longitudinal work on positive youth development, bringing together the needs children have (as described in the beginning of this chapter), culture, and ecology. The 4-H study of positive youth development confirms the value of the "five Cs": competence, confidence, connection, character, and caring (Lerner et al., 2005). Participation in community youth programs builds skills and self-esteem, connects young people to committed adults, and fosters positive values and caring for others.

Implications

The very idea of psychotherapy is a cultural phenomenon, as we know from countless studies of what sorts of models of psychopathology and sources of help different groups and communities adhere to. I have already suggested, slightly tongue in cheek, that being a client is a culturally determined role. In Western industrialized societies we have a definite idea of how clients are supposed to behave—therapists too. I have also argued that what is considered appropriate treatment is defined by standards of evidence and acceptability that are far from universal and are very much determined by the professional and scientific cultural group whose values and standards a professional has internalized. Psychotherapy is especially prone to cultural influences because many treatments are developed to address the needs that exist at a specific time and place in history. Those of us who remember the enthusiastic reception given to Masters and Johnson's or Hartmann and Fithian's sexual therapies know that these treatments are essentially moribund in today's climate of open expressions of sexuality. In the United States it was the Vietnam War that created the need for treatments of posttraumatic stress disorder (PTSD), although identical phenomena were well known after each of the two World Wars. Recently in cognitive–behavioral therapy there has been a resurgence of interest in mindfulness, neglecting, perhaps, the fact that meditation and Eastern philosophies were very prominent in psychotherapy practice and research in the 1970s, but were considered part of the counterculture to mainstream behavioral therapy.

Our foray into cultural influences reminds us again of the importance of context in regulating and changing behavior. The individual, however, is not simply some malleable lump of clay that is shaped by the environment. Individual differences in personality and temperament, as have already been emphasized, determine the effects of environment. To continue the analogy, the type and nature of clay determine what the potter's hands can do with it (Bronfenbrenner & Morris, 2006). Why do we have the concept of cultural identity in psychology? It is because not everyone who might potentially belong to a cultural group—on the basis of ethnicity, upbringing, gender, sexual preferences, and so on—does so with the same degree of interest and dedication. The culture of youth (in

Western societies somewhat dominated by American style) might be far more influential than the culture of an indigenous people. Although we understand that different people have different degrees of identity with a nominated culture, we do not know very much about why these differences come about.

There is a regrettable confound between being a member of a given cultural group and being exposed to potentially negative environmental influences. Indigenous people and ethnic minority cultures all around the world can face considerable economic disadvantage, however vigorously their culture flourishes. Many minority groups are disproportionately exposed to poverty, unemployment, drugs, gangs, violence and crime, and all the other hardships of urban neighborhood decay and less than desirable housing. Lead poisoning, at any level, affects cognitive development, increases behavior problems, and is linked to violence and crime (Stretesky & Lynch, 2004). Childhood lead levels are highest in impoverished environs and among disadvantaged minority groups, yet simple environmental and housing policies can drastically reduce toxic conditions (Nicholson, Schwirian, & Schwirian, 2010). The objective realities of such environments are further filtered by the individual's perceptions of them (Nalls, Mullis, & Mullis, 2009). People who identify strongly with their culture as an affirming experience come under the influence of social forces that promote the positive routines and rituals of that culture. Yet it is still our major responsibility to work against toxic cultures, such as child poverty. By emphasizing the growth of valued behaviors across development, the five Cs, we can better ensure positive adult outcomes and well-being.

12

Conclusions

How and Why People Can Change and Be Changed

I have deliberately resisted the temptation to offer specific advice about how to *do therapy* after discussing a principle of change. The fundamental argument behind this book is that all psychological therapy should be designed to help people change. The effective therapist must, therefore, understand the substantiated principles and processes of change, which can then be *translated* into multiple ingenious, humane, and socially just intervention practices. This is a level of analysis different from what is regarded as evidence-based practice, which often means the implementation of procedures or protocols that have been "validated" in formal outcome research.

I am not at all opposed to well-supported treatment manuals. One of their great advantages is that they do cover a variety of sound change principles. Most of them include psychoeducation—providing a rational account of the client's distress that somewhat normalizes it and creates a common language for negotiation between therapist and client. Most enhance positive motivation by providing expectations of hope and reassurance for a better quality of life. Most include some kind of stress management program. In America, protocols typically encourage self-advocacy and assertiveness and autonomy. If the protocol has to do with interpersonal relationships, such as couples, or parents, teachers, and carers as mediators, it will generally include training to improve communication skills and empathy. Formal manuals often teach problem-solving and self-control, including relapse prevention; they encourage meaningful goal-setting and self-monitoring. And finally they have that extra little bit that makes them distinctive, usually targeting a particular dynamic of psychopathology or a particular kind of distressing symptom for which we have some understanding of cause. If you do not believe me just pick up any two well-developed, empirically supported treatment manuals for totally different problems and compare them side by side—the overlap is striking.

Although we think of these protocols as "treatments," that can be misleading. If an effective treatment is delivered then the problem should be cured or ameliorated. But psychological problems are generally not like infections or physical conditions such as dry rot or condensation in a house. Very influential theorists in the past who have argued that psychotherapy is about change have assumed that it is a process of social influence (Goldstein, Heller, & Sechrest, 1966). However, many things that transpire in therapy are not purely social. Community psychologists, with an ecological bent, emphasize the environmental forces that prevent change or can be mobilized to support it. Their belief is that the therapist does not need to be responsible for delivering a complex treatment. All the therapist has to do is head the client off in the right direction, with the right little map and the proper boots, and the natural environment will take care of the rest of the journey. I think we need a much broader model of change, drawing on many insights from psychological science to understand how and why change happens. The client is never the passive recipient of something called treatment. Change occurs when an interaction is fostered between the individual's psychological structures (make-up) and new, or newly engaged, sources of influence, both close and distant.

One of the most serious scientific problems associated with current efforts to validate treatment procedures is that process understanding is often subordinated to outcome demonstration. For a new treatment approach to be useful we need to know not only the processes of treatment but the processes of change. In other words, we need to understanding more about the trajectory or course of change needed to achieve a desirable outcome for clients. Many demonstrations of treatment efficacy and effectiveness use dubious outcome measures fashioned to the inclusion criteria for the research rather than the positive benefits people seek. We also need to know more about the characteristics of the setting in which the approach is used, which determine its success. We need to know whether the worldviews or cultural presumptions of the clients match those intrinsic to the planned intervention. And most of all, if we want to avoid endless rediscoveries of the same idea, we need to know if the elements named are actually new and special or whether they are simply a creative vehicle or procedure for arranging a few well-worn principles of change.

Finding the Fundamentals

In this chapter I would like to bring together the threads of my thesis and the main points of the previous discussions and suggest the elements common to all successful change efforts. However, I do not want to repeat myself. We have covered a host of principles. Now the task is to take a step back and think about some broad dimensions. If we accept that some therapists are sometimes successful, regardless of what they do, and some therapies are sometimes successful regardless of the style or characteristics of the therapist—or even if there is one—the integration cannot be at the level of formal technique (Miller and

Hubble's "means of production"), but at the level of common, generalizable principles of change: not at the level of kernels but at the level of nuggets.

As such, the integration does not try to unify the different schools of therapy. For one thing, none of us really know what transpires at critical choice points in therapies of different orientations. For another, most schools of therapy are so tied to their own language systems and concepts that they are not easily deconstructed to their basic or common elements. Nor would such deconstruction meet with much favor among their proponents. Schools of therapy, whether behavioral or cognitive or anything else, are really social movements. They develop specialized language systems that are understood and recognized by their adherents and that then serve as essential means of communication—cues to prime or guide therapeutic practices. Schools of psychotherapy develop their own methods of enquiry as well, and establish their own standards of evidence, and when treatments meet these standards they are given legitimacy.

This mildly cynical perspective may seem a little rich coming at the end of many chapters that have drawn largely from what have become known as "cognitive behavioral" therapies, with our own terminology and empirical methodologies. But I have actually tried to keep the discussion *psychological*. Radical behaviorists will appreciate very little of what has been proposed because they eschew internal psychological mechanisms, and cognitive theorists even less so, since they usually adopt the opposite, an intrapsychical model. What goes on consciously inside people's heads is considered what is important by content cognitivists, and what happens unconsciously is considered important by process cognitivists and neuroscientists, all happily ignoring the fundamental attribution error. I have endeavored also to use only principles and concepts that have a sort of general authority within the scientific discipline of psychology. Because of this, if your psychology is spiritual, or magical, or entirely culturally relative, then the present analysis will seem as much an arbitrary set of selected constructs as I am proposing schools of psychotherapy are.

Planful behavior change represents a major intellectual challenge, with so many principles to juggle and so many possible interpretations of how the principles can be translated. Changing your behavior is not like changing your shoes. Simple voluntary, nonhabitual routines are easy enough to change. But ingrained habits, emotional reactions that are not under voluntary control, or thoughts that have been shaped by many years of cultural exposure to linguistic conventions, are much harder to alter. I do not believe that this book offers to make therapy easier—it may actually make it more challenging because the possibilities are so much greater than when following a formal protocol.

Even if accepted, many of the principles I have outlined are not explicitly incorporated into current interventions. I have never really understood why treatments in psychotherapy have become so unidimensional. Everyone knows that the relationship between therapist and client is of major importance, so why would an applied behavior analyst focus only on the trial-by-trial shaping of behavior using materialistic rewards when working with a child with autism? Wouldn't you want to do whatever you can to foster a meaningful emotional relationship or bond with that child? Everyone knows that having a meaningful life involves friendships and positive social networks, so why would a cognitive therapists focus treatment solely on the client's supposedly irrational internal dialogue? I think the cause of this extreme compartmentalization is the attempt to find "the" treatment rather than to assist clients in making the changes that will meet their goals. "Therapies" are tangible; they can be operationalized and made prescriptive. They can be given a brand name and they can be owned by charismatic professional leaders. Changing lives and lifestyles, on the other hand, seems like an intricate, multifaceted, creative, experimental, unproven sort of enterprise. Which indeed it often is, although the core principles derive from hard science. That is the joy of therapy.

Certain forms of theoretical integration involve finding the common underlying change processes. One of the best illustrations of how just one underlying behavioral principle allows for multiple therapeutic possibilities in practice was espoused many years ago by one of the most prominent psychiatrists attracted to emerging behavior therapy, Isaac Marks. Marks (1987) pointed out that research on systematic desensitization had shown it could be carried out therapeutically in many different ways. You could go slowly up the hierarchy or just start right at the top; you could even use a hierarchy generated by a different client. You could use imagined scenes with deep muscle relaxation, or calmness produced by biofeedback or by meditation. You could present stimuli by pictures, or thoughts, or in vivo. Systematic desensitization could be delivered by a skilled therapist, by a novice, or by a computer. None of these things seemed to make much difference in terms of its effectiveness. The reason for this, he concluded, is that the method works through exposure—somehow phobic clients have to be encouraged to confront their fears and to keep doing so until they no longer feel anxiety. The overall lesson for therapy is that to reduce an irrational fear there must be voluntary exposure to the feared situation or its symbolic representation without avoidance in a context experienced as safe and that does not overwhelm the client's emotional system, or if it does there must be high, meaningful levels of social support.

Other forms of theoretical integration ensure instead that a number of essential components are combined. A good example comes from procedures designed to reduce challenging behavior in children with developmental disorders. Negative, harmful, disruptive, and aggressive behaviors have been successfully changed in many ways. We can modify contexts, make the setting more interesting, or remove cues that trigger the negative behavior. We can try to remove all sources of reinforcement for the negative behavior. We can provide negative consequences, such as response cost. We can differentially reward the nonoccurrence of the negative behavior after a certain period of time. We can teach alternative skills that have the same function for the child. We can remove the sources of negative motivation that provide this function. We can enhance communication so that the child's needs and wants are better understood and the child can exercise some control over his or her own life. We can make sure that the clinician or other mediator develops a meaningful relationship with the child, and show his or her parents how to do the same if they are frustrated and bereft of ideas. We can smother the child in love.

Because all of these things have been shown at one time or another to reduce challenging behavior, the integrating concept is that *all* of them should be carried out and at the *same time*. To manage challenging behavior in an autistic child, therefore, the rule is straightforward: within a loving, accepting family environment, change contexts, make the environment more interesting, remove triggers, reward the nonoccurrence of the behavior, make sure the undesirable behavior is not being rewarded and does have appropriate negative consequences or feedback, teach an effective alternative skill, especially social relationships and communication, making sure it is functional (others respond warmly but not overwhelmingly to any communicative bids), and reduce the motivation to perform the negative version of the activity by increasing autonomy and self-control. If *these* are your rules then a whole variety of clever procedures can be designed that will suit the individual child and his or her family and community and that will be acceptable to the relevant culture. Do not formulate an intervention that does just one of those things, do them all.

A Metaphor for Change

To aid in the quite difficult process of bringing together the many themes presented thus far, I am going to start off by drawing on one of the best available books on the nature of psychological change, written by Chip Heath and Dan Heath (2010). Their popular book on change, called *"Switch: How to Change Things When Change Is Hard,"* develops a wonderfully evocative extended metaphor of a Rider steering an Elephant along a jungle Path. The Rider is our intellect, full of ideas, making countless decisions, and prone to analysis and thus indecision. The Elephant is emotion (and motivation) without which the Rider can go nowhere. The Elephant has lots of power and momentum, but needs to be stirred up as well as directed; it prefers the old ways and is slow and lumbering when it comes to change. The Path is the environment and what situations permit the Rider on the Elephant to make its way. If the Path is too steep or has insurmountable barriers no one is going to go anywhere—it does not matter how strong or energized the Elephant might be or how well the Rider makes decisions.

Heath and Heath's metaphor is superb in capturing the big elements controlling behavior: reason, emotion, and opportunity. They also point out, with another analogy I would like to borrow, that *within* each of these broad elements there are many complex interrelationships, not just between them. Thus, as an explanatory system, their model is really like three-dimensional chess. At each level (and by level I do not mean one invariably on top of another), Rider (reason, cognition), Elephant (emotion, motivation, habit), and Path (situation, ecology) have elaborate moves and relationships and rules within each plane as well as between levels. Despite this complexity, the Heaths argue forcefully, solutions need not be overwhelmingly complex. If the Rider were alone, he or she or it would analyze a problem endlessly, the Elephant alone would blunder about with much huffing and puffing but with little direction, and a Path alone would be clear and straight but totally empty. *Together*, however, relatively simple strategies can be forged, and I think that many of these have been proposed, implicitly, throughout this book.

The Elephant, the Rider, and the Path provide an excellent fable for the relationships between emotion-dominated behavior, cognitive reasoning, and environmental context. But even larger relationships must be considered when planning psychological interventions. I have emphasized the importance of self-control of behavior while at the same time (although in different chapters) I have been extolling the enormity of social support for change. Similarly I have emphasized social control of our behavior by others while at the same time proposing that we need self-support. To clarify those four big picture concepts, I will redefine them, following Rutherford (2003), as follows: (1) self-control is when the individual is the source of self-determination and regulation; (2) social control is when other people regulate an individual's behavior; (3) self-support is when an individual's cognitive-emotional networks are sources of sustenance and rejuvenation; and (4) social support is when other people in your social environment are a source of vitality and harmony through affiliative-affective networks.

Expressed this way it can be seen that the four constructs are not incompatible, although they do highlight the difference between determining your own path and being controlled by others, as well as the difference between relying on your own internal resources versus relying on the support of others. Psychological therapy that is directive tends toward social control; when it is nondirective it tends toward a form of social support (the therapeutic relationship). Yet both traditions attempt to foster self-support and self-control as outcomes for clients. This is where there can be much room for a mismatch between the assumptions of Western therapy (of whatever stripe) and non-Western cultural assumptions. Rutherford, for example, proposes that

> Western cultures are, at the behavioral level, organised around 'self-control' in conjunction with 'social support' action tendencies and at the cognitive level organised by 'self support' in conjunction with 'social control' mindsets and belief systems. On the other hand, it is conjectured that Eastern cultural traditions are, at the behavioral level, organised around 'self-support' in conjunction with 'social-control' action tendencies and in a cognitive

level organised around 'self-control' in conjunction with 'social support' mindsets and belief system. (Rutherford, 2003, no page numbers)

This appeals because it is a more sophisticated comparison than that often proposed between "individualistic" (Western) and "collectivist" (Eastern) cultural worldviews.

Simple Fundamentals Illustrated with Two Examples

I have tried to explain that although this book is about changes typically desired in professional psychotherapy, it is not exclusively about psychotherapy itself, or psychotherapeutic theories of change. There has been something of a revolution in the closely relevant world of program evaluation that now extols a "theory of change" approach (Weiss, 1997). Community interventions, such as psychotherapy, have often been designed and evaluated with vague assumptions of the plausible sequence of cause and effect connecting the program to the desired outcomes. Only when the causal expectations underlying the intervention are formally specified is it possible to determine if the expected sequence of steps has unfolded as planned. If you hope to reduce school dropout by using trained home-visitors to support families you cannot really evaluate this program until you have articulated what the causal chain will look like. This might include the following: Home-visitors will enhance positive communication between parents and teachers, teachers will then be more understanding of the difficulties students might be experiencing at home, parents will feel the school is supportive and they will encourage school work and facilitate homework, the child's academic success increases, positive feelings about school are enhanced, engagement and connectedness grow, teachers express optimism for the student's future, and the inevitable setbacks and occasional challenges do not then lead automatically to dropping out (Evans, Okifuji, Engler, Bromley, & Tishelman, 1993). We expect one change to lead to another, and these hypothesized chains of influence need to be described. This is exactly what is intended in good individualized clinical case conceptualization (Persons, 2008)—we develop a logical systems map (Evans, 1985) of causal influences and some or all of these are targeted for intervention.

Many contemporary therapies suggest general intermediate processes such as the client needing to be more accepting, or more compassionate, or more mindful. But these are themselves examples of change—the new skills and traits for the new person. Mindfulness might alter anxiety as a target symptom, but how do we become more mindful? Well, we do so by using a conscious strategy involving attentional shifts. So then how do we acquire that new strategy? There is a slightly disquieting sense here of a sort of infinite regress, possibly ending up at the very reductionist level of neural processes. The challenge, if we are going to avoid such extreme reductionism, is to settle on basic psychological mechanisms with wide generality across a range of clinical and other life phenomena that are commensurate with what neuroscience is revealing about brain substrates.

Causal treatment mechanisms, then, tend to be means–ends relationships. To enhance the quality of life of a child with autism we might want to increase meaningful peer friendships. To bring about that change we might want to teach a few simple social skills, and to acquire these might require teaching a communication repertoire, which in turn might require greater attention to the intentions of others, and that involves understanding that others have minds (theory of mind). This means that changing something specifically desired might first require change in something less obvious. We do not proceed from a static, no-change state to one of change; we change and modify our behavior in an ongoing, dynamic, hierarchical fashion.

But that is not the whole story. First, the learning that takes place in the various steps of the hierarchy needs to be driven by motivation and sustained by available contingencies. The Elephant can learn simple things and make a degree of progress even without the Rider. In terms of motivation, the child with autism who is being taught a social skill is not likely to be aware of the potential benefits for later quality of life. The motivation to acquire social skills, if not preexisting as a sociable human individual, may have to be artificially created, even perhaps by use of material, nonsocial rewards at first. Even so, strategies that engage the child with autism as a participant rather than as a mere recipient would be worth developing, not only ethically but to gain practical traction as well.

A client with agoraphobia who wants to be able to move freely around his or her environment without feeling panic should know and understand that the anxiety management skills being practiced in therapy have the short-term goal of reducing the sense of threat and the long-term goal of being free of the agoraphobia. Good therapists attempt to make these connections highly salient to the client. In terms of contingencies, the acquisition of some prerequisite skills will be sustained only if they are reinforced in some way. The use of relaxation as a self-calming strategy must be reinforced by anxiety reduction if the agoraphobic client is to continue to use it. The communication skills that the child with autism must acquire to enhance social interactions must be ones that the child's environment responds to appropriately, so the child's symbolic, verbal behaviors gain desired outcomes (satisfies needs) more effectively than other overt attempts to control the environment, such as through physical aggression or self-injury.

Second, the preexisting dynamic interrelationships among behaviors determine whether other behaviors in the repertoire interfere with the new learning. The child with autism whose self-stimulation (perhaps flicking fingers in front of his or her eyes) has the function of managing stress from adult demands, will engage in that behavior in a way that interferes with teaching the skill of attending to the communicative signals from others. The person with agoraphobia may have a well-rehearsed belief or verbal rule that it is not safe to venture outside despite the newly acquired ability to manage emotional arousal. This then interferes with the expected progression from improved emotion regulation to practicing more and more adventurous excursions to the mall, to the movies, or to the busy cafeteria. For both clients, increasing competence has benefits. One reason a child, or anyone really, can on occasion be noncompliant is not because of a lack of skill or an oppositional tendency but because they are anxious and do not believe that they can perform the task adequately, or as expected. Bandura (1977) called the interaction between anxiety and confidence "self-efficacy," but the general idea is that with mastery comes reduced anxiety because anxiety is always related to uncertainty.

Third, context and ecological opportunity are critical. There are three specific central contexts in most clinical work that every therapist accepts but does not always place front and centre stage (Shirk & Russell, 1996). These are development (not just child development, but life-course development as well), family (whether child, parent, or extended relatives), and culture (both the client's and the therapist's). We are talking about changing one thing to change another. We recognize that it takes a village to raise a child. Without social capital (people to help, communities that value children, medical and social agencies that can be trusted), parents of a child with autism will be overwhelmed. But as Smyth and Dewar (2009) so cleverly ask, what does it take to raise a village? Communities need to work together, inclusively, with a common purpose.

Even in the absence of basic social skills a child with autism could have real peer friendships if the opportunities existed or are engineered by parents (see Evans & Meyer, 2001). The social context has to be other children who are accepting and tolerant and are willing to include the child with autism in their everyday activities and play. This, in turn, would result in a more socially rich set of everyday routines and hence change to a better quality of life. This is not because of the potential for reward from other children but simply that behavior can occur only in an ecologically relevant context—you cannot exhibit social skills in the absence of other available human beings. Similarly, the individual with agoraphobic tendencies requires ecological opportunities for practicing desired routines; these do not always exist: the client may have no means of transport or family responsibilities may make it difficult to create the space in the daily repertoire to engage in the practice. Neighbors and informal helpers such as tolerant shopkeepers and understanding bus drivers can fill gaps that might exist in more typical, closer social networks. Again, good therapists consider context: the practical opportunities (or sometimes restraints) afforded by existing ecological circumstances.

By using the simple examples of autism and agoraphobia—two completely different patterns of behavioral dysfunction, never conventionally sharing treatment methods—I am hoping to show that at some level of analysis we eventually come to common principles of change. The ability to generalize a concept across clinical phenomena is a good litmus test of whether we have the fundamental principles this book is about. For example, we might want to claim that rapid back and forth movement of the eyes while imagining feared situations eliminates anxiety. If it does, it is an excellent example of a nonreducible change mechanism, as no other known changes are produced by back and forth eye movements. However, if I argued that mindfulness reduces anxiety and mindfulness is an example of an attentional process, then I can think of comparable attentional mechanisms that might result in totally different kinds of change, such as teaching a child to attend to the critical elements of a social situation so as to reduce aggression triggered by erroneous responding to a misinterpreted stimulus. The search for mechanisms of clinical change is the search for generalizable psychological processes, some perhaps tautologically being themselves more microchange mechanisms, but mostly still representing the processes underlying change.

What Is the Client's Role in Change?

One of the strongest philosophical objections to the emergence of behavior therapy in the 1960s was that it seemed to imply that the therapist was some kind of autocratic fascist whose main goal was to manipulate and control the behavior of the client. Perry London's (1969) critique of the field of "behavior modification" had as its cover illustration a wooden puppet. It implied that the client was merely the passive recipient of direction and influence from external sources: the therapist pulling the strings, the client a helpless marionette. There are many social reasons why in the 1960s in Western societies, being an era of social protest against convention, the idea of external control was such an anathema. In an ethos of love and peace and flower power, behavior therapy was poorly marketed, using unpopular language and metaphors. It seemed to be all about control and modification, aversive contingencies, behavioral engineering, and denial of free will. Even self-control was self *control*. Compare that to the language of the new generation cognitive–behavioral therapies, with their quotes from Zen Buddhism and the Dalai Lama: mindfulness, values identification, letting go of angry feelings, compassion (acceptance with kindness), or a life worth living. In reality, everyone in the past knew equally well that all influence was reciprocal. Radical behaviorists themselves widely promulgated the famous cartoon of two rats in a Skinner box, one saying to the other: "Boy, have I got this guy conditioned; every time I press this lever he drops in a pellet of food!" But although things were not quite as bad as painted by the critics of behavior therapy, the fact is that the voice and understanding of the client were greatly neglected topics. When Craig Robinson and I first tried to publish as a case study the very reflective diary of a client who had undergone behavior therapy, we were told firmly by the leading behavior therapy journal that the paper "had no scientific merit." Happily (for us) their view was not shared by Michael Mahoney, the editor of a newly emerged journal much more aware of what it is the client contributes. What our client's diary revealed very poignantly was that her experiences in therapy were nothing like what we thought we were doing in treatment (Evans & Robinson, 1978).

The fact that humans have *agency* changes our understanding of the principles of behavior and how we respond to them. Yes, we are shaped by contingencies of material and social reward and punishment, but not in the way radical behaviorists imply. Once we recognize that, the apparent epistemological gulf between behaviorists and cognitivists is not as wide as it might seem. We do not really have second and third waves of CBT—just a growing understanding of the complexity of influences, with the client's ability to self-regulate a very important feature of this complexity. Nelson Mandela has reported that words from the poem "Invictus" by William Ernest Henley sustained and encouraged him during his long years of imprisonment: "*I am the master of my fate; I am the captain of my soul.*"

Clients, like everyone else, start out with self-knowledge. They have a complex self-concept of who they are and what they are about. The possible selves model (Markus & Nurius, 1986) brings home the added reality that when clients, or anyone who seeks change, presents to therapy, voluntarily or not, they have an idea of what they might become, what they would like to become, and what they are afraid of becoming. But my attempt to analyze change includes people and contexts in which such conscious processes are limited—where the Rider is not very bright. We have no idea what a child with an intellectual disability thinks about being in treatment. What I have tried to convey is that planful change, regardless of the client, abides in the reciprocal exchanges between what the therapist brings and what the client brings, both internally and in terms of the context. When it is argued that client change can and should be self-directed, that is not the same as proposing total client autonomy.

With respect to verbal psychotherapy, when adult clients are asked to think about change they are quite explicit regarding their own experiences. We know this as a result of an interesting study by Carey and colleagues (2007) in which clients identified gradual change as well as sudden moments when things "clicked," with both experienced in much the same way regardless of the type of therapy. They saw how important motivation was, often feeling that they had come to the end of their tether; part of this motivation was facing up to who they were and accepting a need to change. Clients reported the value of tools and strategies they had acquired, and recognized that learning was a critical part of the change process. Their interaction with a therapist who would listen nonjudgmentally was important, and in particular the benefits of talking about issues that had been bottled up for too long.

Planful (Clinical) Change Has Been Preceded by Past Failures

Psychological insights regarding behavior change make it abundantly clear that good therapists need to recognize that the client is not a passive recipient of a treatment. This is the essential message of the constructivist position, which is more a set of values than a school of psychotherapy (Mahoney, 2003). All clients have had the experience of trying to change and the experience of others trying to change them. No client likes to be controlled, although many enjoy the feeling of security that arises from a relationship with someone who seems to understand them and to care about them. Mahoney, knowing there are barriers to change, preferred to understand "resistance" as "expressions of a basic self-protective process by which the adapting person attempts to preserve a precious balance of familiar order (systemic coherence) while exploring changes that necessarily challenge that order" (Mahoney, 2000, p. 199). Echoes of activity settings: old shoes and the front porch.

Because most people change on their own, sometimes using natural supports and opportunities, those who become clients may have experienced past difficulties in facilitating the change they desire. Therapists generally perceive this, especially if clients complain that they have already tried everything, as they often do. It is tempting—I know because I have done it myself—to encourage them and enhance motivation by assuring them that they have now come to the right place, have come to see the right person, armed with the latest scientific evidence, with consummate skills and certificates on the wall to prove it. It is marginally useful to give clients some hope in this way. But because their past failures were probably not caused by lack of positive expectations of success, a therapist's optimism and self-confidence need to be tempered by a good assessment of what has not worked, in addition to knowing what generally works.

Integration: In with the Old

At the start of this book I half-promised a theoretical integration, but this is extremely difficult. Being neither a Newton nor an Einstein, all I can say is that the field of psychotherapy, of deliberate psychological change, is not yet ready for the grand unifying theory based on a few fundamental principles. Psychology itself is extremely fragmented, so much so, as Staats bemoaned, that investigators are doing research on topics that are very similar to each other but nevertheless fail to cite, cross-reference, or even apparently be aware of each other's work. This is somewhat understandable as the range and preciseness of basic research in psychology are very considerable. Examples I have cited were selected partly by chance—studies that struck me as clinically relevant when I read them—not an exhaustive review of the now vast and detailed research literature. Even if we were aware of most of the truly relevant studies, there is no way that a clinical psychologist could derive a therapeutic method from the present corpus of basic research—a derivation, incidentally, that used to be considered the ideal version of the Boulder-model scientist practitioner. Of course we could be au fait with, say, all the studies on hypervigilance to threat cues, which are of interest to understanding the dynamics of certain anxiety disorders. But to actually help someone with an anxiety disorder live a more typical, less distressing, more fulfilling life, the therapist will also need to think about the client's motivation, coping mechanisms, beliefs, alternative skills, social supports, and all of the other psychological processes relevant for change that we have been examining.

It seems slightly odd to me that if indeed the task of the therapist is to bring together a large number of different principles, the history of evidence-based psychological treatment is not to build on good principles but to drop them as quickly as possible when a new one comes along. The rule seems to be: as soon as I can produce evidence for the value of my approach it must mean yours is wrong. Cognitive therapies were founded (erroneously in my opinion) on the apparent shortcomings of conditioning principles, social and cultural perspectives happily dismiss cognition, and constructivists denounce them all when they see that people create their own meanings to contextualize their lives. In such a climate it seems a bit woolly to be bleating on about how all of these ideas have currency and that in order to help people change in meaningful ways all need to be attended to. That is quite a cognitive load for any psychotherapist; it is so much easier to follow a recipe than to create an endless array of new dishes.

A Perspective on Change Aids Translation

Applying psychological principles sensitively to clinical problems is fraught with translation difficulties. As a practical clinical reality it is hard to escape a basic fact: understanding the function of a behavior is a key to changing it. Clinicians should always ask themselves two fundamental questions. First, what is the client getting out of this pattern of (undesirable, inappropriate) behavior, in terms of gaining access to rewards or escape/avoidance from punishment? And second, what are the reinforcement contingencies for the (more desirable, more appropriate) alternative behavior, in terms of the pleasures available or the needs that will be met? Treatment should always involve minimizing the former (the answers to question one) and maximizing the latter (the answers to question two).

The *form* of this treatment, however, will look nothing like the experimental arrangement for studying operant behavior, such as a Skinner box, and the rewards will very rarely be food or water. Reinforcement is undoubtedly a fundamental principle of behavior. Behavior *is* a function of its consequences. Contingencies are powerful controlling variables, but not on their own. Advising a parent or teacher to rely on a simple material reward (or punishment) program for controlling the behavior of a child cannot be good science. There are too many other sources of influence and confounding social and emotional factors to consider reinforcement in isolation from the relationship between the supplier and the recipient—or from the cognitive appraisal of the meaning of the reward, from its symbolic value, from past learning, from cultural acceptability, or even from simple notions of fairness and expectancy. Lettuce just will not work if you were expecting fruit.

Rewards for humans are more commonly social rather than biological and spiritual rather than material. We are more relationship seeking than pleasure seeking. This does not mean that hedonistic pleasures such as food, sex, entertainment, and exciting sports are not powerful reinforcers. It is simply that in our society because basic biological needs are usually taken care of, the analogy between a human client and a rat deprived of food for 24 hours and at 80% of its *ad lib* body weight (the usual state of an experimental animal in operant conditioning studies) is pretty darn tenuous. On the other hand, because human pleasure and pain are so closely tied to emotions, to feeling states, the analogy between a rat behaving to escape fear and a client behaving to reduce fear (anxiety, shame, anger, etc.) is surprisingly close.

Responses Interrelate Dynamically

The way our behavior is regulated by its effects on our own emotions is an important change principle. The idea that we engage in so much of our apparently dysfunctional problematic behavior because it avoids or reduces intensely unpleasant feelings is a very useful one. But it too has limits. The emphasis in our field on such dynamic relationships is a historical influence going back to Freud, who was rather impressed by the technology of his age, with its discovery of forces, hydraulics, and such. We are now in a technological age of information, of social networks and interconnections, and of global systems, and our metaphors allow us to see the importance of relationships as the origin of psychological distress.

One of the great conundrums in changing behavior is to be able to estimate the level at which change must be initiated: is it an immediate problem or underlying personality trait? Once behavior is understood in context and as part of daily living, what features of our everyday circumstances must be addressed to reduce the felt distress? If you are counseling a college student who is anxious and depressed, two phenomena that often go hand in hand, what sort of benefit will accrue if you attempt to change these emotional states, compared with encouraging or facilitating a change in lifestyle, including chance making of new friends, getting more pleasant accommodation, or finding new interests?

We can fully appreciate the fundamental role of context and yet still not know where to start therapeutically. Understanding everyday, comfortable, self-fulfilling routines at least provides us with an understanding of the *content* of typical lives that can then be placed in context. Psychological intervention is not ethereal like Lewin's force fields—it is about what people are doing with their time. There are many barriers to change, from basic personality traits to these external circumstances. Past experiences and well-rehearsed patterns are the major obstacle. As the Duke of Wellington exclaimed: "Habit a second nature? Habit is ten times nature."

It is an important integration to think of real lives in context: behavioral economies (how people spend their time, which patterns of response are incompatible with one another), natural routines and activity settings, and how some competencies enable other aspects of change. A simple example of this can be found in analyzing change when intervening with adolescents. When working with adolescents with anxiety disorders, the key self-management principles are basic emotion regulation abilities such as self-soothing, emotion knowledge, and the ability to delay gratification. However, there are peripheral skills that can be developed that are related to two real life principles. (1) One is that teens who are very anxious often miss out on typical social learning and educational experiences. Thus, they may need to have opportunities to learn about sexual identity (and typical dating experiences that have been disrupted by social anxiety), how to maintain friendships despite the ups and downs of teenagers' relationships, and ensuring that they do not avoid schooling or fall behind academically. (2) The second is that some young people's anxiety is exacerbated by parental anxieties and overprotectiveness that limit their ability to achieve the developmental milestones of adolescence, which require negotiation of emotional and behavioral independence. Albano (2011) has suggested encouraging teens and parents to develop a hierarchy of independent activities that foster an adolescent's sense of mastery and self-competence, such as opening their own bank account, making their own doctor's appointments, cooking their own meals, and arranging their own college applications and interviews. These activities of daily living are presented as weekly development goals, but it must be remembered that there are large cultural differences in how families define and prioritize these steps toward independence.

The Therapeutic Milieu

Therapists' worldviews greatly influences the ethos of change and they are important. Several psychotherapy approaches emphasize "positive psychology": design solutions rather than solve problems, focus on strengths and past successes, and perceive clients as persons of ability looking to the future with hope. Solution-Focused Therapy is self-consciously grounded on these optimistic values (de Shazer et al., 2006), as are ACT and Positive Behavior Support. Although relevant and change oriented, they are not exactly principles of change.

Transactions matter. Disclosing and sharing past distressing experiences is therapeutic. Simply writing down a painful memory makes people feel better; narrative therapists help clients with techniques to reframe their past. Expressing feelings in writing can bring emotional relief (Pennebaker, 2004);

disclosure of traumatic experiences has health benefits (Greenberg & Stone, 1992), although only for selected people in some limited circumstances (Solano, Bonadies, & Di Trani, 2008). When we reminisce with our friends we can relive the pleasures of good times past. With good, honorable, trustworthy friends we can recount bad experiences including both wrongs done to us and wrongs we have perpetrated. Through social acceptance, reinterpretation, and simply reliving in a secure environment we can deactivate the negative associations and reduce the stored memories of pain and shame.

In a safe therapeutic context with a relationship with the clinician that matches the client's personality and coping style, exploration of emotionally unresolved past events seems to allow a sort of extinction process or other type of defusing of the emotion or dismantling the complex emotional schema. What seem to be different therapies, such as implosion (exposure), cognitive restructuring, and mindfulness, may all actually be serving the same general function, meaning that one of them is not the right thing to do and another the wrong thing to do. I started this foray into how and why people change by arguing that our intense professional focus of "the treatment" that must be "empirically validated" has resulted in a professional culture of "mine is better than yours." I am certainly not claiming that all therapies are equally good—far from it; more likely they are equally inadequate. I am suggesting that a variety of beneficial and helpful methods derive their effectiveness from a more limited set of principles of change.

Social Contexts, Social Capital, and Culture

The one truism of psychotherapy and the ace in the hand of the therapist is that coming to therapy is potentially always the start of a change process. To come to the first session means that our anxiety, depression, negative outcome beliefs, and low self-esteem—however you want to identify the range of possible feelings— have been sufficiently overcome, or our distress sufficiently great, that this difficult first step in making change has occurred. Both for the individual on a self-help project, or for the therapist, the trick is to sustain, maintain, and generalize that change, not to leave it as a one hour a week office experience. Intervention needs to serve as the catalyst for a progression of life-altering experiences. We might choose to focus on initial feelings, but only if they are barriers to more substantive life changes. The plan needs to articulate the progression, not simply be a strategy for getting rid of anxiety (or depression, or whatever).

As psychologists these notions are commonplace. Pioneers such as Lewin, or more recently Bronfenbrenner, made these interacting, ecological levels of influence abundantly clear. And most psychologists are quick to understand the interactions that explain behavior: nature/nurture, genetics/environment, and personality/experience. Clinical therapists can easily conceptualize interactions and dynamic response relationships so as to focus change efforts on the emotional responses, keystone behaviors, habits of thought, *and* critical contexts that maintain maladaptive patterns, and I have offered numerous compelling examples from the literature.

What I wanted to show, however, is that thinking of discrete, alternative levels of influence from the one-to-one therapeutic influence to the role of community and culture will not do as a change model. If you are a community psychologist you may assume that the outside (macro-) rings are critical, if you are a behavior therapist you may suppose that the individual in contextual interaction (meso-) is critical, and if you are a cognitive or interpersonal psychotherapist you may judge only the (micro-) interaction between therapist and the client's mind as critical. But these influences cannot be isolated and they cannot be ranked in importance. Experience trumps personality, but personality shapes experiences. People's lives are not first mental events, then social, and then environmental. Mental events are constrained by culture, the very outer, most abstract ring of most such models! Culture determines the rules you take for granted and do not feel the need to question. People's daily activities are regulated by contingencies, some of them physical realities, several determined by social interactions, and many of them planned by enabling behaviors initiated months or years before. So it is not even possible to rely on the person-by-environment interactional models or any of their extensions. There are constant dynamic systems interconnections (Thelen, 2005). Daily routines are as important as emotional schemas; relationships with family, friends, and workmates are as important as the relationships between overt behavior, thoughts, and feelings.

The result of these wonderfully fluid trajectories is not overwhelmingly complex. It is not that difficult to think of placing the client in a nexus of antecedents and consequences, of response interrelationships, of autonomous, self-driven functioning and dependent socially controlled activities, or of fixed reflexive habits intermingled with the expectations and rules of the culture. What I have not been able to do is to place all of these things into one absolutely cohesive and consistent model as I hinted was the aim at the beginning of the book. If you were hoping for a formula, you will be disappointed, but if you keep just a few of these change principles in mind you will be a more helpful therapist.

Summary: Seven Things to Remember

There are probably seven large change principles that encompass much of what has been included in this book. So I will be kind and summarize them.

1. Behavior is context specific, highly influenced by the situations in which we find ourselves. Through processes of association, analogous to classical conditioning, stimuli that serve as cues or primes or triggers or antecedent to emotion

and to thoughts and to actions can be changed and reevaluated—their meaning as well as their emotional significance can be altered.

2. A major part of the context of our lives is also tied up with contingencies, the consequences of our actions, which can produce highly stylized and habitual behaviors that are very hard to change. But because humans have agency they can and do alter these contingencies. Because all behavior is related to approach (appetitive) and withdrawal (punitive) relationships, our motivation, what propels us or draws us into action, is tied to maximizing pleasure and minimizing pain.

3. Contexts, however, are analyzed, judged, and interpreted, and past situations are stored in memory, and all these cognitive processes shape the way we characteristically react, sometimes in ways we would like to change. Automatic thoughts can become more reflective, more mindfully engaged, so that maladaptive habits are weakened.

4. Because we are such social creatures, the pleasures and pains we wish to maximize are rarely simple tangible pleasures and are much more closely tied to needs for acceptance, influence, and closeness, so sustaining social relationships and doing the things that build relationships become very important.

5. Other people influence us in much the same way as the environment: providing cues and consequences and our ability to regulate emotion, imitate and model, and respond to feedback are among the pivotal skills essential for complex development

6. Personality determines how a common context is treated uniquely by every individual. Individual differences refer to repertoires of response interrelationships. When traits have clear causal connections to the change-worthy behavior, general strategies to reset personality dispositions are relevant. This has important implications—change is usually a complex chain of means–ends relationships in which one change leads to another, often in further interaction with components of the environment. Response relationships work internally to the individual, where selected behaviors under voluntary control are able to lead to change in behaviors that are highly reflexive and are not under voluntary control. They also work externally whereby certain competencies, such as problem-solving, communication, or social skills, lead to interactions with parents, family, friends, teachers, peers, and the wider community, whose social responsiveness enables and sustains behavior change.

7. Our wider social networks influence this as well, particularly our culture, which sets the rules for expected behavior: morals, values, and decorum. Within these broader cultural experiences are the routines and rituals that make up a large percentage of people's everyday living: the everyday activity settings—the social furniture of our lives.

These seven general principles seem to be universal and to apply to change processes of all people. But people who are deliberately seeking change through professional means, and especially psychological means, represent a special group—those people who become clients and who receive therapeutic interventions. Whether we just suffer in silence, suffer intrusively, or become a client depends on a myriad of social and economic factors in terms of how so-called mental health services are perceived culturally and offered within a society. Nevertheless, the kinds of problems brought to therapy, although they do fit nicely into categories that we understand to some extent, are often the reflection of larger forces at work—stress, family influences, poverty, disadvantage, and tolerance by others (stigma). It is well known that these social variables contribute to what we call mental illness. Some psychologists work to change society at this level and thus reduce the factors leading to peoples' distress and dysfunction. But there is also value in working with individuals regardless of the distal and immediate causes of their troubles. Here, to be effective and to arrange the conditions of change, the therapist as a facilitator of change needs to have cultural sensitivity and emotional competence, needs to be able to relate to the client, and needs to be able to analyze the barriers to change while at the same time offering strategies leading to solutions.

Within the individual dynamics of certain kinds of disorders are other sets of variables that will be relevant to change. The person trying to give up and desist from a life of crime has different change needs than the person whose obsessional thoughts about germs and cleanliness lead to compulsive hand washing. The teen with anorexia has different needs than the teen with autism. Some behaviors need to be stopped, some need to be started, some are related to traumas from long ago, and some are related to sudden exigencies that have challenged the individuals' coping abilities. In my very general account of change those specific dynamics related to different syndromes have not been addressed in any detail. Most of the procedures called treatments in the psychotherapy field are concerned with those specifics and are not organized around themes of change. But some, usually built into the specific treatment package, are very general: learning better coping methods to manage feelings, learning to solve problems more effectively, coming to understand that in order to change the way you feel you need to change your behavior, and recognizing that in order to make those changes you may need to listen less to your dysfunctional thoughts, to test realities, and to better observe yourself and your own reactions (gain insight).

Therapeutic decisions become more complex when factoring in the conditions affecting neighborhoods and communities that further constrain lifestyles and reduce possibilities and choices for individuals to maximize their opportunities for living fulfilling and meaningful lives. In Western nations these conditions include poverty, discrimination, past losses, and abuses of particular groups. In other parts of the world they include wars, exploitation, natural hazards and disasters, and the stultifying consequences of dictatorial political and religious regimes. Such issues are not typically part of clinical psychology or the expected contribution psychological science can make to mental health and personal fulfillment, but as a few approaches to psychological change now begin to acknowledge, both as process variables and as outcomes (e.g., "lives of value"), it seems an appropriate challenge to our psychotherapy field not to ignore the largest of all pictures: social justice.

Not all psychological interventions are created equal. Some are going to be much more successful than others. Some are going to change the things that really matter in people's lives and some are just going to change their scores on a paper and pencil test. Some are going to alter an individual's life course and some are just going to make them feel a little better for a short period of time. Some are going to stop destructive behavior from ever happening again and some are simply going to delay its next occurrence. Sometimes the therapist—and the client—will be lucky because a small change is the catalyst for a broadly satisfactory outcome relating meaningfully to the client's life goals for a positive possible self, but more usually meaningful change will require intensive treatments that draw on many layered principles of influence. Similar to other protective layers, we need to think of those that can be wrapped around the client from all sides. These principles are complex, but not impossibly so, as I have tried to show in this book, and because in the final analysis it is *experiences* that shape and change behavior, it is rarely the case that suitable experiences cannot be arranged or created or redesigned in order to improve people's lives according to their needs and desires and the expectations of their community.

REFERENCES

Ablon, J. S., Levy, R. A., & Katzenstein, T. (2006). Beyond brand names of psychotherapy: Identifying empirically supported change processes. *Psychotherapy: Theory, Research, Practice, Training, 43,* 216–231.

Ajzen, I. (1991). The theory of planned behavior. *Organizational Behavior and Human Decision Processes, 50,* 179–211.

Ajzen, I., & Fishbein, M. (1973). Attitudinal and normative variables as predictors of specific behavior. *Journal of Personality and Social Psychology, 27,* 41–57.

Albano, A. M. (2011, November). *Targeting developmental milestones in the treatment of anxiety in adolescents.* Paper presented at the 45th annual convention of the Association for Behavioral and Cognitive Therapies, Toronto, Canada.

Albee, G. W. (1990). The futility of psychotherapy. *Mind and Behavior, 11,* 369–384.

Alfano, C. A., Beidel, D. C., & Turner, S. M. (2002). Cognition in childhood anxiety: Conceptual, methodological, and developmental issues. *Clinical Psychology Review, 22,* 1209–1238.

Alloy, L. B., & Abramson, L. Y. (1979). Judgment of contingency in depressed and nondepressed students: Sadder but wiser? *Journal of Experimental Psychology: General, 108,* 441–485.

Alloy, L. B., Abramson, L. Y., Walshaw, P. D., & Neeren, A. M. (2006). Cognitive vulnerability to unipolar and bipolar mood disorders. *Journal of Social and Clinical Psychology, 25,* 726–754.

American Psychiatric Association. (2000). *Diagnostic and statistical manual of mental disorders* (4th ed., text revision). Washington, DC: Author.

Andersen, R. J., Evans, I. M., & Harvey, S. T. (2012). Insider views of the emotional climate of the classroom: What New Zealand children tell us about their teachers' feelings. *Journal of Research in Childhood Education, 26,* 199–220.

Anderson, C. A. (2001). Heat and violence. *Current Directions in Psychological Science, 10,* 33–38.

Annon, J. S. (1977). *Behavioral treatment of sexual problems: Brief therapy.* New York: Joanna Cotler Books.

Apfelbaum, E. P., Pauker, K., Sommers, S. R., & Ambady, N. (2010). In blind pursuit of racial equality? *Psychological Science, 21,* 1587–1592.

Arch, J. J., & Craske, M. G. (2008). Acceptance and commitment therapy and cognitive behavioral therapy for anxiety disorders: Different treatments, similar mechanisms? *Clinical Psychology: Science and Practice, 15,* 263–279.

Argyris, C, (1970). *Intervention theory and method: A behavioral science view.* Reading, MA: Addison-Wesley.

Ariely, D., Kamenica, E., & Prelec, D. (2008). Man's search for meaning: The case of Legos. *Journal of Economic Behavior and Organization, 67,* 671–677.

Aron, A. R., & Verbruggen, F. (2008). Stop the presses: Dissociating a selective from a global mechanism for stopping. *Psychological Science, 19,* 1146–1153.

Aronfreed, J. (1968). *Conduct and conscience: The socialization of internalized control over behavior*. New York: Academic Press.

Aye, A. M., Guerin, B., Evans, I. M., & Ho, E. (2000, August). Autonomy and parental monitoring in Asian households with the father absent or present. Paper presented at the annual conference of the New Zealand Psychological Society, Hamilton, NZ.

Azar, S. T., Nix, R. L., & Makin-Byrd, K. N. (2005). Parenting schemas and the process of change. *Journal of Marital and Family Therapy, 31*, 45–58.

Bacon, L., & Aphramor, L. (2011). Weight science: Evaluating the evidence for a paradigm shift. *Nutrition Journal, 10*, doi: 10.1186/1475-2891-10-9.

Baer, D. M. (1997). Some meanings of antecedent and environmental control. In D. M. Baer & E. M. Pinkston (Eds.), *Environment and behavior* (pp. 15–29). Boulder, CO: Westview Press.

Baer, R. A. (Ed.) (2010). *Assessing mindfulness and acceptance processes in clients*. Oakland, CA: Context Press.

Baker, T. B., McFall, R. M., & Shoham, V. (2009). Current status and future prospects of clinical psychology: Toward a scientifically principled approach to mental and behavioral health care. *Psychological Science in the Public Interest, 9*, 67–103.

Banaji, M. R., & Kihlstrom, J. F. (1996). The ordinary nature of alien abduction memories. *Psychological Inquiry, 7*, 132–135.

Bandura, A. (1971). *Psychological modeling*. Chicago: Aldine-Atherton.

Bandura, A. (1977). Self-efficacy: Toward a unifying theory of behavior change. *Psychological Review, 84*, 191–215.

Bandura, A. (1997). Editorial: The anatomy of stages of change. *American Journal of Health Promotion, 12*, 8–10.

Bandura, A. (2006). Toward a psychology of human agency. *Perspectives on Psychological Science, 1*, 164–180.

Barkham, M. (1989). Brief prescriptive therapy in two-plus-one sessions: Initial cases from the clinic. *Behavioural Psychotherapy, 17*, 161–175.

Barlow, D. H., Farchione, T. J., Fairholme, C. P., Ellard, K. K., Boisseau, C. L., Allen, L. B., & Ehrenreich May, J. T. (2010). *Unified protocol for transdiagnostic treatment of emotional disorders: Therapist guide*. New York: Oxford University Press.

Barlow, J., & Coren, E. (2004). Parent-training programmes for improving maternal psychosocial health. *Cochrane Data Base Systematic Reviews, 2004*(1), CD002020.

Barnard, P., & Teasdale, J. D. (1991). Interacting cognitive subsystems: A systemic approach to cognitive-affective interaction and change. *Cognition and Emotion, 5*, 1–39.

Barnett, S. M., & Ceci, S. J. (2002). When and where do we apply what we learn? A taxonomy for far transfer. *Psychological Bulletin, 128*, 612–637.

Baron-Cohen, S., Leslie, A. M., & Frith, U. (1985). Does the autistic child have a "theory of mind"? *Cognition, 21*, 37–46.

Barth, R. S. (2002). The culture builder. *Beyond Instructional Leadership, 59*(8), 6–11.

Bateman, A. W., & Fonagy, P. (Eds.) (2011). *Handbook of mentalizing in mental health practice*. Arlington, VA: American Psychiatric Publishing.

Beaudry, J., Sanders, W., Gibbons, M., & Coffey, A. (1995). The university visit: A mosaic of futures. In I. M. Evans, T. Cicchelli, M. Cohen, & N. Shapiro (Eds.), *Staying in school: Partnerships for educational change* (pp. 135–148). Baltimore, MD: Paul H. Brookes.

Beck, A. T. (1976). *Cognitive therapy and the emotional disorders*. New York: International University Press.

Beck, A. T., Epstein, N., Harrison, R. P., & Emery, G. (1983). *Development of the Sociotropy-Autonomy Scale: A measure of personality factors in depression*. Unpublished manuscript, University of Pennsylvania Center for Cognitive Therapy, Philadelphia, PA.

Bellack, A. S., Mueser, K. T., Gingerich, S., & Agresta, J. (2004). *Social skills training for schizophrenia: A step-by-step guide* (2nd ed.). New York: Guilford.

Belsky, J., & Pluess, M. (2009). Beyond diathesis stress: Differential susceptibility to environmental influences. *Psychological Bulletin, 135*, 885–908.

Bentall, R. P. (2003). *Madness explained: Psychosis and human nature*. London, UK: Penguin Books.

Bergin, A. (1967). Some implications of psychotherapy research for therapeutic practice. *International Journal of Psychiatry, 3*, 136–160.

Best, J., & Horiuchi, G. T. (1985). The razor blade in the apple: The social construction of urban legends. *Social Problems, 32*, 488–499.

Bevins, R. A., & Palmatier, M. I. (2004). Extending the role of associative learning processes in nicotine addiction. *Behavioral and Cognitive Neuroscience Reviews, 3*, 143–158.

Bijou, S. (1968) Child behavior and development: A behavioral analysis. *International Journal of Psychology, 3*, 221–238.

Bitterman, M. E. (2006). Classical conditioning since Pavlov. *Review of General Psychology, 10*, 365–376.

Blakemore, S. J., & Frith, C. D. (2005). The role of motor contagion in the prediction of action. *Neuropsychologia, 43*, 260–267.

Blandy, M. (1971). *Harvest from rotten apples. Experimental work with detached youth.* London, UK: Gollancz.

Blume, B. D., Ford, J. K., Baldwin, T. T., & Huang, J. L. (2010). Transfer of training: A meta-analytic review. *Journal of Management, 36*, 1065–1105.

Bootzin, R. R., Epstein, D., & Wood, J. M. (1991). Stimulus control instructions. In P. J. Hauri (Ed.), *Case studies in insomnia* (pp. 19–28). New York: Plenum.

Bordin, E. (1994). Theory and research on the therapeutic working alliance: New directions. In A. O. Horvath & L. S. Greenberg (Eds.), *The working alliance: Theory, research, and practice* (pp. 13–37). Oxford, UK: Wiley.

Borkovec, T. D., Robinson, E., Pruzinsky, T., & DePree, J. A. (1983). Preliminary exploration of worry: Some characteristics and processes. *Behaviour Research and Therapy, 21*, 9–16.

Bowlby, J. (1969). *Attachment and loss.* New York: Basic Books.

Braithwaite, J. (1989). *Crime, shame and reintegration.* New York: Cambridge University Press.

Bransford, J. D., & Schwartz, D. L. (1999). Rethinking transfer: A simple proposal with multiple implications. *Review of Research in Education, 24*, 61–100.

Brehm, S., & Brehm, J. W. (1981). *Psychological reactance: A theory of freedom and control.* New York: Academic Press.

Briesmeister, J. M., & Schaefer, C. E. (Eds.) (2007). *Handbook of parent training: Helping parents prevent and solve problem behaviors* (3rd ed.). New York: Wiley.

Brodberg, D. J., & Bernstein, I. L. (1987). Candy as a scapegoat in the prevention of food aversions in children receiving chemotherapy. *Cancer, 60*, 2344–2347.

Bronfenbrenner, U. (1977). Toward an experimental ecology of human development. *American Psychologist, 32*, 513–531.

Bronfenbrenner, U., & Morris, P. (2006). The bioecological model of human development. In R. M. Lerner (Ed.), *Handbook of child psychology: Vol. 1. Theoretical models of human development* (6th ed., pp. 793–893). New York: Wiley.

Brown, A. L., & Campione, J. C. (1986). Psychological theory and the study of learning disabilities. *American Psychologist, 47*, 1059–1068.

Brown, F., Evans, I. M., Weed, K. A., & Owen, V. (1987). Delineating functional competencies: A component model. *Journal of the Association for Persons with Severe Handicaps, 12*, 117–124.

Bryant, F. B., & Veroff, J. (2007). *Savoring: A new model of positive experience.* Mahwah, NJ: Lawrence Erlbaum.

Burke, E. (1759/1909). *On taste.* The Harvard Classics, Vol. XXIV. New York: P. F. Collier & Son.

Busch, C. J., & Evans, I. M. (1977). The effectiveness of electric shock and foul odor as unconditioned stimuli in classical aversive conditioning. *Behaviour Research and Therapy, 15*, 167–175.

Busseri, M. A., & Sadava, S. W. (2011). A review of the tripartite structure of subjective well-being: Implications for conceptualization, operationalization, analysis, and synthesis. *Personality and Social Psychology Review, 15*, 290–314.

Buttle, H. (2011). Attention and working memory in mindfulness-meditation practices. *Journal of Mind and Behavior, 32*, 123–134.

Campos, P., Saguy, A., Ernsberger, P., Oliver, E., & Gaesser, G. (2006). The epidemiology of overweight and obesity: Public health crisis or moral panic? *International Journal of Epidemiology, 35*, 55–60.

Capaldi, E. J., Martins, A. P. G., & Altman, M. (2009). Memories of reward and nonreward regulate the extinction and reacquisition of both excitatory and inhibitory associations. *Learning and Motivation, 40*, 259–273.

Carey, T. A., Carey, M., Stalker, K., Mullan, R. J., Murray, L. K., & Spratt, M. B. (2007). Psychological change from the inside looking out: A qualitative investigation. *Counselling and Psychotherapy Research, 7*, 178–187.

Carr, E. G. (1994). Emerging themes in the functional analysis of problem behavior. *Journal of Applied Behavior Analysis, 27*, 393–399.

Carr, E. G., Dunlap, G., Horner, R. H., Koegel, R. L., Turnbull, A. P., Sailor, W., Anderson, J. L., Albin, R. W., Koegel, L. K., & Fox, L. (2002). Positive behavior support: Evolution of an applied science. *Journal of Positive Behavior Interventions, 4*, 4–16.

Carr, E. G., & Durand, V. M. (1985). Reducing behavior problems through functional communication training. *Journal of Applied Behavior Analysis, 18*, 111–126.

Carroll, P. J., Shepperd, J. A., & Arkin, R. M. (2009). Downward self-revision: Erasing possible selves. *Social Cognition, 27*, 550–578.

Carter, T. J., Ferguson, M. J., & Hassin, R. R. (2011). A single exposure to the American flag shifts support towards Republicanism up to 8 months later. *Psychological Science, 22*, 1011–1018.

Carver, C. S., & White, T. L. (1994). Behavioral inhibition, behavioral activation, and affective responses to impending reward and punishment: The BIS/BAS scales. *Journal of Personality and Social Psychology, 67*, 319–333.

Casey, B. J., Jones, R. M., & Hare, T. A. (2008). The adolescent brain. *Annals of the New York Academy of Sciences, 1124*, 111–126.

Casey, R. J., & Berman, J. (1985). The outcome of psychotherapy with children. *Psychological Bulletin, 98*, 388–400.

Castelnuovo, G., Faccio, E., Molinari, E., Nardone, G., & Salvini, A. (2005). Evidence based approach in psychotherapy: The limitations of current Empirically Supported Treatments paradigms and of similar theoretical approaches as regards establishing efficient and effective treatments in psychotherapy. *Brief Strategic and Systemic Therapy European Review, 2*, 229–248.

Castonguay, L. G., & Beutler, L. E. (Eds.). (2006). *Principles of psychotherapeutic change that work.* New York: Oxford University Press.

Cataldo, M. F. (1991). The effects of punishment and other behavior reducing procedures on the destructive behaviours of persons with developmental disabilities. In National Institutes of Health (Ed.), *Treatment of destructive behaviors in persons with developmental disabilities* (pp. 231–343). (NIH Publication No. 91-2410.) Washington, DC: U.S. Government Printing Office.

Cautela, J. R. (1977). *Behavior analysis forms for clinical intervention.* Champaign, IL: Research Press.

Centers for Disease Control and Prevention. (2010). State-specific trends in fruit and vegetable consumption among adults—United States, 2000–2009. *Morbidity and Mortality Weekly Report, 59*(35), 1125–1130.

Chamberlain, K. (2000). Methodolatry and qualitative health research. *Journal of Health Psychology, 5*, 285–296.

Chambless, D. L., Baker, M. J., Baucom, D. H., Beutler, L. E., Calhoun, K. S., Crits-Christoph, P., et al. (1998). Update on empirically validated therapies, II. *The Clinical Psychologist, 51*(1), 3–16.

Chambless, D. L., & Hollon, S. D. (1998). Defining empirically supported therapies. *Journal of Consulting and Clinical Psychology, 66*, 7–18.

Chambless, D. L., & Hollon, S. D. (2012). Treatment validity for intervention studies. In H. Cooper (Ed.), *APA handbook of research methods in psychology. Vol. 2. Quantitative, qualitative, neuropsychological, and biological.* Washington, DC: American Psychological Association.

Chorpita, B. F., et al. (2011). Evidence-based treatments for children and adolescents: An updated review of indicators of efficacy and effectiveness. *Clinical Psychology: Science and Practice, 18*, 154–172.

Christakis, N. A., & Fowler, J. H. (2009). *Connected: The surprising power of our social networks and how they shape our lives.* New York: Little, Brown & Company.

Clark, D. M., & Wells, A. (1995). A cognitive model of social phobia. In R. Heimberg, M. Liebowitz, D. A. Hope, & F. R. Schneier (Eds.), *Social phobia: Diagnosis, assessment and treatment* (pp. 69–93). New York: Guilford.

Clearfield, M. W., Feng, J., & Thelen, E. (2007). The development of reaching across the first year in twins of known placental type. *Motor Control, 11,* 29–53.

Cohen, A. B. (2009). Many forms of culture. *American Psychologist, 64,* 194–204.

Cole, M. (1985). The zone of proximal development: Where culture and cognition create each other. In J. V. Wertsch (Ed.), *Culture, communication, and cognition: Vygotskian perspectives* (pp. 146–161). Cambridge, UK: Cambridge University Press.

Comstock, D. L., Hammer, T. R., Strentzsch, J., Cannon, K., Parsons, J., & Salazar, G., II. (2008). Relational-cultural theory: A framework for bridging relational, multicultural, and social justice competencies. *Journal of Counseling & Development, 86,* 279–287.

Cone, J. D. (1979). Confounded comparisons in triple response mode assessment research. *Behavioral Assessment, 1,* 85–95.

Congiu, M., Whelan, M., Oxley, J., Charlton, J., D'Elia, A., & Muir, M. (2008). *Child pedestrians: Factors associated with ability to cross roads safely and development of a training package.* Report No. 23, Accident Research Centre, Monash University, Australia.

Connelly, M. L. (2001). *New direction for treating parent-adolescent conflict: Comparison of problem solving skills training and social cognitive development training.* Unpublished doctoral dissertation, Department of Psychology, University of Waikato, Hamilton, New Zealand.

Conner, M., & Norman, P. (Eds.) (1995). *Predicting health behaviour.* Buckingham, UK: Open University Press.

Corcoran, K., & Fischer, J. (2000). *Measures for clinical practice: A sourcebook* (3rd ed.). New York: Free Press.

Corr, P. J., & McNaughton, N. (2008). Reinforcement sensitivity theory and personality. In P. J. Corr (Ed.), *The reinforcement sensitivity theory of personality* (pp. 155–187). Cambridge, UK: Cambridge University Press.

Corrigan, P. W., & Penn, D. L. (1999). Lessons from social psychology on discrediting psychiatric stigma. *American Psychologist, 54,* 765–776.

Couch, C. M., & Evans, I. M. (2011). Relationship focused parent training within a dialectical framework: A case study. *Clinical Child Psychology and Psychiatry.* Published online before print September 28, 2011, doi: 10.1177/1359104511415639.

Crisp, R. J., Husnu, S., Meleady, R., Stathi, S., & Turner, R. N. (2010). From imagery to intention: A dual route model of imagined contact effects. In W. Stroebe & N. Hewstone (Eds.), *European review of social psychology* (Vol. 21, pp. 188–236). Hove, UK: Psychology Press.

Currie, J., DellaVigna, S., Moretti, E., & Pathania, V. (2009). *The effect of fast food restaurants on obesity* (NBER Working Paper No. W14721). Cambridge, MA: National Bureau of Economic Research.

Curry, J., et al. (2010). Recovery and recurrence following treatment for adolescent major depression. *Archives of General Psychiatry,* published online November 1, 2010. doi: 10.1001/archgenpsychiatry.2010.150.

Cyders, M. A., & Smith, G. T. (2007). Mood-based rash action and its components: Positive and negative urgency and their relations with other impulsivity-like constructs. *Personality and Individual Differences, 43,* 839–850.

Dannahy, L., & Stopa, L. (2007). Post-event processing in social anxiety. *Behaviour Research and Therapy, 45,* 1207–1219.

Dawes, R. M. (1994). *House of cards: Psychology and psychotherapy built on myth.* New York: Free Press.

Dawson, S. A., Grant, B. F., Stinson, F. S., Chou, P. S., Huang, B., & Ruan, W. J. (2005). Recovery from DSM-IV alcohol dependence: United States, 2001–2002. *Addiction, 100,* 281–292.

De Houwer, J., Thomas, S., & Baeyens, F. (2001). Associative learning of likes and dislikes: A review of 25 years of research on human evaluative conditioning. *Psychological Bulletin, 127,* 853–869.

De Jong, P., & Berg, I. K. (2008). *Interviewing for solutions* (3rd ed.). Belmont, CA: Brooks/Cole.

de Shazer, S., Dolan, Y. M., Korman, H., Trepper, T. S., McCollum, E. E., & Berg, I. K. (2006). *More than miracles: The state of the art of solution focused therapy*. Binghamton, NY: Haworth Press.

Diamond, A. (2005). Attention-deficit disorder (attention-deficit/hyperactivity disorder without hyperactivity): A neurobiologically and behaviorally distinct disorder from attention-deficit/hyperactivity disorder (with hyperactivity). *Development and Psychopathology, 17,* 807–825.

Diamond, A., Barnett, W. S., Thomas, J., & Munro, S. (2007). Preschool program improves cognitive control. *Science, 318,* 1387–1388.

Diener, E., Oishi, S., & Lucas, R. E. (2003). Personality, culture, and subjective well-being: Emotional and cognitive evaluations of life. *Annual Review of Psychology, 54,* 403–425.

Dodge, K. A. (2011). Social information processing models of aggressive behavior. In M. Mikulncer & P. R. Shaver (Eds.), *Understanding and reducing aggression, violence, and their consequences* (pp. 165–186). Washington, DC: American Psychological Association.

Doherty, R. W. (1997). The Emotional Contagion Scale: A measure of individual differences. *Journal of Nonverbal Behavior, 21,* 131–154.

Doleys, D. M. (1977). Behavioral treatment for nocturnal enuresis in children: A review of the recent literature. *Psychological Bulletin, 84,* 20–54.

Doss, B. D. (2004). Changing the way we study change in psychotherapy. *Clinical Psychology: Science and Practice, 11,* 368–386.

Drayton, M., Birchwood, M., & Trower, P. (1998). Early attachment experience and recovery from psychosis. *British Journal of Clinical Psychology, 37,* 269–284.

Dunlap, K. (1932). *Habits: Their making and unmaking*. New York: Liveright.

Dunsmoor, J. E., Mitroff, S. R., & LaBar, K. S. (2009).Generalization of conditioned fear along a dimension of increasing fear intensity. *Learning & Memory, 16,* 460–469.

Duran, E., Firehammer, J., & Gonzalez, J. (2008). Liberation psychology as the path toward healing cultural soul wounds. *Journal of Counseling & Development, 86,* 288–295.

Durand, V. M. (1990). *Severe behavior problems: A functional communication approach*. New York: Guilford.

Dutra, L., Stathopoulou, G., Basden, S. L., Leyro, T. M., Powers, M. B., & Otto, M. W. (2008). A meta-analytic review of psychosocial interventions for substance use disorders. *American Journal of Psychiatry, 165,* 179–187.

Dweck, C. S. (1999). Caution: Praise can be dangerous. *American Educator, 23*(1), 4–9.

D'Zurilla, T. J., & Goldfried, M. R. (1971). Problem solving and behavior modification. *Journal of Abnormal Psychology, 78,* 107–126.

Eifert, G. H., Evans, I. M., & McKendrick, V. G. (1990). Matching treatments to client problems not diagnostic labels: A case for paradigmatic behavior therapy. *Journal of Behavior Therapy and Experimental Psychiatry, 21,* 163–172.

Eifert, G. H., & Wilson, P. H. (1991). The triple response approach to assessment: A conceptual and methodological reappraisal. *Behaviour Research and Therapy, 29,* 283–292.

Eisenberg, N., Fabes, R. A., Shepard, S. A., Murphy, B. C., Jones, S., & Guthrie, I. K. (1998). Contemporaneous and longitudinal prediction of children's sympathy from dispositional regulation and emotionality. *Developmental Psychology, 34,* 910–924.

Eisenberger, R. (1992). Learned industriousness. *Psychological Review, 99,* 248–267.

Eisler, I., Dare, C., Hodes, M., Russell, G., Dodge, E., & Le Grange, D. (2000). Family therapy for adolescent anorexia nervosa: The results of a controlled comparison of two family interventions. *Journal of Child Psychology and Psychiatry, 41,* 727–736.

Elgar, F. J., & McGrath, P. J. (2008). Self-help therapies for childhood disorders. In P. L. Watkins & G. A. Clum (Eds.), *Handbook of self-help therapies* (pp. 129–161). New York: Taylor & Francis/Routledge.

Elliot, A. J., & Church, M. A. (2002). Client-articulated avoidance goals in the therapy context. *Journal of Counseling Psychology, 49,* 243–254.

Ellis, A. (1962). *Reason and emotion in psychotherapy*. New York: Lyle Stuart.

Ellis, A. (1971). *Growth through reason*. Palo Alto, CA: Science and Behavior Books.

Elster, J. (1989). *Nuts and bolts for the social sciences.* Cambridge, UK: Cambridge University Press.

Embry, D. D. (2004). Community-based prevention using simple, low-cost, evidence-based kernels and behavior vaccines. *Journal of Community Psychology, 32,* 575–591.

Embry, D. D., & Biglan, A. (2008). Evidence-based kernels: Fundamental units of behavioral influence. *Clinical Child and Family Psychology Review, 11,* 75–113.

Emmons, R. A. (1986). Personal strivings: An approach to personality and subjective well-being. *Journal of Personality and Social Psychology, 51,* 1058–1068.

Epstein, S. (1994). Integration of the cognitive and the psychodynamic unconscious. *American Psychologist, 49,* 709–724.

Evans, G. W., & Kutcher, R. (2011). Loosening the link between childhood poverty and adolescent smoking and obesity: The protective effects of social capital. *Psychological Science, 22,* 3–7.

Evans, I. M. (1972). A conditioning model of a common neurotic pattern—fear of fear. *Psychotherapy: Theory, Research and Practice, 9,* 238–241.

Evans, I. M. (1985). Building systems models as a strategy for target behavior selection in clinical assessment. *Behavioral Assessment, 7,* 21–32.

Evans, I. M. (1986). Response structure and the triple-response-mode concept. In R. O. Nelson & S. C. Hayes (Eds.), *Conceptual foundations of behavioral assessment* (pp. 131–155). New York: Guilford.

Evans, I. M. (1996). Individualizing therapy, customizing clinical science. *Journal of Behavior Therapy and Experimental Psychiatry, 27,* 99–105.

Evans, I. M. (2005). Applied behavior analysis. In M. Hersen, A. M. Gross, & R. S. Drabman (Eds.), *Encyclopedia of behavior modification and cognitive behavior therapy. Vol. 2: Child clinical applications* (pp. 666–674). Thousand Oaks, CA: Sage.

Evans, I. M. (2007). Getting to the South Pole: A fable for excrement-free treatment outcome research. *The Behavior Therapist, 30,* 132–134.

Evans, I. M. (2010). Positive affective priming: A behavioral technique to facilitate therapeutic engagement by families, caregivers, and teachers. *Child & Family Behavior Therapy, 32,* 257–271.

Evans, I. M., & Berryman, J. S. (1998). Supervising support staff in naturalistic behavioural interventions: Process and outcome. *New Zealand Journal of Psychology, 27,* 10–21.

Evans, I. M., Eifert, G. H., & Corrigan, S. A. (1990). A critical appraisal of paradigmatic behaviorism's contribution to behavior therapy. In G. H. Eifert & I. M. Evans (Eds.), *Unifying behavior therapy: Contributions of paradigmatic behaviorism* (pp. 293–317). New York: Springer.

Evans, I. M., & Galyer, K. (2009). Are you sure there isn't a monster in the closet? Regulation of children's worrying in uncertain contexts. *Child & Family Behavior Therapy, 31,* 38–53.

Evans, I. M., Galyer, K. T., & Smith, K. J. H. (2001). Children's perceptions of unfair reward and punishment. *Journal of Genetic Psychology, 162,* 212–227.

Evans, I. M., & Harvey, S. T. (2012). *Warming the emotional climate of the primary school classroom.* Auckland, NZ: Dunmore.

Evans, I. M., Harvey, S. T., Buckley, L., & Yan, E. (2009). Differentiating classroom climate concepts: Academic, management, and emotional environments. *Kotuitui: The New Zealand Journal of Social Science, 4,* 131–146.

Evans, I. M., Herbert, A. M. L., Fitzgerald, J. M., & Harvey, S. T. (2010). Cultural competence and power sharing: An international perspective on training clinical child psychologists. *Journal of Mental Health Training, Education and Practice, 5,* 34–42.

Evans, I. M., & Meyer, L. H. (1990). Toward a science in support of meaningful outcomes: A response to Horner et al. *Journal of the Association for Persons with Severe Handicaps, 15,* 133–135.

Evans, I. M., & Meyer, L. H. (2001). Having friends and Rett syndrome: How social relationships create meaningful contexts for limited skills. *Disability & Rehabilitation, 23,* 167–176.

Evans, I. M., Meyer, L. M., Kurkjian, J. A., & Kishi, G. S. (1988). An evaluation of behavioral interrelationships in child behavior therapy. In J. C. Witt, S. N. Elliott, & F. N. Gresham (Eds.), *Handbook of behavior therapy in education* (pp. 189–215). New York: Plenum.

Evans, I. M., & Moltzen, N. L. (2000). Defining effective community support for long-term psychiatric patients according to behavioural principles. *Australian and New Zealand Journal of Psychiatry, 34*, 637–644.

Evans, I. M., & Nelson, R. O. (1977). Assessment of child behavior problems. In A. R. Ciminero, K. S. Calhoun, & H. E. Adams (Eds.), *Handbook of behavioral assessment* (pp. 603–682). New York: Wiley.

Evans, I. M., Okifuji, A., Engler, L., Bromley, K., & Tishelman, A. (1993). Home-school communication in the treatment of childhood behavior problems. *Child & Family Behavior Therapy, 15*, 37–60.

Evans, I. M., & Pechtel, P. (2010). Phagophobia: Behavioral treatment of a complex case involving fear of fear. *Clinical Case Studies, 10*, 37–52.

Evans, I. M., & Robinson, C. R. (1978). Behavior therapy observed: The diary of a client. *Cognitive Therapy and Research, 2*, 335–355.

Evans, I. M., Salisbury, C. L, Palombaro, M. M., Berryman, J., & Hollowood, T. M. (1992). Peer interactions and social acceptance of elementary-age children with severe disabilities in an inclusive school. *Journal of The Association for Persons with Severe Handicaps, 17*, 205–212.

Eysenck, H. J. (1952). The effects of psychotherapy: An evaluation. *Journal of Consulting Psychology, 16*, 319–324.

Eysenck, H. J. (1967). *The biological basis of personality.* Springfield, IL: Charles C Thomas.

Eysenck, H. J. (1968). A theory of the incubation of anxiety/fear responses. *Behaviour Research and Therapy, 6*, 309–321.

Farkas, G. M., Evans, I. M., Sine, L. F., Eifert, G., Wittlieb, E., & Vogelmann-Sine, S. (1979). Reliability and validity of the mercury-in-rubber strain gauge measure of penile circumference. *Behavior Therapy, 10*, 555–561.

Fenz, W., & Epstein, S. (1967). Gradients of physiological arousal in parachutists as a function of an approaching jump. *Psychosomatic Medicine, 29*, 33–55.

Festinger, L. (1957). *A theory of cognitive dissonance.* Stanford, CA: Stanford University Press.

Fiese, B. H. (2006). *Family routines and rituals.* New Haven, CT: Yale University Press.

Fiske, A. P., Kitayama, S., Markus, H. R., & Nisbett, R. E. (1998). The cultural matrix of social psychology. In D. T. Gilbert, S. Fiske, & G. Lindzey (Eds.), *Handbook of social psychology* (4th ed. Vol. 2, pp. 915–981). Boston, MA: McGraw-Hill.

Fitzgerald, J. (2002). *Depression and self-concept: The role of self perceptions in understanding, assessing, and intervening with depressed adolescents.* Unpublished doctoral thesis, School of Psychology, University of Waikato, Hamilton, NZ.

Fogarty, J. S. (1997). Reactance theory and patient noncompliance. *Social Science & Medicine, 45*, 1277–1288.

Fonagy, P. (1998). Moments of change in psychoanalytic theory: Discussion of a new theory of psychic change. *Infant Mental Health Journal, 19*, 346–353.

Forbes, D. L. (2011). Toward a unified model of human motivation. *Review of General Psychology, 15*, 85–98.

Frank, J. D. (1961). *Persuasion and healing.* Baltimore, MD: Johns Hopkins University Press.

Frankl, V. E. (1967). *Psychotherapy and existentialism.* Harmondsworth, UK: Pelican.

Frazer, J. A., Shennan, J., Evans, I. M., & Sumpter, C. E. (2002, August). *Psychological intervention in complex Regional Pain Syndrome.* Paper presented at the 10th World Congress on Pain, San Diego, CA.

Freud, S. (1920). *A general introduction to psychoanalysis.* New York: Horace Liveright.

Friedman, A. G., Campbell, T. A., & Evans, I. M. (1993). Multi-dimensional child behavior therapy in the treatment of medically-related anxiety: A practical illustration. *Journal of Behavior Therapy and Experimental Psychiatry, 24*, 241–247.

Froján, M. X., Montaño, M., & Calero, A. (2010). Therapists' verbal behavior analysis: A descriptive approach to the psychotherapeutic phenomenon. *The Spanish Journal of Psychology, 13*, 914–926.

Frost, J. (2006). *Ask Supernanny. What every parent wants to know.* London, UK: Hodder & Stoughton.
Fu, F., Rosenbloom, D. I., Wang, L., & Nowak, M. A. (2010). Imitation dynamics of vaccination behaviour on social networks. *Proceedings of the Royal Society.* Published online 28 July 2010. doi: 10.1098/rspb.2010.1107.
Fuchs, C., & Rehm, L. (1977). A self-control behavior therapy program for depression. *Journal of Consulting and Clinical Psychology, 45,* 206-215.
Fulmer, C. A., Gelfand, M. J., Kruglanski, A. W., Kim-Prieto, C., Diener, E., Pierro, A., & Higgins, E. T. (2010). On "feeling right" in cultural contexts: How person-culture match affects self-esteem and subjective well-being. *Psychological Science, 21,* 1563-1569.
Galbicka, G. (1992). Editorial: The dynamics of behavior. *Journal of the Experimental Analysis of Behavior, 57,* 243-248.
Gallimore, R. (2005). Behavior change in the natural environment: Everyday activity settings as a workshop of change. In C. R. O'Donnell & L. A. Yamauchi (Eds.), *Culture and context in human behavior change* (pp. 207-232). New York: Peter Lang.
Galyer, K. T., & Evans, I. M. (2001). Pretend play and the development of emotion regulation in preschool children. *Early Child Development and Care, 166,* 93-108.
Gawande, A. (2010). *The checklist manifesto: How to get things right.* London, UK: Profile Books.
Gershkoff-Stowe, L., & Thelen, E. (2004). U-shaped changes in behavior: A dynamic systems perspective. *Journal of Cognition and Development, 5,* 11-36.
Gilbert, D. T., & Malone, P. S. (1995). The correspondence bias. *Psychological Bulletin, 117,* 21-38.
Gilbert, P. (2009). *The compassionate mind: A new approach to life's challenges.* Oakland, CA: New Harbinger Publications.
Gilford, T. T., & Reynolds, A. (2010). "My mother's keeper": The effects of parentification on Black female college students. *Journal of Black Psychology,* published online June 7th 2010 as doi: 10.1177/0095798410372624.
Glasgow, R. E., Toobert, D. J., & Gillette, C. D. (2001). Psychosocial barriers to diabetes self-management and quality of life. *Diabetes Spectrum, 14*(1), 33-41.
Goldfried, M. R. (1980). Toward the delineation of therapeutic change principles. *American Psychologist, 35,* 991-999.
Goldiamond, I. (1974). Toward a constructional approach to social problems: Ethical and constitutional issues raised by applied behavior analysis. *Behaviorism, 2,* 1-84.
Goldstein, A. P., Glick, B., & Gibbs, J. C. (1998). *Aggression Replacement Training: A comprehensive intervention for aggressive youth* (rev. ed.). Champaign, IL: Research Press.
Goldstein, A. P., Heller, K., & Sechrest, L. B. (1966). *Psychotherapy and the psychology of behavior change.* New York: Wiley.
Gollwitzer, P. M., Sheeran, P., Trötschel, R., & Webb, T. L. (2011). Self-regulation of priming effects on behavior. *Psychological Science, 22,* 901-907.
Goodman, S. H., & Gotlib, I. H. (1999). Risk for psychopathology in the children of depressed mothers: A developmental model for understanding mechanisms of transmission. *Psychological Review, 106,* 458-490.
Gray, J. A. (1982). *The neuropsychology of anxiety: An enquiry into the functions of the septo-hippocampal system.* New York: Oxford University Press.
Gray, J. A., & McNaughton, N. (2000). *The neuropsychology of anxiety: An enquiry into the functions of the septo-hippocampal system* (2nd ed.). New York: Oxford University Press.
Greenberg, M. A., & Stone, A. A. (1992). Emotional disclosure about traumas and its relation to health: Effects of previous disclosure and trauma severity. *Journal of Personality and Social Psychology, 63,* 75-84.
Greenberg, M. T., & Kusché, C. A., (2006). Building social and emotional competence: The PATHS Curriculum. In S. R. Jimerson & M. J. Furlong (Eds.), *Handbook of school violence and school safety: From research to practice* (pp. 395-412). Mahwah, NJ: Erlbaum.
Grilo, C. M., Masheb, R. M., & Wilson, G. T. (2006). Rapid response to treatment for binge eating disorder. *Journal of Consulting and Clinical Psychology, 74,* 602-613.
Guerin, B. (2001). Replacing catharsis and uncertainty reduction theories with descriptions of historical and social context. *Review of General Psychology, 5,* 44-61.

Guerin, B. (2003). Language use as social strategy: A review and an analytic framework for the social sciences. *Review of General Psychology, 7*, 251–298.

Guerra, N. G., & Bradshaw, C. P. (2008). Linking the prevention of problem behavior and positive youth development: Core competencies for positive youth development. *New Directions in Child and Adolescent Development, 122*, 1–17.

Guinote, A. (2007). Power affects basic cognition: Increased attentional inhibition and flexibility. *Journal of Experimental Social Psychology, 43*, 685–697.

Guthrie, E. R. (1935). *The psychology of learning*. New York: Harper.

Hagan, R., & Turkington, D. (2011). Introduction. CBT for psychosis: A symptom-based approach. In R. Hagan, D. Turkington, T. Berge, & R. W. Gråwe (Eds.), *CBT for psychosis: A symptom-based approach* (pp. 3–11). Hove, East Sussex, UK: Routledge.

Hamm, L. (2010). Alexa Ray Joel: "I hit rock bottom." *People, 73*(19), 78–80.

Hansen, N. B., & Lambert, M. J. (2003). An evaluation of the dose-response relationship in naturalistic treatment settings using survival analysis. *Mental Health Services Research, 5*, 1–12.

Hardeman, W., Johnston, M., Johnston, D. W., Bonetti, D., Wareham, N., & Kinmonth, A. L. (2002). Application of the theory of planned behavior in behavior change interventions: A systematic review. *Psychology and Health, 17*, 123–158.

Harris, G. T., & Rice, M. E. (1997). Risk appraisal and management of violent behavior. *Psychiatric Services, 48*, 1168–1176.

Harvey, S. T., Boer, D., Meyer, L. H., & Evans, I. M. (2009). Updating a meta-analysis of intervention research with challenging behaviour: Treatment validity and standards of practice. *Journal of Intellectual and Developmental Disabilities, 34*, 1–14.

Hatfield, E., Cacioppo, J., & Rapson, R. L. (1994). *Emotional contagion*. New York: Cambridge University Press.

Hatzigeorgiadis, A., Zourbanos, N., Galanis, E., & Theodorakis, Y. (2011). Self-talk and sports performance: A meta-analysis. *Perspectives on Psychological Science, 6*, 348–356.

Hawkins, R. P. (1974, March). *Who decided "that" was the problem? Two stages of responsibility for applied behavior analysis*. Paper presented at the Drake Conference on Professional Issues in Behavior Analysis, Des Moines, IO.

Hayes, A. M., Feldman, G. C., Beevers, C. G., Laurenceau, J. P., Cardaciotto, L., & Lewis-Smith, J. (2007). Discontinuities and cognitive changes in an exposure-based cognitive therapy for depression. *Journal of Consulting and Clinical Psychology, 75*, 409–421.

Hayes, S. C. (1989). A contextual approach to therapeutic change. In N. S. Jacobson (Ed.), *Psychotherapists in clinical practice: Cognitive and behavioral perspectives* (pp. 327–386). New York: Guilford.

Hayes, S. C. (2004). Acceptance and commitment therapy, relational frame theory, and the third wave of behavioral and cognitive therapies. *Behavior Therapy, 35*, 639–665.

Hayes, S. C., Barnes-Holmes, D., & Roche, B. (Eds.) (2001). *Relational Frame Theory: A post-Skinnerian account of human language and cognition*. New York: Kluwer.

Hayes, S. C., Luoma, J., Bond, F., Masuda, A., & Lillis, J. (2006). Acceptance and Commitment Therapy: Model, processes, and outcomes. *Behaviour Research and Therapy, 44*, 1–25.

Hayes, S. C., Strosahl, K. D., & Wilson, K. G. (1999). *Acceptance and commitment therapy: An experiential approach to behavior change*. New York: Guilford.

Heath, C., & Heath, D. (2010). *Switch: How to change things when change is hard*. New York: Broadway Books.

Heiby, E. M. (1982). A self-reinforcement questionnaire. *Behaviour Research and Therapy, 20*, 397–401.

Higginbotham, H. N., West, S. G., & Forsyth, D. R. (1988). *Psychotherapy and behavior change: Social, cultural and methodological perspectives*. New York: Pergamon.

Higgins, S. T., Alessi, S. M., & Dantona, R. L. (2002). Voucher-based incentives: A substance abuse treatment innovation. *Addictive Behaviors, 27*, 887–910.

Hill-Briggs, F. (2003). Problem solving in diabetes self-management: A model of chronic illness self-management behavior. *Annals of Behavioral Medicine, 25*, 182–193.

Hiss, T. (2010). *In motion: The experience of travel.* New York: Alfred A. Knopf.

Hodal, K. (2012). Indonesia's smoking epidemic—an old problem getting younger. *The Guardian*, Friday, 23 March, p. 21, UK.

Hofmann, S. G. (2007). Cognitive factors that maintain social anxiety disorder: A comprehensive model and its treatment implications. *Cognitive Behavior Therapy, 36,* 193–209.

Hofmann, S. G., Schulz, S. S., Meuret, A. E., Moscovitch, D. A., & Suvak, M. (2006). Sudden gains during therapy of social phobia. *Journal of Consulting and Clinical Psychology, 74,* 687–697.

Hogan, R., & Bond, M. H. (2009). Culture and personality. In P. J. Corr & G. Matthews (Eds.), *The Cambridge handbook of personality psychology* (pp. 570–588). Cambridge, UK: Cambridge University Press.

Holland, P. C. (2008). Cognitive versus stimulus-response theories of learning. *Learning & Behavior, 36,* 227–241.

Hong, Y. Y., & Mallorie, L. M. (2004). A dynamic constructivist approach to culture: Lessons learned from personality psychology. *Journal of Research in Personality, 38,* 59–67.

Hooley, J. M. (1985). Expressed emotion: A review of the critical literature. *Clinical Psychology Review, 5,* 119–139.

Hooley, J. M., & Hillier, J. B. (2000). Personality and expressed emotion. *Journal of Abnormal Psychology, 109,* 40–44.

Houben, K., Wiers, R. W., & Jansen, A. (2011). Getting a grip on drinking behavior: Training working memory to reduce alcohol abuse. *Psychological Science, 22,* 968–975.

Howard, K. I., Kopte, S. M., Krause, M. S., & Orlinsky, D. E. (1986). The dose-effect relationship in psychotherapy. *American Psychologist, 41,* 159–164.

Howes, M., Hokanson, J., & Lowenstein, D. (1985). Induction of depressive affect after prolonged exposure to a mildly depressed individual. *Journal of Personality and Social Psychology, 49,* 110–113.

Hsee, C. K., Yang, A. X., & Wang, L. (2010). Idleness aversion and the need for justifiable busyness. *Psychological Science, 21,* 926–930.

Hsu, S. H., Grow, J., & Marlatt, G. A. (2008). Mindfulness and addiction. *Recent Developments in Alcoholism, 18,* 229–250.

Hull, C. L. (1943). *Principles of behavior.* New York: Appleton-Century-Crofts.

Ilardi, S. S., & Craighead, W. E. (1999). Rapid early response, cognitive modification, and nonspecific factors in cognitive behavior therapy for depression: A reply to Tang and DeRubeis. *Clinical Psychology: Science and Practice, 6,* 295–299.

Ipsos MORI, & Nairn, A. C. (2011). *Children's well-being in UK, Sweden and Spain: The role of inequality and materialism.* UNICEF commissioned report. London, UK: Ipsos MORI Social Research Institute.

Ivanović, E. M., Vuletić, Z., & Bebbington, P. (1994). Expressed emotion in the families of patients with schizophrenia and its influence on the course of illness. *Social Psychiatry and Psychiatric Epidemiology, 29,* 61–65.

Izard, C. E. (2009). Emotion theory and research: Highlights, unanswered questions, and emerging issues. *Annual Review of Psychology, 60,* 1–25.

Jacobson, N. S., & Christensen, A. (1996). *Acceptance and change in couple therapy.* New York: Norton.

Jacobson, N. S., Dobson, K. S., Truax, P. A., Addis, M. E., Koerner, K., Gollan, J. K., Gortner, E., & Prince, S. E. (1996). A component analysis of cognitive-behavioral treatment for depression. *Journal of Consulting and Clinical Psychology, 64,* 295–304.

Jacobson, N. S., & Truax, P. (1991). Clinical significance: A statistical approach to defining meaningful change in psychotherapy research. *Journal of Consulting and Clinical Psychology, 59,* 12–19.

James, W. (1890/1950). *Principles of psychology* (Vol. 1). New York: Dover Publications.

Jarrett, R. B., & Nelson, R. O. (1987). Mechanisms of change in cognitive therapy of depression. *Behavior Therapy, 18,* 227–241.

Jones, M. C. (1924). A laboratory study of fear: The case of Peter. *Pedagogical Seminary, 31,* 308–315.

Jourdain, R. (2010). *Treating the psychological effects of exposure to nuclear testing in the South Pacific in the 1950s*. Unpublished doctoral dissertation, Massey University, Palmerston North, New Zealand.

Judge, T. A., & Bono, J. E. (2001). Relationship of core self-evaluations traits—self-esteem, generalized self-efficacy, locus of control, and emotional stability—with job satisfaction and job performance: A meta-analysis. *Journal of Applied Psychology, 86*, 80–92.

Judge, T. A., & Kammeyer-Mueller, J. D. (2010). Implications of core self-evaluations for a changing organizational context. *Human Resources Management Review*, published on line, doi: 10.1016/j.hmr.2010.10.003.

Kabat-Zinn, J. (2003). Mindfulness-based interventions in context: Past, present, and future. *Clinical Psychology: Science and Practice, 10*, 144–156.

Kadera, S. W., Lambert, M. J., & Andrews, A. A. (1996). How much therapy is really enough? A session-by-session analysis of the psychotherapy dose-effect relationship. *Journal of Psychotherapy Practice and Research, 5*, 132–151.

Kahn, P. H., Jr. (1999). *The human relationship with nature: Development and culture*. Cambridge, MA: MIT Press.

Kanfer, F. H., & Goldstein, A. P. (Eds.) (1991). *Helping people change: A textbook of methods* (4th ed.). Elmsford, NY: Pergamon.

Kanfer, F. H., & Schefft, B. K. (1988). *Guiding the process of therapeutic change*. Champaign, IL: Research Press.

Kantor, J. R. (1969). *The scientific evolution of psychology*. Chicago: Principia Press.

Karoly, P. (1993). Goal systems: An organizing framework for clinical assessment and treatment planning. *Psychological Assessment, 5*, 273–280.

Karoly, P. (1999). A goal systems—self-regulatory perspective on personality, psychopathology, and change. *Review of General Psychology, 3*, 264–291.

Kazantzis, N., Deane, F. P., Ronan, K. R., & L'Abate, L. (Eds.) (2005). *Using homework assignments in cognitive behavior therapy*. London, UK: Routledge.

Kazdin, A. E. (1977). *The token economy: A review and evaluation*. New York: Plenum.

Kazdin, A. E. (2007). Mediators and mechanisms of change in psychotherapy research. *Annual Review of Clinical Psychology, 3*, 1–27.

Kazdin, A. E. (2009a). Psychological science's contributions to a sustainable environment: Extending our reach to a grand challenge of society. *American Psychologist, 64*, 339–356.

Kazdin, A. E. (2009b). Understanding how and why psychotherapy leads to change. *Psychotherapy Research, 19*, 418–428.

Kazdin, A. E., & Blase, S. (2011). Rebooting psychotherapy research and practice to reduce the burden of mental illness. *Perspectives on Psychological Science, 6*, 21–37.

Keene, N. A., Isler, R. B., Evans, I. M., Herd, D., Moltzen, N., McAnulty, K., & Hedge, B. (2003). An examination of caregiver influences on child distress during an invasive medical procedure. *Bulletin of the New Zealand Psychological Society, 101*, 36–41.

Kendall, P. C. (2009). Principles of therapeutic change circa 2010. *Applied and Preventive Psychology, 13*, 19–21.

Kendall, P. C., & Hedtke, K. A. (2006). *Coping cat workbook* (2nd ed.). Ardmore, PA: Workbook Publishing.

Kendler, K. S., Gardner, C. O., & Prescott, C. A. (2001). Toward a comprehensive developmental model for major depression in women. *American Journal of Psychiatry, 159*, 1133–1145.

Kenney, M., Ninness, C., Rumph, R., Bradfield, A., & Cost, H. (2004). Paradoxical patterns in the measurement of hyperactivity. *Behavior and Social Issues, 13*, 69–81.

Kipling, R. (1919/2008). *Rudyard Kipling's verse: Inclusive edition 1885–1918*. Facsimile reprint, 2008. Whitefish, MT: Kessinger Publishing.

Kitzmann, K. M., & Howard, K. M. (2011). Emotion socialization by early childhood educators: Conceptual models from psychology. *Asia-Pacific Journal of Research in Early Childhood Education, 5*, 23–44.

Klump, K. L., McGue, M., & Iacono, W. G. (2002). Genetic relationships between personality and eating attitudes and behaviors. *Journal of Abnormal Psychology, 111*, 380–389.

Koegel, R. L., & Koegel, L. K. (2006). *Pivotal response treatment for autism: Communication, social, and academic development.* Baltimore, MD: Paul H. Brookes.

Kohlenberg, R. J., & Tsai, M. (1991). *Functional analytic psychotherapy.* New York: Plenum.

Kohn, A. (1993). *Punished by rewards: The trouble with gold stars, incentive plans, A's, praise, and other bribes.* Boston, MA: Houghton Mifflin.

Krasner, L., & Ullmann, L. P. (1969). *A psychological approach to abnormal behavior.* New York: Prentice-Hall.

Kubany, E. S., & Ralston, T. C. (2008). *Treating PRSD in battered women: A step-by-step manual for therapists and counselors.* Oakland, CA: New Harbinger.

Kuppens, P., Allen, N. B., & Sheeber, L. B. (2010). Emotional inertia and psychological maladjustment. *Psychological Science, 21,* 984–991.

Laborda, M. A., McConnell, B. L., & Miller, R. R. (2011). Behavioral techniques to reduce relapse after exposure therapy: Applications of studies of experimental extinction. In T. R. Schachtman & S. S. Reilly (Eds.), *Associative learning and conditioning theory: Human and non-human applications* (pp. 79–103). New York: Oxford University Press.

Laborda, M. A., & Miller, R. R. (2011). S-R associations, their extinction and recovery in an animal model of anxiety: A new associative account of phobias without recall of the original trauma. *Behavior Therapy, 42,* 153–169.

Lakoff, G., & Johnson, M. (1980). *Metaphors we live by.* Chicago, IL: University of Chicago Press.

Lang, P. J. (1968). Fear reduction and fear behavior: Problems in treating a construct. *Research in Psychotherapy, 3,* 90–102.

Lang, P. J. (1994). The varieties of emotional experience: A meditation on James-Lange theory. *Psychological Review, 101,* 211–221.

Latané, B. (1996). Dynamic social impact: The creation of culture by communication. *Journal of Communication, 46,* 13–25.

Lazarus, R. S., & Folkman, S. (1984). *Stress, appraisal, and coping.* New York: Springer.

Lazev, A. B., Herzog, T. A., & Brandon, T. H. (1999). Classical conditioning of environmental cues to cigarette smoking. *Experimental and Clinical Psychopharmacology, 7,* 56–63.

Leahy, R. L. (2008). A closer look at ACT. *The Behavior Therapist, 31,* 148–150.

Léduc, A., Dumais, A., & Evans, I. M. (1990). Social behaviorism, rehabilitation, and ethics: Applications for people with severe disabilities. In G. H. Eifert & I. M. Evans (Eds.), *Unifying behavior therapy: Contributions of paradigmatic behaviorism* (pp. 268–289). New York: Springer.

Lee, D. A. (2005). The perfect nurturer: A model to develop a compassionate mind within the context of cognitive therapy. In P. Gilbert (Ed.), *Compassion: Conceptualisations, research and use in psychotherapy* (pp. 326–351). Hove, East Sussex, UK: Routledge.

Lee, H., & Kwon, S. (2003). Two different types of obsession: Autogenous obsessions and reactive obsessions. *Behaviour Research and Therapy, 41,* 11–29.

Leenders, R. T. A. J. (2003). *Structure and influence: Statistical models for the dynamics of actor attributes, network structure and their interdependence.* West Lafayette, IN: Purdue University Press.

Le Grange, D. (2005). The Maudsley family-based treatment for adolescent anorexia nervosa. *World Psychiatry, 4,* 142–146.

Lerner, R. M., Lerner, J. V., et al. (2005). Positive youth development, participation in community youth development programs, and community contributions to fifth-grade adolescents: Findings from the first wave of the 4-H study of positive youth development. *Journal of Early Adolescence, 25,* 17–71.

Lepper, M. R., Greene, D., & Nisbett, R. E. (1973). Undermining children's intrinsic interest with extrinsic reward: A test of the "overjustification" hypothesis. *Journal of Personality and Social Psychology, 28,* 129–137.

Levis, D. J. (1991). A clinician's plea for a return to the development of nonhuman models of psychopathology: New clinical observations in need of laboratory study. In M. R. Denny (Ed.), *Fear, avoidance, and phobias: A fundamental analysis* (pp. 395–427). Hillsdale, NJ: Erlbaum.

Levis, D. J., & Malloy, P. F. (1982). Research in infrahuman and human conditioning. In G. T. Wilson & C. M. Franks (Eds.), *Contemporary behavior therapy: Conceptual and empirical foundations* (pp. 65–118). New York: Guilford.

Lewin, K. (1931). The conflict between Aristotelian and Galilean modes of thought in contemporary psychology. *Journal of General Psychology, 5*, 141–177.

Lilienfeld, S. O. (2007). Psychological treatments that cause harm. *Perspectives on Psychological Science, 2*, 53–70.

Linscheid, T. R., Iwata, B. A., Ricketts, R. W., Williams, D. E., & Griffin, J. D. (1990). Clinical evaluation of the self-injurious behavior inhibiting system (SIBIS). *Journal of Applied Behavior Analysis, 23*, 53–78.

Lindsley, O. R. (1992). Precision teaching: Discoveries and effects. *Journal of Applied Behavior Analysis, 25*, 51–57.

Linehan, M. M. (1994). Acceptance and change: The central dialectic in psychotherapy. In S. C. Hayes, N. S. Jacobson, V. M. Follette, & M. J. Dougher (Eds.), *Acceptance and change: Content and context in psychotherapy* (pp. 73–86). Reno, NV: Context Press.

Lock, J., Le Grange, D., Agras, W. S., & Dare, C. (2001). *Treatment manual for anorexia nervosa: A family-based approach*. New York: Guilford.

Lohr, J. M., & Hamberger, L. K. (1990). Verbal, emotional, and imagery repertoires in the regulation of dysfunctional behavior: An integrative conceptual framework for cognitive-behavioral disorders and interventions. In G. H. Eifert & I. M. Evans (Eds.), *Unifying behavior therapy: Contributions of paradigmatic behaviorism* (pp. 153–172). New York: Springer.

London, P. (1969). *Behavior control*. New York: Harper & Row.

Lovett, H. (1996). *Learning to listen: Positive approaches and people with difficult behavior*. Baltimore, MD: Paul H. Brookes.

Luborsky, L., Rosenthal, R., Diguer, L., Andrusyna, T. P., Berman, J. S., Levitt, J. T., Seligman, D. A., & Krause, E. D. (2002). The Dodo bird verdict is alive and well—mostly. *Clinical Psychology: Science and Practice, 9*, 2–12.

Ludwig, T. D. (2002). On the necessity of structure in an arbitrary world: Using concurrent schedules of reinforcement to describe response generalization. *Journal of Organizational Behavior Management, 21*, 13–38.

Lutz, R. S., Karoly, P., & Okun, M. A. (2008). The *why* and the *how* of goal pursuit: Self-determination, goal process cognition, and participation in physical exercise. *Psychology of Sport and Exercise, 9*, 559–575.

Lutz, W., Martinovich, Z., & Howard, K. I. (1999). Patient profiling: An application of random coefficient regression models to depicting the response of a patient to outpatient psychotherapy. *Journal of Consulting and Clinical Psychology, 67*, 571–577.

Mahoney, M. J. (1976). *Scientist as subject: The psychological imperative*. Cambridge, MA: Ballinger.

Mahoney, M. J. (2000). Behaviorism, cognitivism, and constructivism: Reflections on persons and patterns in my intellectual development. In M. R. Goldfried (Ed.), *How therapists change: Personal and professional reflections* (pp. 183–200). Washington, DC: American Psychological Association.

Mahoney, M. J. (2003). *Constructive psychotherapy: Theory and practice*. New York: Guilford.

Makrygianni, M. K., & Reed, P. (2010). A meta-analytic review of the effectiveness of behavioral early intervention programs for children with Autistic Spectrum Disorders. *Research in Autism Spectrum Disorders, 4*, 577–593.

Mann, T., Tomiyama, A. J., Westling, E., Lew, A-M., Samuels, B., & Chatman, J. (2007). Medicare's search for effective obesity treatments: Diets are not the answer. *American Psychologist, 62*, 220–233.

Marks, I. M. (1987). *Fears, phobias and rituals*. Oxford, UK: Oxford University Press.

Markus, H., & Nurius, P. (1986). Possible selves. *American Psychologist, 41*, 954–969.

Marlatt, G. A., & Gordon, J. R. (Eds.) (1985). *Relapse prevention: Maintenance strategies in the treatment of addictive behaviors*. New York: Guilford.

Martin, I., & Levey, A. B. (1978). Evaluative conditioning. *Advances in Behaviour Research and Therapy, 1,* 57–101.

Maruna, S. (2001). *Making good: How ex-convicts reform and rebuild their lives.* Washington, DC: American Psychological Association.

McCleery, J., & Evans, I. M. (2001, November). *Cognitive behavior therapy with schizophrenia: Is it more than a validated wet noodle?* Poster presented at the 35th annual conference of the Association for Advancement of Behavior Therapy, Philadelphia, PA.

McClintock, K., Hall, S., & Oliver, C. (2003). Risk markers associated with challenging behaviours in people with intellectual disabilities: A meta-analytic study. *Journal of Intellectual Disability Research, 47,* 405–416.

McEvedy, C. P., & Beard, A. W. (1970). Royal free epidemic of 1955: A reconsideration. *British Medical Journal, 1,* 7–11.

McGlashan, T. H. (1987). Recovery style from mental illness and long-term outcome. *Journal of Nervous and Mental Disorders, 175,* 681–685.

McGraw, M. (1935). *Growth: A study of Johnny and Jimmy.* New York: Appleton-Century-Crofts.

McIvor, J. (2011, August). *Will the needle make me bleed to death? Cognitions of chronically ill children.* Paper presented at the annual conference of the New Zealand Psychological Society, Queenstown, NZ.

McMahon, R. J., & Forehand, R. L. (2003). *Helping the noncompliant child: Family-based treatment for oppositional behavior* (2nd ed.). New York: Guilford.

McNaughton, N., & Corr, P. J. (2008). The neuropsychology of fear and anxiety: A foundation for reinforcement sensitivity theory. In P. J. Corr (Ed.), *The reinforcement sensitivity theory of personality* (pp. 44–94). Cambridge, UK: Cambridge University Press.

Mdaka, S. L. (1994). *A comparison of the relative efficacy of rational behavior therapy and study skills training with middle school adolescents at risk for academic failure.* Unpublished doctoral dissertation, State University of New York at Binghamton.

Meichenbaum, D. (1977). *Cognitive-behavior modification: An integrative approach.* New York: Plenum.

Meichenbaum, D. J., & Goodman, J. (1971). Training impulsive children to talk to themselves: A means of developing self-control. *Journal of Abnormal Psychology, 77,* 115–126.

Melamed, B. G. (1983). The effects of preparatory information on adjustment of children to medical procedures. In M. Rosenbaum, C. M. Franks, & Y. Jaffe (Eds.), *Perspectives on behavior therapy in the eighties* (pp. 344–362). New York: Springer.

Metcalf, J., & Mischel, W. (1999). A hot/cool-system analysis of delay of gratification: Dynamics of willpower. *Psychological Review, 106,* 3–19.

Meyer, L. H., & Evans, I. M. (1989). *Non-aversive intervention for behavior problems: A manual for home and community.* Baltimore, MD: Paul H. Brookes.

Michie, S., van Stralen, M. M., & West, R. (2011). The behaviour change wheel: A new method for characterising and designing behaviour change interventions. *Implementation Science, 6,* 42–53.

Miller, N. E. (1948). Studies of fear as an acquired drive: I. Fear as motivation and fear-reduction as reinforcement in the learning of new responses. *Journal of Experimental Psychology, 38,* 89–101.

Miller, N. E. (1959). Liberalization of basic S-R concepts: Extensions to conflict behavior, motivation and social learning. In S. Koch (Ed.), *Psychology: A study of a science, Vol.2* (pp. 196–292). New York: McGraw-Hill.

Miller, S. D., Duncan, B. L., Brown, J., Sorrell, R., & Chalk, M. B. (2006). Using formal client feedback to improve retention and outcome: Making ongoing, real-time assessment feasible. *Journal of Brief Therapy, 5,* 5–22.

Miller, S. D., & Hubble, M. A. (2004). Further archeological and ethnological findings on the obscure, late 20th century, quasi-religious Earth group known as "the therapists" (a fantasy about the future of psychotherapy). *Journal of Psychotherapy Integration, 14,* 38–65.

Miller, W. R. (1983). Motivational interviewing with problem drinkers. *Behavioural Psychotherapy, 11,* 147–172.

Miller, W. R., & Rollnick, S. (2002). *Motivational interviewing: Preparing people for change* (2nd ed.). New York: Guilford.

Mischel, W. (1968). *Personality and assessment*. New York: Wiley.

Mischel, W. (1973). Toward a cognitive social learning reconceptualization of personality. *Psychological Review, 80*, 252–283.

Mischel, W. (2004). Toward an integrative science of the person. *Annual Review of Psychology, 55*, 1–22.

Mischel, W., & Shoda, Y. (1995). A cognitive-affect system theory of personality: Reconceptualizing situations, dispositions, dynamics, and invariance in personality structure. *Psychological Review, 102*, 246–268.

Mischel, W., Shoda, Y., & Rodriguez, M. L. (1989). Delay of gratification in children. *Science, 244*, 933–938.

Mowrer, O. H. (1939). A stimulus-response analysis of anxiety and its role as a reinforcing agent. *Psychological Review, 46*, 553–565.

Mowrer, O. H. (1960). *Learning theory and the symbolic processes*. New York: Wiley.

Mulick, J. A., & Butter, E. (2005). Positive behavior support: A paternalistic utopian delusion. In J. W. Jacobson, R. M. Foxx, & J. A. Mulick (Eds.), *Controversial therapies for developmental disabilities: Fads, fashion, and science in professional practice* (pp. 385–404). Mahwah, NJ: Erlbaum.

Najmi, S., Riemann, B. C., & Wegner, D. M. (2009). Managing unwanted intrusive thoughts in obsessive-compulsive disorder: Relative effectiveness of suppression, focused distraction, and acceptance. *Behaviour Research and Therapy, 47*, 494–503.

Nalls, A. M., Mullis, R. L., & Mullis, A. K. (2009). American Indian youths' perceptions of their environment and their reports of depressive symptoms and alcohol/marijuana use. *Adolescence, 44*, 965–978.

Nardone, G. (2004). Constructivist theory and therapy. In J. Sommers-Flanagan & R. Sommers-Flanagan (Eds.), *Counseling and psychotherapy theories in context and practice* (pp. 376–392). Chichester, UK: Wiley.

Nardone, G., & Salvini, A. (2007). *The strategic dialogue: Rendering the diagnostic interview a real therapeutic intervention*. London, UK: Karnac Books.

Neal-Barnett, A., Stadulis, R., Murray, M., Payne, M. R., Thomas, A., & Salley, B. B. (2011). Sister circles as a culturally relevant intervention for anxious Black women. *Clinical Psychology: Science and Practice, 18*, 266–273.

Nelson, R. O., & Hayes, S. C. (1981). Theoretical explanations for reactivity in self-monitoring. *Behavior Modification, 5*, 3–14.

New Zealand Herald. (2010). *Drink-driver fails to learn from daughter's accident, say police*. Sunday, August 1. http://www.nzherald.co.nz/nz/news/article.cfm?c_id=1&objectid=10643874.

Nezu, A. M., Nezu, C. M., & D'Zurilla, T. J. (2007). *Solving life's problems: A 5-step guide to enhanced well-being*. New York: Springer.

Nicholson, L. M., Schwirian, K. P., & Schwirian, P. M. (2010). Childhood lead poisoning laws in New York City: Environment, politics and social action. *Children, Youth and Environments, 20*, 178–199.

O'Donnell, C. R., & Yamauchi, L. A. (Eds.) (2005). *Culture and context in human behavior change: Theory, research, and applications*. New York: Peter Lang.

Oishi, S., & Graham, J. (2010). Social ecology: Lost and found in psychological science. *Perspectives on Psychological Science, 5*, 356–377.

Okifuji, A., & Friedman, A. G. (1992). Experimentally induced taste aversion in humans: Effects of overshadowing on acquisition. *Behaviour Research and Therapy, 30*, 23–32.

Olfati-Saber, R. (2007, December). Evolutionary dynamics of behavior in social networks. *Proceedings of the 46th Institute of Electrical and Electronics Engineers Conference on Decision and Control*, New Orleans. Available at http://engineering.dartmouth.edu/~Reza_Olfati_Saber/papers/cdc07_evolution.pdf.

O'Leary, S. G., & Dubey, D. R. (1979). Applications of self-control procedures by children: A review. *Journal of Applied Behavior Analysis, 12*, 449–464.

Orbach, S. (2005). The psychotherapy relationship. In J. Ryan (Ed.), *How does psychotherapy work?* (pp. 69–84). London, UK: Karnac.

Oreg, S. (2003). Resistance to change: Developing an individual differences measure. *Journal of Applied Psychology, 88*, 680–693.

Oreg, S. (2006). Personality, context, and resistance to organizational change. *European Journal of Work and Organizational Psychology, 15*, 73–101.

Oreg, S., Bayazıt, M., Vakola, M., Arciniega, L., Armenakis, A., Barkauskiene, R., et al. (2008). Dispositional resistance to change: Measurement equivalence and the link to personal values across 17 nations. *Journal of Applied Psychology, 93*, 935–944.

Orelus, P. (2011). *Rethinking race, class, language, and gender*. Lanham, MD: Rowman & Littlefield.

Overton, W. F., & Horowitz, H. A. (1991). Developmental psychopathology: Integrations and differentiations. In D. Cicchetti & S. L. Toth (Eds.), *Rochester symposium on developmental psychopathology. Vol. 3: Models and integrations* (pp. 1–42). Rochester, NY: University of Rochester Press.

Patterson, G. R. (1974). Interventions for boys with conduct problems: Multiple settings, treatments, and criteria. *Journal of Consulting and Clinical Psychology, 42*, 471–481.

Patterson, G. R. (1982). *Coercive family process*. Eugene, OR: Castalia.

Paul, G. L., & Menditto, A. A. (1992). Effectiveness of inpatient treatment programs for mentally ill adults in public psychiatric facilities. *Applied & Preventive Psychology, 1*, 41–63.

Pavlov, I. P. (1927). *Conditioned reflexes*. Oxford, UK: Oxford University Press.

Pear, J. J., & Eldridge, G. D. (1984). The operant-respondent distinction: Future directions. *Journal of the Experimental Analysis of Behavior, 42*, 453–467.

Pechtel, P., Evans, I. M., & Podd, J. (2011). Conceptualization of the complex outcomes of sexual abuse: A signal detection analysis. *Journal of Child Sexual Abuse, 20*, 1–18.

Pennebaker, J. W. (2004). *Writing to heal: A guided journal for recovering from trauma and emotional upheaval*. Oakland, CA: New Harbinger.

Persons, J. B. (2008). *The case formulation approach to cognitive-behavior therapy*. New York: Guilford.

Pessin, S. (2010). Solomon Ibn Gabirol [Avicebron]. In E. N. Zalta (Ed.), *The Stanford Encyclopedia of Philosophy*. Available at http://plato.stanford.edu/archives/win2010/entries/ibn-gabirol/.

Pinel, E. C., & Constantino, M. J. (2003). Putting self psychology to good use: When social and clinical psychologists unite. *Journal of Psychotherapy Integration, 13*, 9–32.

Pogarsky, G., & Piquero, A. R. (2003). Can punishment encourage offending? Investigating the "resetting" effect. *Journal of Research in Crime and Delinquency, 40*, 95–120.

Price, M., & Anderson, P. L. (2011). Latent growth curve analysis of fear during a speech task before and after treatment for social phobia. *Behaviour Research and Therapy, 49*, 763–770.

Prizant, B. M., & Wetherby, A. M. (1998). Understanding the continuum of discrete trial traditional behavioral to social-pragmatic, developmental approaches in communication enhancement for young children with ASD. *Seminars in Speech and Language, 19*, 329–353.

Prochaska, J. O., & DiClemente, C. C. (1982). Transtheoretical therapy: Toward a more integrative model of change. *Psychotherapy: Theory, Research, and Practice, 19*, 276–288.

Prochaska, J. O., & DiClemente, C. C. (1983). Stages and processes of self-change of smoking: Toward an integrative model of change. *Journal of Consulting and Clinical Psychology, 51*, 390–395.

Pryor, T., & Wiederman, M. W. (1996). Measurement of nonclinical personality characteristics of women with anorexia nervosa or bulimia nervosa. *Journal of Personality Assessment, 67*, 414–421.

Puhl, R. M., & Heuer, C. A. (2010). Obesity stigma: Important considerations for public health. *American Journal of Public Health, 100*, 1019–1028.

Pyszczynski, T., Greenberg, J., Solomon, S., & Maxfield, M. (2006). On the unique psychological import of the human awareness of mortality: Theme and variations. *Psychological Inquiry, 17*, 328–356.

Rataemane, S. T., Rataemane, L. U. Z., & Mohlahle, J. S. (2002). Mass hysteria among learners at Mangaung schools in Bloemfontein, South Africa. *International Journal of Psychosocial Rehabilitation, 6,* 61–67.

Read, J., Mosher, L., & Bentall, R. (Eds.) (2005). *Models of madness: Psychological, social and biological approaches to schizophrenia.* New York: Brunner-Routledge.

Reisberg, D., & Hertel, P. (Eds.) (2004). *Emotion and memory.* Oxford, UK: Oxford University Press.

Reiss, S. (2004). Multifaceted nature of intrinsic motivation: The theory of 16 basic desires. *Review of General Psychology, 8,* 179–193.

Rescorla, R. A. (1988). Pavlovian conditioning: It's not what you think it is. *American Psychologist, 43,* 151–160.

Richeson, J. A., & Nussbaum, R. J. (2004). The impact of multiculturalism versus color-blindness on racial bias. *Journal of Experimental Social Psychology, 40,* 417–423.

Rittel, H., & Webber, M. (1973). Dilemmas in a general theory of planning. *Policy Sciences, 4,* 155–169.

Roelofs, K., Hagenaars, M. A., & Stins, J. (2010). Facing freeze: Social threat induces bodily freeze in humans. *Psychological Science, 21,* 1575–1581.

Roemer, L., & Borkovec, T. D. (1994). Effects of suppressing thoughts about emotional material. *Journal of Abnormal Psychology, 103,* 467–474.

Rogers, C. R. (1958). A process conception of psychotherapy. *American Psychologist, 13,* 142–149.

Rosales-Ruiz, J., & Baer, D. M. (1997). Behavioral cusps: A developmental and pragmatic concept for behavior analysis. *Journal of Applied Behavior Analysis, 30,* 533–544.

Rosen, G. M., Barrera, M., Jr., & Glasgow, R. E. (2008). Good intentions are not enough: Reflections on past and future efforts to advance self-help. In P. L. Watkins & G. A. Clum (Eds.), *Handbook of self-help therapies* (pp. 25–39). New York: Taylor & Francis/Routledge.

Rosen, G. M., & Davison, G. C. (2003). Psychology should list empirically supported principles of change (ESPs) and not credential trademarked therapies or other treatment packages. *Behavior Modification, 27,* 300–312.

Rosenbaum, M. (1990). A model for research on self-regulation: Reducing the schism between behaviorism and general psychology. In G. H. Eifert & I. M. Evans (Eds.), *Unifying behavior therapy: Contributions of paradigmatic behaviorism* (pp. 126–149). New York: Springer.

Rosenberg, T. (2011). *Join the club: How peer pressure can transform the world.* London, UK: Icon Books.

Rosenzweig, S. (1936). Some implicit common factors in diverse methods of psychotherapy: "At last the Dodo said, 'Everybody has won and all must have prizes.'" *American Journal of Orthopsychiatry, 6,* 412–415.

Rosner, R., Beutler, L. E., & Daldrup, R. J. (2000). Vicarious emotional experience and emotional expression in group psychotherapy. *Journal of Clinical Psychology, 56,* 1–10.

Ross, L. (1977). The intuitive psychologist and his shortcomings. In L. Berkowitz (Ed.), *Advances in experimental social psychology* (Vol. 10, pp. 173–220). San Diego, CA: Academic Press.

Rotter, J. B. (1954). *Social learning and clinical psychology.* New York: Prentice-Hall.

Rozin, P. (2003). Five potential principles for understanding cultural differences in relation to individual differences. *Journal of Research in Personality, 37,* 273–283.

Rozin, P., Kabnick, K., Pete, E., Fischler, C., & Shields, C. (2003). The ecology of eating: Smaller portion sizes in France than in the United States help explain the French paradox. *Psychological Science, 14,* 450–454.

Rutherford, G. D. (2003). A flow theory of behavioral dynamics. *Dynamical Psychology, 8,* Available at http://www.goertzel.org/dynapsyc/2003/flow.htm.

Rutter, M., & Rutter, M. (1993). *Developing minds: Challenge and continuity across the life span.* New York: Basic Books.

Safran, J. D., & Muran, J. C. (1996). The resolution of ruptures in the therapeutic alliance. *Journal of Consulting and Clinical Psychology, 64,* 447–458.

Saguy, A. C., & Gruys, J. (2010). Morality and health: News media constructions of overweight and eating disorders. *Social Problems, 57,* 231–250.

Salkovskis, P. M. (1996). The cognitive approach to anxiety: Threat beliefs, safety seeking behaviour, and the special case of health anxiety and obsessions. In P. M. Salkovskis (Ed.), *Frontiers of cognitive therapy* (pp. 48–74). New York: Guilford.

Salmon, K., Dadds, M. R., Allen, J., & Hawes, D. (2009). Can emotion language be taught during parent training for conduct problem children? *Child Psychiatry and Human Development, 40,* 485–498.

Salmon, K., Evans, I. M., Moskowitz, D., Parkes, F., & Miller, J. D. (2012). *The elements of young children's emotion knowledge. What are enhanced by adult talk?* Unpublished manuscript, School of Psychology, Victoria University of Wellington, New Zealand.

Salzinger, K. (2008). Waves and ripples. *The Behavior Therapist, 31,* 147–148.

Salzinger, K., & Pisoni, S. (1958). Reinforcement of affect responses of schizophrenics during the clinical interview. *Journal of Abnormal and Social Psychology, 57,* 84–90.

Sameroff, A. J. (1991). The social context of development. In M. Woodhead, R. Carr, & P. Light (Eds.), *Becoming a person* (pp. 167–189). Florence, KY: Taylor & Francis/Routledge.

Sanders, M. R. (1982). The generalization of parent responding to community settings: The effects of instructions, plus feedback, and self-management training. *Behavioural Psychotherapy, 10,* 273–287.

Sarason, S. B. (1974). *The psychological sense of community. Prospects for a community psychology.* San Francisco, CA: Jossey-Bass.

Schachter, S. (1968). Obesity and eating. *Science, 161,* 751–756.

Scotti, J. R., Evans, I. M., Meyer, L. H., & Walker, P. (1991). A meta-analysis of intervention research with problem behavior: Treatment validity and standards of practice. *American Journal on Mental Retardation, 96,* 233–256.

Segal, Z. V., Williams, J. M. G., & Teasdale, J. D. (2002). *Mindfulness-based cognitive therapy for depression: A new approach to preventing relapse.* New York: Guilford.

Seligman, L. D., Wuyek, L. A., Geers, A. L., Hovey, J. D., & Motley, R. L. (2009). The effects of inaccurate expectations on experiences with psychotherapy. *Cognitive Therapy and Research, 33,* 139–149.

Seligman, M. E. P. (1975). *Helplessness: On depression, development and death.* San Francisco, CA: W. H. Freeman.

Seligman, M. E. P. (2002). *Authentic happiness: Using the new positive psychology to realize your potential for lasting fulfillment.* New York: The Free Press.

Semple, K. (2010). The movie that made a Justice. *The New York Times,* Monday October 18, p. A23.

Serin, R. C., & Lloyd, C. D. (2009). Examining the process of offender change: The transition to crime desistance. *Psychology, Crime & Law, 15,* 347–364.

Shepperd, J. A., Ouellette, J. A., & Fernandez, J. K. (1996). Abandoning unrealistic optimism: Performance estimates and the temporal proximity of self-relevant feedback. *Journal of Personality and Social Psychology, 70,* 844–855.

Sherman, D. K., & Cohen, G. L. (2006). The psychology of self-defense: Self-affirmation theory. In M. P. Zanna (Ed.), *Advances in experimental social psychology* (Vol. 38, pp. 183–242). San Diego, CA: Academic Press.

Shirk, S. R., & Russell, R. L. (1996). *Change processes in child psychotherapy: Revitalizing treatment and research.* New York: Guilford.

Shure, M. B., & Spivack, G. (1982). Interpersonal problem-solving in young children: A cognitive approach to prevention. *American Journal of Community Psychology, 10,* 341–356.

Sidman, M. (1960). *Tactics of scientific research: Evaluating experimental data in psychology.* New York: Basic Books.

Sieverding, M., Decker, S., & Zimmerman, F. (2010). Information about low participation in cancer screening demotivates other people. *Psychological Science, 21,* 941–943.

Skinner, B. F. (1938). *The behavior of organisms: An experimental analysis.* New York: Appleton-Century.

Skinner, B. F. (1953). *Science and human behavior.* New York: Macmillan.

Skinner, B. F. (1958). Reinforcement today. *American Psychologist, 13*, 94–99.

Smetana, J. G. (2002). Culture, autonomy, and personal jurisdiction in adolescent-parent relationships. In H. W. Reese & R. Kail (Eds.), *Advances in child development and behavior* (Vol. 29, pp. 51–87). New York: Academic Press.

Smetana, J. G. (2011). *Adolescents, families, and social development: How teens construct their worlds.* New York: Wiley.

Smith, A. F., Jobe, J. B., & Mingay, D. J. (1991). Retrieval from memory of dietary information. *Applied Cognitive Psychology, 5,* 269–296.

Smith, E. R., & DeCoster, J. (2000). Dual-process models in social and cognitive psychology: Conceptual integration and links to underlying memory system. *Personality and Social Psychology Review, 4,* 108–131.

Smyth, T., & Dewar, T. (2009). *Raising the village: How individuals and communities can work together to give our children a stronger start in life.* Toronto, Canada: BPS Books.

Sobell, L. C., Sobell, M. B., Leo, G. I., Agrawal, S., Johnson-Young, L., & Cunningham, J. A. (2002). Promoting self-change with alcohol abusers: A community-level mail intervention based on natural recovery studies. *Alcoholism: Clinical and Experimental Research, 26,* 936–948.

Solano, L., Bonadies, M., & Di Trani, M. (2008). Writing for all, for some, or for no one? Some thoughts on the applications and evaluations of the writing technique. In A. J. J. M. Vingerhoets, I. Nyklicek, & J. Denollet (Eds.), *Emotion regulation: Conceptual and clinical issues* (pp. 234–246). New York: Springer.

Spagnola, M., & Fiese, B. H. (2007). Family routines and rituals: A context for development in the lives of young children. *Infants & Young Children, 20,* 284–299.

Spellerberg, A. (2001). *Framework for the measurement of social capital in New Zealand.* Wellington, NZ: Statistics New Zealand.

Spence, K. W. (1950). Cognitive versus stimulus-response theories of learning. *Psychological Review, 57,* 159–172.

Spirito, A., Simon, V., Cancilliere, M. K., Stein, R., Norcott, C., Loranger, K., & Prinstein, M. J. (2011). Outpatient psychotherapy practice with adolescents following psychiatric hospitalization for suicide ideation or a suicide attempt. *Clinical Child Psychology and Psychiatry, 16,* 53–64.

Staats, A. W. (1968). *Learning, language and cognition.* New York: Holt, Rinehart & Winston.

Staats, A. W. (1972). Language behavior therapy: A derivative of social behaviorism. *Behavior Therapy, 3,* 165–192.

Staats, A. W. (1975). *Social behaviorism.* Homewood, IL: Dorsey Press.

Staats, A. W. (1981). Social behaviorism, unified theory, unified theory construction methods, and the zeitgeist of separatism. *American Psychologist, 36,* 239–256.

Staats, A. W. (1990). Paradigmatic behavior therapy: A unified framework for theory, research, and practice. In G. H. Eifert & I. M. Evans (Eds.), *Unifying behavior therapy: Contributions of paradigmatic behaviorism* (pp. 14–54). New York: Springer.

Staats, A. W., & Hammond, O. R. (1972). Natural words as physiological conditioned stimuli: Food-word elicited salivation and deprivation effects. *Journal of Experimental Psychology, 96,* 206–208.

Stampfl, T. G., & Levis, D. J. (1976). Implosive therapy: A behavioral therapy. In J. T. Spence, R. C. Carson, & J. W. Thibaut (Eds.), *Behavioral approaches to therapy* (pp. 86–110). Morristown, NJ: General Learning Press.

Steel, P. (2007). The nature of procrastination: A meta-analytic and theoretical review of quintessential self-regulatory failure. *Psychological Bulletin, 133,* 65–94.

Steele, C. M. (1997). A threat in the air: How stereotypes shape intellectual identity and performance. *American Psychologist, 52,* 613–629.

Stern, D. N. (2004). *The present moment: In psychotherapy and everyday life.* New York: W. W. Norton.

Stiles, W. B., Elliott, R., Llewelyn, S. P., Firth-Cozens, J. A., Margison, F. R., Shapiro, D. A., & Hardy, G. (1990). Assimilation of problematic experiences by clients in psychotherapy. *Psychotherapy, 27,* 411–420.

Stokes, T. F., & Baer, D. M. (1977). An implicit technology of generalization. *Journal of Applied Behavior Analysis, 10,* 349–367.

Stott, R., Mansell, W., Salkovskis, P., Lavender, A., & Cartwright-Hatton, S. (2010). *Oxford guide to metaphors in CBT: Building cognitive bridges.* Oxford, UK: Oxford University Press.

Strack, F., & Deutsch, R. (2004). Reflective and impulsive determinants of social behavior. *Personality and Social Psychology Review, 8,* 220–247.

Stretesky, P., & Lynch, M. J. (2004). The relationship between lead and crime. *Journal of Health and Social Behavior, 45,* 213–229.

Stricker, G. (2010). A second look at psychotherapy integration. *Journal of Psychotherapy Integration, 20,* 397–405.

Strong, S. R., & Claiborn, C. D. (1982). *Change through interaction: Social psychological processes of counseling and psychotherapy.* New York: Wiley.

Strong, S. R., & Matross, R. P. (1973). Change processes in counseling and psychotherapy. *Journal of Counseling Psychology, 20,* 25–37.

Strupp, H. (1986). The nonspecific hypothesis of therapeutic effectiveness: A current assessment. *American Journal of Orthopsychiatry, 56,* 513–520.

Sue, S. (1998). In search of cultural competence in psychotherapy and counseling. *American Psychologist, 53,* 440–448.

Suls, J., Green, P., & Hillis, S. (1998). Emotional reactivity to everyday problems, affective inertia, and neuroticism. *Personality and Social Psychology Bulletin, 24,* 127–136.

Swann, W. B. (1984). Quest for accuracy in person perception: A matter of pragmatics. *Psychological Review, 91,* 457–477.

Tang, T. Z., & DeRubeis, R. J. (1999). Sudden gains and critical sessions in cognitive–behavioral therapy for depression. *Journal of Consulting and Clinical Psychology, 67,* 894–904.

Tannen, D. (1990). *You just don't understand.* New York: William Morrow & Company.

Taylor, J. E., & Harvey, S. T. (2009). Effects of psychotherapy with people who have been sexually assaulted: A meta-analysis. *Aggression and Violent Behavior, 14,* 273–285.

Taylor, J. G. (1963). A behavioural interpretation of obsessive-compulsive neurosis. *Behaviour Research and Therapy, 1,* 237–244.

Tchanturia, K., Davies, H., & Campbell, I. C. (2007). Cognitive remediation therapy for patients with anorexia nervosa: Preliminary findings. *Annals of General Psychiatry, 6,* doi: 10.1186/1744–859X-6-14.

Teasdale, J. D. (1999). Emotional processing, three modes of mind, and the prevention of relapse in depression. *Behaviour Research and Therapy, 37,* 53–77.

Tee, J., & Kazantzis, N. (2011). Collaborative empiricism in cognitive therapy: A definition and theory of the relationship construct. *Clinical Psychology: Science and Practice, 18,* 47–61.

Tharp, R. G., & Gallimore, R. (1988). *Rousing minds to life: Teaching, learning, and schooling in social context.* Cambridge, UK: Cambridge University Press.

Tharp, R. G., & Wetzel, R. J. (1969). *Behavior modification in the natural environment.* New York: Academic Press.

Thelen, E. (2005). Dynamic systems theory and the complexity of change. *Psychoanalytic Dialogues, 15,* 255–283.

Thomas, R., & Zimmer-Gembeck, M. J. (2007). Behavioral outcomes of Parent-Child Interaction Therapy and Triple P-Positive Parenting Program: A review and meta-analysis. *Journal of Abnormal Child Psychology, 35,* 475–495.

Thompson, R. A. (2001). Childhood anxiety disorders from the perspective of emotion regulation and attachment. In M. W. Vasey & M. R. Dadds (Eds.), *The developmental psychopathology of anxiety* (pp. 160–182). Oxford, UK: Oxford University Press.

Thorndike, E. L. (1898). Animal intelligence: An experimental study of the associative process in animals. *Psychological Review, Monograph Supplements, No. 8.*

Thorndike, E. L. (1932). *The fundamentals of learning.* New York: Teachers College, Columbia University.

Tinklepaugh, O. L. (1928). An experimental study of representative factors in monkeys. *Journal of Comparative Psychology, 8,* 197–236.

Todes, D. (2000). *Ivan Pavlov: Exploring the animal machine.* New York: Oxford University Press.

Tolman, E. C. (1932). *Purposive behavior in animals and men.* New York: Century.

Tomasello, M. (1999). *The cultural origins of human cognition.* Cambridge, MA: Harvard University Press.

Tsukayama, E., Toomey, S. L., Faith, M. S., & Duckworth, A. L. (2010). Self-control as a protective factor against overweight status in the transition from childhood to adolescence. *Archives of Pediatrics and Adolescent Medicine, 164,* 631–635.

Turkington, D., et al. (2009). *Back to life, back to normality: Recovery, cognitive therapy and psychosis.* Cambridge, UK: Cambridge University Press.

Turner, R. K., Young, G. C., & Rachman, S. (1970). Treatment of nocturnal enuresis by conditioning techniques. *Behaviour Research and Therapy, 8,* 367–381.

Tversky, A., & Kahneman, D. (1974). Judgment under uncertainty: Heuristics and biases. *Science, 185,* 1124–1131.

Tyrer, P., Duggan, C., Cooper, S., Crawford, M., Seivewright, H., Rutter, D., Maden, T., Byford, S., & Barrett, B. (2010). The successes and failures of the DSPD experiment: The assessment and management of severe personality disorder. *Medicine, Science and the Law, 50,* 95–99.

Ullrich, S., & Coid, J. (2011). Protective factors for violence among released prisoners—Effects over time and interactions with static risk. *Journal of Consulting and Clinical Psychology, 79,* 381–390.

Unger, W., Evans, I. M., Rourke, P., & Levis, D. J. (2003). The S-S construct of expectancy versus the S-R construct of fear: Which motivates the acquisition of avoidance behavior? *The Journal of General Psychology, 130,* 131–147.

Van Bergen, P., Salmon, K., Dadds, M. R., & Allen, J. (2009). Training mothers in emotion-rich elaborative reminiscing: Facilitating children's autobiographical memory and emotion knowledge. *Journal of Cognition and Development, 10,* 162–187.

Vancil, M. (Ed.) (2005). *Driven from within: Michael Jordan.* New York: Atria Books.

Van Houten, R., Axelrod, S., Bailey, J. S., Favell, J. E., Foxx, R. M., Iwata, B. A., & Lovaas, O. I. (1988). The right to effective behavioral treatment. *Journal of Applied Behavior Analysis, 21,* 381–384.

Vaughn, C. E., & Leff, J. P. (1976). The influence of family and social factors on the course of psychiatric illness: A comparison of schizophrenic and depressed neurotic patients. *British Journal of Psychiatry, 129,* 125–137.

Vasey, M. W., & Dadds, M. R. (2001). An introduction to the developmental psychopathology of anxiety. In M. W. Vasey & M. R. Dadds (Eds.), *The developmental psychopathology of anxiety* (pp. 3–26). Oxford, UK: Oxford University Press.

Vermeiren, R., Schwab-Stone, M., Deboutte, D., Leckman, P. E., & Ruchkin, V. (2005). Violence exposure and substance use in adolescents: Findings from three countries. *Pediatrics, 111,* 535–540.

Villegas, A. M. (1991). *Culturally responsive pedagogy for the 1990s and beyond* (Trends and Issues Paper No. 6). Washington, DC: ERIC Clearinghouse on Teacher Education.

Voeltz, L. M., & Evans, I. M. (1982). The assessment of behavioral interrelationships in child behavior therapy. *Behavioral Assessment, 4,* 131–165.

Voeltz, L. M., & Evans, I. M. (1983). Educational validity: Procedures to evaluate outcomes in programs for severely handicapped learners. *Journal of The Association for the Severely Handicapped, 8,* 3–15.

Vollmann, M., Scharloo, M., Salewski, C., Dienst, A., Schonauer, K., & Renner, B. (2010). Illness representations of depression and perceptions of the helpfulness of social support: Comparing depressed and never-depressed persons. *Journal of Affective Disorders, 125,* 213–220.

Wahler, R. G. (1980). The insular mother: Her problems in parent-child treatment. *Journal of Applied Behavior Analysis, 13,* 207–219.

Wahler, R. G., Winkel, G. H., Peterson, R. F., & Morrison, D. C. (1965). Mothers as behavior therapists for their own children. *Behaviour Research and Therapy, 3,* 113–124.

Wakefield, J. C. (2006). Is behaviorism becoming a pseudo-science? Power versus scientific rationality in the eclipse of token economies by biological psychiatry in the treatment of schizophrenia. *Behavior and Social Issues, 15,* 202–221.

Waldron, I., Hughes, M. E., & Brooks, T. L. (1996). Marriage protection and marriage selection—prospective evidence for reciprocal effects of marital status and health. *Social Science and Medicine, 43,* 113–123.

Walitzer, K. S., Dermen, K. H., & Connors, G. J. (1999). Strategies for preparing clients for treatment: A review. *Behavior Modification, 23,* 129–151.

Walsh, R. (2011). Lifestyle and mental health. *American Psychologist, 66,* 579–592.

Wampold, B. E. (2001). *The great psychotherapy debate: Models, methods, and findings.* New York: Routledge.

Ward, T., Mann, R. E., & Gannon, T. A. (2007). The good lives model of offender rehabilitation: Clinical implications. *Aggression and Violent Behavior, 12,* 87–107.

Ward, T., & Marshall, W. L. (2004). Good lives, aetiology and the rehabilitation of sex offenders: A bridging theory. *Journal of Sexual Aggression, 10,* 153–169.

Watkins, P. L., & Clum, G. A. (Eds.) (2008). *Handbook of self-help therapies.* New York: Taylor & Francis/Routledge.

Watson, D. L., & Tharp, R. G. (1977). *Self-directed behavior: Self-modification for personal adjustment.* Monterey, CA: Brooks/Cole.

Watson, J. B., & Rayner, R. (1920). Conditioned emotional reactions. *Journal of Experimental Psychology, 3,* 1–14.

Weersing, V. R., Weisz, J. R., & Donenberg, G. R. (2002). Development of the therapy procedures checklist: A therapist-report measure of technique use in child and adolescent treatment. *Journal of Clinical Child and Adolescent Psychology, 31,* 168–180.

Wegner, D. M. (1989). *White bears and other unwanted thoughts: Suppression, obsession, and the psychology of mental control.* New York: Viking/Penguin.

Weingarten, H. P. (1983). Conditioned cues elicit feeding in sated rats: A role for learning in meal initiation. *Science, 220*(4595), 431–433.

Weisner, T. S., Gallimore, R., & Jordan, C. (1988). Unpackaging cultural effects on classroom learning: Native Hawaiian peer assistance and child-generated activity. *Anthropology & Education Quarterly, 19,* 327–353.

Weiss, C. H. (1997). How can theory-based evaluation make greater headway? *Evaluation Review, 21,* 501–524.

Weisz, J., Weiss, B., Alicke, M., & Klotz, M. (1987). Effectiveness of psychotherapy with children and adolescents: A meta-analysis for clinicians. *Journal of Consulting and Clinical Psychology, 55,* 542–549.

Weisz, J. R., Ugueto, A. M., Herren, J., Afienko, S. R., & Rutt, C. (2011). Kernels vs. ears, and other questions for a science of treatment dissemination. *Clinical Psychology: Science and Practice, 18,* 41–46.

Weld, E. M., & Evans, I. M. (1990). Effects of part versus whole instructional strategies on skill acquisition and excess behavior. *American Journal on Mental Retardation, 94,* 377–386.

Wells, A. (1999). A metacognitive model and therapy for generalized anxiety disorder. *Behavioural and Cognitive Psychotherapy, 23,* 301–320.

White, O. (2005). Trend lines. In G. Sugai & R. Horner (Eds.), *Encyclopedia of behavior modification and cognitive behavior therapy, Volume 3: Educational applications.* Thousand Oaks, CA: Sage.

Whitelaw, S., Baldwin, S., Bunton, R., & Flynn, D. (2000). The status of evidence and outcomes in Stages of Change research. *Health Education Research: Theory and Practice, 15,* 707–718.

Wilson, F. E., & Evans, I. M. (1983). The reliability of target behavior selection in behavioral assessment. *Behavioral Assessment, 5,* 33–54.

Wilson, G. T., & Evans, I. M. (1977). The therapist-client relationship in behavior therapy. In A. S. Gurman & A. M. Razin (Eds.), *The therapist's contribution to effective psychotherapy: An empirical approach* (pp. 544–565). New York: Pergamon.

Wilson, G. T., Fairburn, C. C., Agras, W. S., Walsh, B. T., & Kraemer, H. (2002). Cognitive-behavioral therapy for bulimia nervosa: Time course and mechanisms of change. *Journal of Consulting and Clinical Psychology, 70,* 267–274.

Wilson, G. T., Hannon, A. E., & Evans, I. M. (1968). Behavior therapy and the therapist-patient relationship. *Journal of Consulting and Clinical Psychology, 32,* 103–109.

Wilson, G. T., & Vitousek, K. (1999). Self-monitoring in the assessment and treatment of eating disorders. *Psychological Assessment, 11,* 480–489.

Wilson, N., & Evans, I. M. (2002). Relationship between reward-dominant response style and ratings of boys' conduct problems. *New Zealand Journal of Psychology, 31,* 59–64.

Winett, R. A., & Winkler, R. C. (1972). Current behavior modification in the classroom: Be still, be quiet, be docile. *Journal of Applied Behavior Analysis, 5,* 499–504.

Wolpe, J. (1958). *Psychotherapy by reciprocal inhibition.* Palo Alto, CA: Stanford University Press.

Wonderlich-Tierney, A. L., & Vander Wal, J. S. (2010). The effects of social support and coping on the relationship between social anxiety and eating disorder symptomatology. *Eating Behaviors, 11,* 85–91.

Wittgenstein, L. (1980). *Culture and value.* (Translated by P. Winch.) Oxford, UK: Blackwell.

Wright, C. (1992). *Race relations in the primary school.* London, UK: David Fulton.

Wykes, T., Reeder, C., Landau, S., Everitt, B., Knapp, M., Patel, A., & Romeo, R. (2007). Cognitive remediation therapy in schizophrenia: Randomised controlled trial. *British Journal of Psychiatry, 190,* 421–427.

Young, J. E. (1999). *Cognitive therapy for personality disorders: A schema-focused approach* (rev. ed.). Sarasota, FL: Professional Resource Press.

Young, M. A., Meaden, P. M., Fogg, L. F., Cherin, E. A., & Eastman, C. I. (1997). Which environmental variables are related to the onset of seasonal affective disorder? *Journal of Abnormal Psychology, 106,* 554–562.

Zajonc, R. B. (1980). Feeling and thinking: Preferences need no inferences. *American Psychologist, 35,* 151–175.

Zentall, T. R. (2010). Justification of effort by humans and pigeons: Cognitive dissonance or contrast? *Psychological Science, 19,* 296–300.

Zettle, R. D. (2011). The evolution of a contextual approach to therapy: From comprehensive distancing to ACT. *The International Journal of Behavioral Consultation and Therapy, 7,* 78–84.

Zimring, F. E., & Hawkins, G. J. (1973). *Deterrence: The legal threat in crime control.* Chicago, IL: University of Chicago Press.

Zinbarg, R. E. (1998). Concordance and synchrony in measures of anxiety and panic reconsidered: A hierarchical model of anxiety and panic. *Behavior Therapy, 29,* 301–323.

Zuroff, D. C., & Blatt, S. J. (2002). Vicissitudes of life after the short-term treatment of depression: Roles of stress, social support, and personality. *Journal of Social and Clinical Psychology, 21,* 473–496.

INDEX

ABA. *See* applied behavior analysis
acceptance, 21–22, 170, 177, 213–14
Acceptance and Commitment Therapy (ACT), 146, 152, 163, 172, 175
active avoidance learning, 106–9
active coping strategies, 181
activities, 237, 238
activity settings, 237–39
actor-observer bias, 88
addictions, behaviors as, 57
ADHD. *See* attention deficit hyperactivity disorder
adolescents
  anxiety of, 263
  behavior of, 133
  parents' conflict with, 78
  parents' harmony with, 217
  skills of, 133
  treatments, 12
afferent input, 159
Aggression Replacement Training, 75
agoraphobia, 256–68
Ajzen, I., 59, 157
Albee, George, 198
alcoholism, 42, 228
anger, 196
animals, electric shock applied to, 106–7
Annon, Jack, 2
anorexia nervosa, 81, 192, 219
anxiety, 47–48
  of adolescents, 263
  behaviors influencing, 151
  images influencing, 169–70
  learning extinguishing, 108
  manifestations of, 139–40, 154–55
  parents influencing, 221
  social support influencing, 221
  treatment of, 152
  worry influencing, 86
anxiety sensitivity, 81, 103, 107
applied behavior analysis (ABA), 9

approach, 98–99
approach-avoidance conflict, 75
A-R-D Stimulus. *See* Attitude-Reinforcement-Discriminative Stimulus
aspiration, 70–71, 71*t*
attention deficit hyperactivity disorder (ADHD), 6–7
Attitude-Reinforcement-Discriminative Stimulus, 123
autism, 18, 143, 206–7, 256, 257–58
automatic processes, 158
automatic thoughts, 125, 159
autoshaping, 126–27
aversives controversy, 130–32
avoidance, 98–99, 106–7, 129
Baer, Don, 15

Bandura, Albert
  on change, 57
  human agency articulated by, 161
  modeling considered by, 233
  self-efficacy and, 59–60, 79, 80, 257
  studies of, 230–31
BAS. *See* Behavioral Activation System
Beck, A. T., 159, 162, 163, 165–66, 177
bedwetting, 44, 45, 186
Behavioral Activation System (BAS), 84–85, 86
behavioral assessment, 49
Behavioral Inhibition System (BIS), 84, 85, 86, 139–40
behavioral psychology, change and, 5–7
behavioral regularities, 226
behaviorism, 13
behaviors. *See also* response
  activity settings influencing, 237–38
  as addictions, 57
  of adolescents, 133
  agency changing understanding of, 259
  agents changing, 212
  aggressive, 140–41
  anxiety influenced by, 151

behaviors (*cont.*)
  behaviors influenced by, 138, 181
  beliefs, 59
  caregivers influencing, 215
  causes of, 62–63
  chains of, 142–43, 183
  challenging, 62, 63, 93–94, 130–32, 252–53
  change at cost of, 34
  changing, 41–42, 56–57, 62–63, 99, 144
  cognitive therapy influencing, 177
  communication skill as alternative to, 63
  consequences influencing, 115, 116–17
  context influencing, 87, 120, 123–24
  contingencies influencing, 134
  criminal, 71–72, 207
  cultures and abnormal, 241–42
  cultures influencing, 235, 241
  cusp, 143–44
  desires driving, 71
  dreams influencing, 66–67
  emotion influencing, 148
  enabling, 180, 226
  environments controlled by, 100, 131
  environments influencing, 89–90, 91, 185–86
  experiences shaping, 268
  familiarity of, 119
  feelings influencing, 107, 150
  feelings reduced by, 150
  as functional, 61, 62–63, 134–35, 137, 142
  incompatible, 147–49
  inner speech controlling, 164, 165
  keystone, 143, 144
  learning interfered with by, 256–57
  meaningful, 148
  memories influencing, 167–68
  modeling influencing patterns of, 231
  motivation influencing, 72
  motivation sustaining, 53–54
  needs met by, 63
  negative, 62, 63
  negative reinforcement influencing, 107
  parents influencing, 215–16
  punishment influencing, 39, 115, 127, 128–29
  reinforcement of, 127–28
  relationships of, 142–43, 256–57, 264–65
  in response class, 141–42
  as response sequences, 149
  rewards for, 79–80, 115–16
  rewards influencing, 115, 119–20
  safety-seeking, 103–4, 150–51, 235
  self different from, 180
  situations influencing, 92–94
  social networks influencing, 231–32
  species-specific, 117–18
  stimuli influencing, 37, 42–43, 92, 123
  stimuli produced by, 124
  study, 116
  targeted, 87
  therapeutic alliance shaping, 203–4, 206

  therapists, 190
  therapy, 14, 206, 258–59
  treatment influenced by, 138
  variation in, 122
  words regarding, 115–16
behavior theory, 13
beliefs, 59–60, 79, 161, 236
biases, 161, 167
Big Five personality model, 82
Bijou, S., 144
binge drinking, 226–27
BIS. *See* Behavioral Inhibition System
blame, 77, 217, 218, 219
Bootzin, Richard, 45, 187
Borderline Personality Disorder (BPD), 168
BPD. *See* Borderline Personality Disorder
bracing, 68
Brehm, Jack, 77–79
Brehm, Sharon, 77–79
Bronfenbrenner, Urie, 95, 264
Burke, Edmund, 187–88

caregivers, 213–14, 215
Carla (client), 53–54
catharsis, 26
CBT. *See* cognitive-behavioral therapy
change. *See also* motivation; self-change
  acceptance's dialectic with, 21–22
  of activities, 238
  barriers to, 75–76
  behavioral, 41–42, 56–57, 62–63, 99, 144
  at behavioral cost, 34
  behavioral psychology and, 5–7
  causes and, 17–19
  causes of, ix
  as challenge, 251
  client's role in, 258–59
  clients seeking, 266–67
  clients' trouble with, 55, 57, 73–74
  clients undergoing, 69
  clinical significance of, 30
  cognitive therapies creating principles of, 176–77
  commitments to, 209
  competence and, 45–47
  content and, 262–63
  context and, 262, 263
  cultural groups influenced by, 228
  in cultures, 246
  defining, 153–54
  dispositional resistance to, 81–82
  effect size of, 29–30
  environment influencing, 250
  failure to, 260
  features of, 28–30
  of feelings, 112
  as harm reduction, 27
  identifying, 30
  measurement determining, 32, 33, 44–45,

47–48, 191
metaphor for, 253–54
methods of, 2
model of, 250, 265
motivation to, 53–54
nature of, 50–51
permanence of, 33–35
personality as target of, 153
pivotal skills leading to, 144–45
planful, 18–19, 70, 164–65
planning focusing, 149
positive psychology applied to, 171
principles of, xi–xii, xiii, 3–4, 250–51, 257–58, 265–68
professionals writing on, xii
psychology and, xi–xii
psychotherapy and, x–xi, 2, 5, 7, 19–20, 23, 264
public's understanding of, 2–3
questions regarding, 33–34
reasons for, 1–2, 14–15
relapses integral in process of, 44
of relationships, 201
research determining, 32
as response class, 63–64
rewards for, 64
societies undergoing, x, 55
stages of, 56–57
statistical significance of, 29–30
syndromes revealing, 17
target behavior selection and, 29
theory of, 255
therapists influencing, 14, 64, 263, 267
therapists on, 4
of thought experiencing, 168
treatment objectives met by, 33
in treatments, 250
types of, 28
unified theory of, 3
value judgments and, 32–33
variables influencing, 16–17, 267–68
variants accommodated by, xi
change agents, 36
childhood aggression, 140–41, 159
Christakis, N. A., 229, 231–33
classical conditioning, 99, 103–4, 107–8, 111, 112
clients, xi. *See also* therapeutic alliance
as agents, 94
change presenting trouble for, 55, 57, 73–74
change role of, 258–59
change sought by, 266–67
changing, 69
in comfort zone, 244–45
criterion reference for, 30–31
effect size model used by, 31–32
expectations of, 208
feedback needed by, 204
mediator's relationship with, 213
memory escape of, 111
motivation of, 53

problem solving and, 146
in psychotherapy, 210–12
psychotherapy benefiting, 13, 26, 97–98, 219–20
psychotherapy sought by, 7–8, 14–16
punishment benefiting, 129
rewards focused on by, 188
role of, 207, 208
as scientists, 182–83
self-change practiced by, 182, 187
social networks pressuring, 222
therapists and relationships of, 214–15
therapists asked for advice by, 78–79
therapists assessing, 211–12
therapists confronting, 76–77
therapists influencing changes of, 81–82
therapists influencing tasks of, 93–94
therapists interacting with, 202–3
therapists measuring satisfaction of, 49
therapists on future of, 181–82
therapist's relationship with, 5, 7–8, 13, 21, 58, 76, 79, 201
therapists setting goals for, 65–66
therapists shaping, 204
treatment ability of, 11–12
well-being of, 50
clinical change, xi
Clum, G. A., 198–99
cocaine, 120–21
coercive trap, 127–28
cognitions, 155, 157–58, 159, 162–64, 167–68
cognitive-behavioral therapy (CBT), 3, 171
for depression, 193
evolution of, 8–9
for hand-washing, 148–49
history of, 11
problem solving in, 145
self-recording in, 193
therapists, 211–12
cognitive dissonance, 119, 187–88
cognitive flexibility, 82–83
cognitive processing, 159
cognitive-processing therapy, 167
cognitive remediation therapy, 83
cognitive restructuring, 125
cognitive rigidity, 83
cognitive skills, 157
cognitive therapy, 158, 161–63, 165–66, 176–77, 210
cognitive triad, 166
collaborative empiricism, 166
collateral effects, 137–38
color blindness, 243
comfort zone, 244–45
communication, 63, 154, 174, 175, 236–37
competence, 45–47
conditioned response (CR), 103
conditioned stimulus (CS), 100, 101, 102–3, 104
conditioned suppression, 127

conditioning, basic, 106
conscience, punishment developing, 128
consequences, behavior influenced by, 115, 116–17
constructivist theory, 94, 260
content, 163–64, 262–63
contexts
   behavior influenced by, 87, 120, 123–24
   change and, 262, 263
   in clinical work, 257
   personality intertwined with, 87–88
   therapists considering, 257
contingencies
   behavior influenced by, 134
   in learning situations, 123
   relationships specifying, 120
   response cost, 121
   response influenced by, 117, 118
   rules, 141
controlled processing, 158
coping, 107
   active strategies for, 181
   emotion-focused, 146
   problem-focused, 146
   as self-change, 196–98
   social support matching, 221
   strategies, 196–98
core self-evaluations, 80
correspondence bias, 88–89
counterconditioning, valence influenced by, 105–6
covert punishment, 43, 173
covert sensitization, 43, 172–73
CR. *See* conditioned response
credulous-skeptical continuum, 7
crime
   behavior of, 71–72, 207
   environments influencing, 89–90
   rewards influencing, 41
   violent, 40
   youth, 19
criterion reference, 30–31
CS. *See* conditioned stimulus
cueing, 199, 200
cultural competence, 242
culturally responsive pedagogy, 243
culturally responsive therapy, 243–47
cultures
   behavior, abnormal, and, 241–42
   behavioral, 226–27
   behavior influenced by, 235, 241
   challenged, 246–47
   change in, 246
   description of, 225–26
   Eastern, 254–55
   environments and, 248
   of family, 225
   groups, 227–29, 237
   identity in, 247–48
   personality styles valued by, 229
   psychotherapy influenced by, 245, 247
   psychotherapy recognizing importance of, 242
   scientific method shaped by, 245
   shock, 229
   smoking influenced by, 229
   therapeutic alliance influenced by, 242
   Western, 254, 255
cutting, 128

daydreaming, 158
decentering, 168
delay of gratification, 195
depression
   CBT for, 193
   information processing influencing, 163–64
   possible selves influencing, 68
   social networks influencing, 227–28
   social support influencing, 221, 228
   thoughts influencing, 163
   treating, 177
depression spike, 50
desires, 71, 192
desistance, 41–42
deterioration effect, 32
Diagnostic and Statistical Manual of Mental Disorders, 7
DiClemente, C. C., 56–57, 189
discrimination, 92
dispositional resistance to change, 81–82
dissociation, 158
distress, 161, 170, 197
Dodge, K. A., 159
dogs, 97, 100
dreams, behavior influenced by, 66–67
drive theory, 54–55
driving, 142
drunk driving, 2–3
Durand, V. Mark, 62, 63, 142
dynamic predictors, 40
Dynamic Social Impact Theory, 236–37
D'Zurilla, T. J., 145

eating, 90, 141
effect size, clients using model of, 31–32
efferent output, 159
effort, rewards influenced by, 119
Eifert, G. H., 4, 10, 140
electric shock, 106–7
Ellis, Albert, 162–63, 166, 223
emotion. *See also* feelings
   approach yielding, 99
   avoidance yielding, 99
   behavior influenced by, 148
   cognition influencing, 155
   control, 111
   as functional, 61–62
   images regulating, 197
   manifestations of, 139–40, 154–55

Index

memories, 109–11
physiological expressions of, 183
in psychotherapy, 212
punishment generating, 128–29
self-regulation of, 181
in stimuli, 112–13
emotional contagion, 232–34
emotional inertia, 74
emotional intelligence, 82
emotion talk, 4–5
empathy, 233
enabling behaviors, 180, 226
engagement as motivational variable, 203
enuresis. *See* bedwetting
environments
 behavior influenced by, 89–90, 91, 185–86
 behaviors controlling, 100, 131
 change influenced by, 250
 classroom, 91
 crime influenced by, 89–90
 cultures and, 248
 deficit, 91
 eating influenced by, 90
 fantasies regulated by, 169
 reactance influenced by, 93
 thoughts regulated by, 169
 threats from, 150–51
equifinality, 4
ethics in treatment, 131–32
etic position, 246
evaluative conditioning, 104–5
executive functions, 193, 195–96
expectations, 99
experiences, 110, 121, 158, 263–64, 268
experiential avoidance, 74, 107, 151, 172, 206
experimental neurosis, 97
expressed emotion, 221–22
extinction, 36–37
 avoidance influencing, 106–7
 of fear, 108
 of habits, 186
 memories influencing, 110
 to stimuli, 38
 stimuli causing, 102
Eysenck, Hans, 10, 32, 84, 103
Eysenck/Gray theory, 84–86

familiarity, 119
family, culture of, 225
fantasies, environment regulating, 169
fear, 86. *See also* anxiety; phobias
 avoidance and, 106
 classical conditioning of, 103–4, 107–8
 CS eliciting, 102–3
 extinguishing of, 108
 of fear, 103, 109
 of flying, 109
 information influencing, 161
 phases of, 48

punishment eliciting, 128
stimuli evoking, 104
stimuli generalized to by, 38
feedback, 199–200, 204
feelings, 107, 112, 150, 158, 160
FFFS. *See* Flight-Fight-Freeze System
five Cs, 247
flexibility, 82–83
Flight-Fight system, 85
Flight-Fight-Freeze System (FFFS), 85, 86
follow-up assessments, 29, 34, 35
Fonagy, P., 168
Forbes, D. L., 70–71
Fowler, J. H., 229, 231–33
frame, 120
Frankl, Victor, 170
freedom, 77–78
Freud, Sigmund, xiii, 26, 209–10, 262
functional analytic psychotherapy, 211–12
fundamental attribution error, 88–89
Gallimore, R., 237, 238

general case instruction, 38
generalization, 35, 37–39, 149–50
Gibson, James, 74
Gilbert, D. T., 88–89
global brake, 194
Gloria (client), 20–21
goals
 activity settings influenced by, 238
 life, 8, 64–65
 measurable, 65
 of psychotherapy, 7–8, 15, 20–21, 31
 in self-change, 184–85
 self-recording defining, 191
 setting, 65–66, 184–85
goal theories, 54–55
Goldfried, Marvin, 4, 145
Goldiamond, Israel, 58–59
Good Lives Model, 71–72, 207
Gray, Jeffrey, 84–85
group therapy, 222–23
Guerin, B., 26, 222, 226, 236
guilt, 128, 167
Guthrie, E. R., 124, 159

habilitation, 28
habits, 124, 125, 186
habits of the mind, 97–98
habit strength, 141–42
hand-washing, compulsive, 148–49
harm reduction, change as, 27
Hawkins, Robert, 29
Hayes, S. C., 82, 176–77
Health Belief Model, 60
Heath, Chip, 253–54
Heath, Dan, 253–54
hindsight bias, 167
homeostatic control, 183

homework, 124–25, 166
Hull, Clark, 104, 118
human agency, 161

"I Can Problem Solve" protocol, 147
images, 169–70, 172–74, 197
imaginary game, 61–62
imitation, 231, 234
implicit attitudes, 242
impulsive system, 193
impulsivity, 85, 86–87, 151–52
increased incentive salience, 101–2
incubation, 103, 109
individual difference variables, 90–91
industriousness, reinforcement promoting, 133–34
information, 60, 161, 163–64, 165, 167
informed consent, 131
inhibition, 193–96
inner speech, 164, 165
innovation, 238
insomnia, 187
instrumental conditioning, 99, 133
intentions, 189
interventions. *See* treatments
introspection, 158
Introverts (Eysenck's theory), 84
itching, 233–34

Jacobson, N. S., 177
James, William, 124
Jones, Mary Cover, 102
Jordan, Michael, 54–55
Joshua (client), 45–47

Karoly, P., 23, 25, 66
Kazdin, Alan, x
Kendall, P. C., 4, 194–95
kernels, 13–14
kindling effect, 35
King, Martin Luther, Jr., 157
Kohlenberg, R. J., 211–12
Kohn, A., 121–22
Krasner, L., 7
Kubany, E. S., 167
language, 174, 234–37

lapses, 42
Law of Effect, 123, 125
Law of Exercise, 123–25, 124
Lazarus, R. S., 146
learned helplessness, 80
learned resourcefulness, 199
learning, 97–98. *See also* active avoidance learning
  anxiety extinguished by, 108
  behaviors interfering with, 256–57
  contingencies in situations of, 123
  definition of, 116

to learn, 145
modeling as, 230–31
situations, 123
skills, 116
learning curve, 116
lever pressing, 116–17
Levis, D. J., 110, 112, 150
Lewin, Kurt, 95, 264
Linehan, Marsha, 21, 176, 211
low behavior potential, 79–80

Mahoney, Michael, 182, 259, 260
maintenance, 35–37
Marks, Isaac, 252
marriage, 143
Maudsley approach, 219
McGraw, Myrtle, 47
McNaughton, Neil, 85–86, 152
meaning making, 161
measuring
  change determined by, 32, 33, 44–45, 47–48, 191
  goals, 65
  human performance, 48
  probability, 116
mediators, xi, 194, 201, 212–13
meditation, 171–72
Meichenbaum, D. J., 164, 194
memories
  behavior influenced by, 167–68
  clients escaping, 111
  in cognitive therapy, 210
  CS and, 104
  emotional, 109–11
  episodic, 109
  extinction influenced by, 110
  of situations, 109–10
  in therapeutic alliance, 210
  unconscious, 210
  working, 172, 196
mental illness, stigma of, 221
mental images. *See* images
meta-cognition, 164
metaphors, 174–75, 253–54
meta-worry, 108–9
methodological individualism, x
Meyer, L. H. (Voeltz), 137-138, 239
Miller, N. E., 75, 106–7, 150
Miller, S. D., 19
mindfulness, 171, 176–77
mindfulness training, 12, 168, 172, 186–87
miracle question, 66–67
Mischel, Walter
  hot cognitions and, 163
  personality and, 87, 88
  planning and, 184
  reward and, 188
  self-control and, 195

self-regulation and, 184
modeling, 143, 230–31, 232–34
mood disorders, 35
moral reasoning, 75
motivation
 behavior influenced by, 72
 behavior sustained by, 53–54
 to change, 53–54
 of clients, 53
 engagement as variable of, 203
 planful change as, 70
 psychotherapy influenced by, 53
 rewards as, 121, 189
motivational interviewing, 57–59
Mowrer, O. H., 106–7, 150
multifinality, 4

needle distress, 161
needs, behavior meeting, 63
negative reinforcement, 106, 107, 127
Nelson-Gray, Rosemery, 191, 193
Neuroticism (Eysenck's theory), 84
New Zealand, 185, 235, 240–41, 243–44
Nezu, Arthur, 145–46, 157, 200
noncompliance, 76

obesity, 6, 7
obsessive-compulsive disorder (OCD), 16
operant response, 48
organisms, biologically prepared, 105
overshadowing, 101

pain, self-inflicted, 128
panic, sensations prior to, 111
paradoxical intention, 170
parents
 adolescents' conflict with, 78
 adolescents' harmony with, 217
 anxiety influenced by, 221
 behaviors influenced by, 215–16
 blaming, 217, 218, 219
 therapist's similarity to, 224
 training, 42, 215–19
partial reinforcement effect (PRE), 36
patients, deinstitutionalization of, 12–13
Patterson, Gerald, 127
Pavlov, Ivan, 97, 100, 164
Pavlovian conditioning. *See* classical
 conditioning
PBS. *See* positive behavior support
personalities
 attractor sensitivity reflected by, 86
 as change target, 153
 context intertwined with, 87–88
 cultures valuing, 229
 deficit repertoires of, 91
 dimensions, 84
 disorders, 74–75, 153
 fixed aspects of, 87

repulsor sensitivity reflected by, 86
 resetting, 152
 as response classes, 151–52
 treatments changing, 152–53
phobias, 102
pigeons, 117
pivotal skills, 143, 144–45, 147
planning, 149–50
plasticity, 83
play therapy, 207
pleasure, 118–19, 121, 170–71
positive behavior support (PBS), 9
positive psychology, 171, 263
positivity strivings, 90
possible selves, 67–70
PRE. *See* partial reinforcement effect
prechange-postchange model, 32
precision teaching, 190
predictors, 40
prisoners, 39–41
probability, 115–16, 126
problem-focused paradigm, 7
problem solving, 145–47, 157
processes, 159, 163–64
processing, 110–11
process studies, 1
Prochaska, J. O., 56–57, 189
procrastination, 189–90
psychological flexibility, 82
psychology, xi–xii, 10, 171, 260–61, 263
psychopathology, treatments influenced by,
 16–17
psychopathy, 153
psychotherapy. *See also* clients; therapists;
 treatments
 change and, x–xi, 2, 5, 7, 19–20, 23, 264
 clients benefiting from, 13, 26, 97–98,
 219–20
 clients in, 210–12
 clients seeking, 7–8, 14–16
 cultural groups influencing, 237
 culture influencing, 245, 247
 culture's importance recognized by, 242
 description of, 25–26, 204, 210–11
 effectiveness of, 1
 emotion in, 212
 as emotion talk, 4–5
 experiences interacting with, 110
 features of, 20
 goals of, 7–8, 15, 20–21, 31
 as limited resource, 198
 mediators managing, 212–13
 metaphorical language used in, 174
 motivation influencing, 53
 outcomes of, 25–26
 paradoxical intention in, 170
 perception of, 208
 schools of, xiii, 3, 251
 scientific method in, 182–83

psychotherapy (*cont.*)
  skills in, 132
  as social influence process, 207–8
  stimuli and, 37–38
  techniques, 12
  therapists and, 10–11, 205
  verbal, 259
  women's liberation promoted in, 228
public, change understood by, 2–3
public policy, 22, 23
Punished by Rewards (Kohn), 121–22
punishment
  agent of, 128
  avoidance's similarities to, 129
  behavior influenced by, 39, 115, 127, 128–29
  challenging behavior and, 130–32
  in classroom, 218
  clients benefiting from, 129
  conscience developed by, 128
  corporal, 129
  covert, 43, 173
  as discriminative stimulus, 126
  emotions generated by, 128–29
  fear elicited by, 128
  probability influenced by, 126
  response elicited by, 126
  response influenced by, 125–26
  results of, 129
  in treatment, 129–32

rational-emotive therapy (RET), 162–63
rats, 116–17
Rayner, Rosalie, 102
reactance, 77–79, 93
reactive outcomes, 153–54
reading, 134
rebound effect, 170
recovery, 14, 26–27, 28, 36–37
reflective system, 193
reinforcement, 118, 127–28, 133–34, 256. *See also* negative reinforcement; rewards
reinforcement expectancy, 79
reinforcement sensitivity, 85
Reiss, Steven, 71
relapse prevention, 42–44
relapses, 34–35, 42, 43
Relational Frame Theory, 120
relationships
  avoiding, 153
  of behaviors, 142–43, 256–57, 264–65
  changing, 201
  in cognitive therapy, 210
  conditional, 120
  contingencies specified by, 120
  if A, then B, 120
  language sustaining, 236
  parenting, 209–10, 215, 216
  response, 138–39, 141–42
  social, 236

  social-emotional, 153
  therapeutic alliance as attachment, 206
Rescorla, R. A., 101
research
  change determined by, 32
  studies, 31
resistance, 76–77, 260
response
  behavior as sequences of, 149
  cognitions and, 159
  contingencies influencing, 117, 118
  continuum of, 159–60
  disproportionate, 161
  personalities as classes of, 151–52
  punishment eliciting, 126
  punishment influencing, 125–26
  rate of, 117
  relationships, 138–39, 141–42
  reward eliciting, 126
  stimuli influencing, 125–26
response class, 141–42
response generalization, 38
response latency, 116
restraint, description of, 194
RET. *See* rational-emotive therapy
rewards. *See also* self-reward
  behavior influenced by, 115, 119–20
  for behaviors, 79–80, 115–16
  for change, 64
  in classroom, 121
  clients focusing on, 188
  conditioned, 122–23
  crime influenced by, 41
  deserved, 188
  desires satisfied by, 192
  dominance, 85
  effort influencing, 119
  extrinsic, 121
  immediacy of, 122, 195
  intrinsic, 121
  as motivation, 121, 189
  pleasure of, 118–19
  program, 188–89
  response elicited by, 126
  secondary, 122–23
  self-recording of progress as, 191
  Skinner on, 115
  spontaneous, 120
  stimuli predicting, 123
  treatment influencing, 36
  in treatment programs, 120–21, 261–62
rituals, 239–40
Robinson, Craig, 258–59
Rogers, Carl, 13
role playing, skills taught by, 173–74
Rosenbaum, M., 199
Ross, Lee, 88
Rotter, J. B., 79
routines, 239, 240

rule-governed behavior, 120
rules, 120, 141
ruminating, 158
Rutherford, G. D., 254–55
Rutter, M., 28

savoring, 170–71
scarring effect, 35
Schachter, S., 81
schema, 163, 173
school dropouts, 255
school phobia, 100
scientific method, 182–83, 245
Seasonal Affective Disorder, 90
second signal system, 164
self, behavior different from, 180
self-change
    active coping strategies as, 181
    clients practicing, 182, 187
    contracts in, 185
    coping strategies as, 196–98
    description of, 179–80
    goals in, 184–85
    principles of, 183, 184
    scientific method in, 182–83
    self-recording influencing, 190–93
    self-reward influencing, 187–89
    stimuli influencing, 185–87
    therapists promoting, 181–83
self-control, 180–81, 195, 254
self-control strategy, 43
self-efficacy, 59–60, 79, 80, 257
self-help, 14, 183–84, 198–99
self-influence, 180
self-modification. *See* self-change
self-monitoring. *See* self-recording
self-recording, 190–93
self-report, 49–50, 190
self-reward, 187–89
self-support, 254
self-talk, 194–95
Seligman, Martin, 80, 150, 176
sensations, 111–12
sexual abuse, 26
sexual arousal, 155
Shure, M. B., 147
Sidman, M., 33
sister circle, 222–23
situations, 92–94, 109–10, 123, 197. *See also* stimuli
skills. *See also* pivotal skills
    of adolescents, 133
    alcoholism influenced by, 228
    autism and, 143
    cognitive, 157
    communication, 63, 154
    deficit, 132–33
    description of, 132
    executive function, 195–96

imagery teaching self-management, 173–74
    learning, 116
    performing, 116
    in psychotherapy, 132
    reinforcement of, 256
    road crossing, 132–33
    role playing teaching self-management, 173–74
    self-control, 131
Skinner, B. F.
    on behavior, 62–63
    environment and, 100
    operant response and, 48
    reinforcement defined by, 118
    on reward, 115
    shaping introduced by, 45
    skills and, 46
    Walden Two, 73, 77
Skinner chamber, 116–17
sleeping disorders, 45
smoking, 18, 101–2, 123–24, 229
social behaviorism, 10
social capital, 201–2
social change, x
social connectedness, social support different from, 220
social control, 254
social networks, 222, 227–28, 231–32
social support, 219–23, 228, 254
societies, x, 6, 55, 227, 231
Solution-Focused Brief Therapy, 58–59, 72
spanking, 129
Spence, K. W., 104
Spivack, G., 147
spontaneous recovery, 14, 36–37
S-R connection. *See* stimulus-response connection
Staats, A. W.
    on behaviors, 138
    images and, 163
    model of, 91, 123
    on psychology, 10, 260
    words and, 105, 163
static predictors, 40
Steele, Claude, 236
stereotypes, 236, 242–43
Stiles, W. B., 25
stimuli. *See also* conditioned stimulus; unconditioned stimulus
    aversive, 111–12
    behavior influenced by, 37, 42–43, 92, 123
    behavior producing, 124
    controlling, 185–87
    discriminative, 92, 120, 123, 126
    emotion in, 112–13
    extinction caused by, 102
    extinction to, 38
    fear evoked by, 104
    fear generalizing to, 38

stimuli (*cont.*)
  hedonic value of, 104–5
  images as, 172–73
  liked, 118
  metaphors influencing, 175
  psychotherapy and, 37–38
  in relapse prevention, 43
  response influenced by, 125–26
  reward predicted by, 123
  self-change influenced by, 185–87
  sensations as, 111–12
  therapeutic procedures and, 37–38
  words as, 165, 195
stimulus equivalence, 104
stimulus generalization, 37–38
stimulus-response (S-R) connection, 104
stimulus-stimulus connections, 104
strategic dialogue, 57–58
stream of consciousness, pleasure and, 170
stress, anger influenced by, 196
subjective report, 49
substance abuse, mindfulness training influencing, 186–87
Supernanny, 179–80
symbols, schema activated by, 173
symptom substitution, 137–38
syndromes, change revealed by, 17
systematic desensitization, 165, 169–70, 172, 252

talking therapies, 13
talk story, 222
target behavior selection, 65–66
task analysis, 132
Teasdale, J. D., 176
television watching, 141–42
tension release, 26
terror management theory, 105
Tharp, R. G., 36, 184, 212, 237
theory of planned behavior, 59–60, 157
theory of self-efficacy, 79, 80
therapeutic alliance
  as attachment relationship, 206
  autism influenced by, 206–7
  behaviors shaped by, 203–4, 206
  criminal behavior influenced by, 207
  cultures influencing, 242
  description of, 202, 223–24
  experiential avoidance counteracted by, 206
  importance of, 204–7, 208
  influence of, 204
  memory in, 210
  parenting relationships influencing, 209–10
  treatment influencing, 206
  as treatment vehicle, 206
therapeutic framework, 181
therapists. *See also* therapeutic alliance
  activity settings found out about by, 238–39
  behavior, 190
  behavior principle used by, 63
  on change, 4
  change failures and, 260
  change influenced by, 14, 64, 263, 267
  clients asking advice from, 78–79
  clients assessed by, 211–12
  client satisfaction measured by, 49
  clients' changes influenced by, 81–82
  clients confronted by, 76–77
  on clients' future, 181–82
  client's goals set by, 65–66
  clients interacting with, 202–3
  client's relationships and, 214–15
  client's relationship with, 5, 7–8, 13, 21, 58, 76, 79, 201
  clients shaped by, 204
  clients' tasks influenced by, 93–94
  cognitive-behavioral, 211–12
  context considered by, 257
  credulous, 7
  cultural competence of, 242
  marital, 143
  metaphors used by, 175
  parent's similarity to, 224
  possible selves described by, 69–70
  psychotherapy and, 10–11, 205
  role of, 207–8
  self-change promoted by, 181–83
  skeptical, 7
  stereotypes and, 243
  supply of, 198
therapy. *See* psychotherapy
thinking errors, 162
Thorndike, Edward, 115, 116, 123, 124
thoughts
  automatic, 125, 159
  change of experiencing of, 168
  cognitive therapy and, 161–62
  compound, 160
  content of, 162
  depression influenced by, 163
  ego-dystonic, 160
  environment regulating, 169
  errors, 163
  feelings influenced by, 158
  irrational, 160–61, 162–63
  rebound effect and, 170
  stopping, 160
  unconstrained, 160
threats, 68
time-out, 131
Tinklepaugh, O. L., 134
token economy, 12–13
Tolman, E. C., 100, 159
Tools of the Mind, 195–96
training, 42, 87, 142, 177, 215–19
transdiagnostic treatment, xii
transference, 209–10
transfer of learning, 38–39, 149–50
Transtheoretical Model, 56–57

treatments, 255–56
　adolescent, 12
　of anxiety, 152
　behaviors influencing, 138
　change in, 250
　change meeting objectives of, 33
　child, 12
　clients' ability to follow, 11–12
　in clinical practice, 15
　correspondence bias influencing, 88
　depression, 177
　description of, 249–50
　ethics in, 131–32
　gains loss prevention, 39–41
　iatrogenic effects of, 25–26
　manuals, 249
　outcome studies, 15
　personality changed by, 152–53
　psychopathology influencing, 16–17
　punishment in, 129–32
　purpose of, 7
　reward influenced by, 36
　rewards in, 120–21, 261–62
　right to effective, 131–32
　similarities among, 264
　stimulus control of behavior influencing, 124
　therapeutic alliance and, 206
　unidimensional, 251–52
trichotillomania, 186
triple response concept, 139–40
Tsai, M., 211–12
two-factor theory, 106–9, 150

UCS. *See* unconditioned stimulus
Ullmann, L. P., 7
unconditioned stimulus (UCS), 100, 101, 105, 172–73
UNICEF, 225
United Kingdom (UK), 225
unlearning, 97–98
urban legends, 235
U-shaped development, 45

vaccination, imitation influencing, 234
valence, 104–6
value-diversity message, 243
verbal mediators, 194
verification strivings, 90
violence, 17–18, 40

Wahler, Robert, 220
Wampold, B. E., 206
Ward, T., 71–72, 207
Watkins, P. L., 198–99
Watson, D. L., 184
Watson, John B., 102
Wegner, Daniel, 160, 170
weight loss, 191–92
well-being, 50
Wetzel, R. J., 36, 212
wicked problems, 22–23
Wilson, Nick, 39–40, 90, 153, 227
Wilson, G. Terence, 13, 33, 50, 191, 206
Winett, R. A., 32
Winkler, R. C., 32
withdrawal. *See* avoidance
Wittgenstein, L., 21
women, 228, 241
words, 105, 115–16, 165, 195
worry, 86, 108–9, 158
Wright, C., 242

Zajonc, R. B., 159
Zentall, T. R., 119